Cardiac
Arrhythmias

Commissioning Editor: Anne Lenehan
Project Development Manager: Sheila Black
Project Manager: Glenys Norquay
Illustration Manager: Mick Ruddy
Design Manager: Jayne Jones
Illustrator: Martin Woodward

Cardiac Arrhythmias

Gregory Y H Lip MD FRCP DFM FACC FESC
Professor of Cardiovascular Medicine
University Department of Medicine
City Hospital
Birmingham
UK

John Godtfredsen MD FESC
Senior Research Associate
Department of Cardiology
Herlev University Hospital
Herlev
Denmark

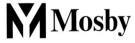

Edinburgh   London   New York   Oxford   Philadelphia   St Louis   Sydney   Toronto   2003

Mosby

An affiliate of Elsevier Limited

First published 2003

ISBN 0 323 02476 9

British Library Cataloguing in Publication Data
A catalogue record for this book is available from the British Library

Library of Congress Cataloging in Publication Data
A catalog record for this book is available from the Library of Congress

Note
Medical knowledge is constantly changing. Standard safety precautions must be followed, but as new research and clinical experience broaden our knowledge, changes in treatment and drug therapy may become necessary or appropriate. Readers are advised to check the most current product information provided by the manufacturer of each drug to be administered to verify the recommended dose, the method and duration of administration, and contraindications. It is the responsibility of the practitioner, relying on experience and knowledge of the patient, to determine dosages and the best treatment for each individual patient. Neither the Publisher nor the editors/contributors assumes any liability for any injury and/or damage to persons or property arising from this publication.
The Publisher

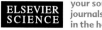 your source for books, journals and multimedia in the health sciences
www.elsevierhealth.com

The
Publisher's
policy is to use
**paper manufactured
from sustainable forests**

Printed in China

Contents

SECTION VI MANAGEMENT

Contributors

Vytautas Abraitis MD
Cardiologist
Centre for Cardiology and Angiology
Vilnius University Hospital Santariskiu Klinikos
Vilnius, Lithuania

Audrius Aidietis PhD
Associate Professor of Cardiology
Head of Department of Cardiac Arrhythmias
Centre for Cardiology and Angiology
Vilnius University Hospital Santariskiu Klinikos
Vilnius, Lithuania

Dwayne S G Conway MRCP
Research Fellow and Specialist Registrar in
Cardiology
University Department of Medicine
City Hospital
Birmingham, UK

Mads D M Engelmann MD PhD
Senior Fellow in Cardiology
Department of Cardiology
Herlev University Hospital
Herlev, Denmark

Rodney H Falk MD FRCP FACC FAHA
Professor of Medicine
Associate Director
Amyloidosis Treatment & Research Program
Boston University School of Medicine
Boston Medical Center
Boston, Massachusetts, USA

Bethan Freestone MBChB MRCP
Research Fellow in Cardiology
University Department of Medicine
City Hospital
Birmingham, UK

John Godtfredsen MD FESC
Senior Research Associate
Department of Cardiology
Herlev University Hospital
Herlev, Denmark

Arjun V Gururaj MD
Instructor in Medicine (Arrhythmia and
Electrophysiology)
Division of Cardiac Electrophysiology
Boston Medical Center
Boston, Massachusetts, USA

Melanie Hümmelgen MD
Fellow
Department of Cardiology
Universitätsklinikum Hamburg-Eppendorf
Hamburg, Germany

Ernest W Lau MD MA MRCP(UK)
Fellow in Clinical Electrophysiology
Department of Clinical Electrophysiology
University of Ottawa Heart Institute
Ottawa, Ontario, Canada

Aleksandras Laucevičius PhD FESC FACC
Professor of Cardiology
Chairman of Heart Clinic
Centre for Cardiology and Angiology
Vilnius University Hospital Santariskiu Klinikos
Vilnius, Lithuania

Gregory Y H Lip MD FRCP DFM FACC FESC
Professor of Cardiovascular Medicine
University Department of Medicine
City Hospital
Birmingham, UK

Germanas Marinskis PhD
Associate Professor of Cardiology
Consultant Electrophysiologist
Centre for Cardiology and Angiology
Vilnius University Hospital Santariskiu Klinikos
Vilnius, Lithuania

Thomas Meinertz MD
Professor of Medicine
Department of Cardiology
Universitätsklinikum Hamburg-Eppendorf
Hamburg, Germany

Preface

The seeds for this book were sown on a beautiful summers day in Finland 1997 during the biennial Nordic Congress of Cardiology. Steen Juul-Möller and John Godtfredsen, attending from Sweden and Denmark, respectively, met the distinguished guest speaker, the late Professor Ronnie Campbell, and suggested forming a European team with the purpose of teaching courses in atrial fibrillation (and other arrhythmias) to a broader audience of internists and cardiologists in training.

The idea was confirmed later in the same year at the European Cardiology Congress in Stockholm, where it was rather easy to persuade Gregory Lip of Birmingham and Rodney Falk of Boston University to join the team. Successful expansions to the faculty occurred later.

Under the aegis of the European Society of Cardiology, the first course was held in January 1999 at the European Heart House in Nice, and because of its very favorable reception repeats were to follow every year thereafter, in Vilnius (Lithuania), Nice (again!) and Kiev (Ukraine). In 2003, the course goes to Shanghai (China) and Thessaloniki (Greece).

Broadly speaking, it is the constantly updated syllabus from these courses which forms the core content of this textbook. In many major textbooks on arrhythmias, the scope is comprehensive and background details on physiology and pathophysiology are abundant, with lots of ECGs and treatment options listed to exhaustion - the patient may sometimes almost disappear in the wealth of information.

Our approach - we think - is different. This textbook is certainly not an ECG atlas of arrhythmias and not a book on clinical pharmacology. Rather, we have tried to synthesize and integrate the many pieces of data that are needed to manage a particular clinical situation effectively. We hope to present a patient-oriented guide with relevant information from clinical epidemiology, bedside diagnostics, common sense clinical judgment and evidence-based treatment options.

We are aware that between the chapters there is much overlap of conceptual facts, but this is deliberate for two reasons: it is intended that each chapter should be independently readable in its own right, and repetition is the mother of all good teaching. Thus, even though the sections on epidemiology and pathophysiology / electrophysiology are mainly theoretical in their scope, they still contain a lot of clinically relevant information.

Our target readers are physicians who care for acute patients presenting with cardiac arrhythmias as the main problem. These patients are certainly not rare and, in many emergency departments, atrial fibrillation and other acute cardiac arrhythmias are common.

We thank our good colleagues for their contributions and the European Society of Cardiology for excellent logistic backup during our academic odyssey around the world.

John Godtfredsen
Gregory Y H Lip

Copenhagen and Birmingham, 2003.

Acknowledgments

We thank all our helpful colleagues and contributors who have helped put this book together so effectively and efficiently. We also acknowledge the help and support of the European Society of Cardiology in organizing, administrating and planning our educational courses, without which this book would not have materialized. Finally, we thank the team at Elsevier, whose persistence has helped make this book a permanent reality.

EPIDEMIOLOGY

Epidemiology and costs of cardiac arrhythmias

Bethan Freestone MBChB MRCP
City Hospital, Birmingham, UK

Gregory Y H Lip MD FRCP DFM FACC FESC
City Hospital, Birmingham, UK

Incidence and prevalence of arrhythmias - particularly AF and VT - are currently increasing with a steep age gradient

Introduction

Many arrhythmias confer a significant morbidity and mortality. For example, many patients with supraventricular arrhythmias present with palpitations and on occasion, complications such as heart failure and thromboembolism. Many patients with ventricular arrhythmias present with sudden death, and this represents a substantial cause of mortality in patients with poor cardiac function and ischemic heart disease.

Arrhythmias also represent an important cause for hospital admissions and longer hospital stays. For example, atrial fibrillation (AF) was present in 6% of acute medical admissions to a Scottish district general hospital.[1] The development of arrhythmias postoperatively often results in morbidity (including heart failure, thromboembolism, etc.), longer inpatient stays and greater hospital costs. The aim of this chapter is to provide an overview of the epidemiology and costs of cardiac arrhythmias.

ATRIAL FIBRILLATION

AF is the commonest sustained cardiac arrhythmia. In one study in the USA, AF was the commonest arrhythmia causing hospitalization (Fig. 1.1).[2] Indeed, AF can occur in association with a wide variety of cardiac and non-cardiac conditions, ranging from ischemic heart disease to thyroid disease and may occur with any pyrexial illness. AF may also occur asymptomatically in an otherwise fit elderly 85-year-old man, but equally can present in an unwell young 20-year-old with Wolff-Parkinson-White syndrome with a fast rate of 200 beats/min who is too lightheaded even to stand.

Most of the epidemiological data for AF comes from observation of predominantly white populations. An estimated 2.2 million of the population in the USA have AF.[3] The prevalence of AF has been estimated in four major population based studies (Cardiovascular Health Study, Framingham Study, Mayo Clinic Study, W Australia

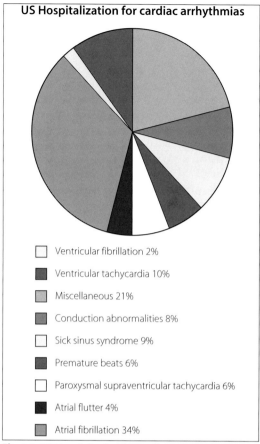

US Hospitalization for cardiac arrhythmias

- Ventricular fibrillation 2%
- Ventricular tachycardia 10%
- Miscellaneous 21%
- Conduction abnormalities 8%
- Sick sinus syndrome 9%
- Premature beats 6%
- Paroxysmal supraventricular tachycardia 6%
- Atrial flutter 4%
- Atrial fibrillation 34%

Fig. 1.1 US Hospitalization for cardiac arrhythmias. Reproduced with permission from Bialy et al. J Am Coll Cardiol 1992; 19:41A.[2] © 1992 The American College of Cardiology Foundation.

Study) (Fig. 1.2).[4–7] These showed an overall prevalence of AF in Western communities of 1.5–6.2% in patients aged between 35 and 80-plus years group in the Framingham and Cardiovascular Health Study. In the Renfrew-Paisley cohort, the prevalence of AF was 8/1000 in males and 5/1000 in females (Fig. 1.3).[8]

Incidence of AF amongst older adults, studied over a 3-year follow-up period in the Cardiovascular Health Study population, was 19.2/1000 person-years among adults > 65 years old.[9] An increased incidence was associated with age, sex and presence of other cardiovascular disease at baseline. In the Renfrew-Paisley cohort, the incidence of AF was 0.9 new cases/1000 patient-years in males and 0.2 new cases/1000 patient-years in females.[8]

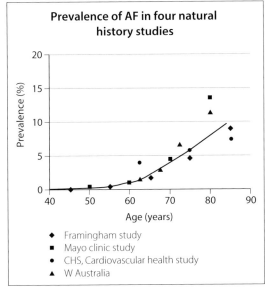

Fig. 1.2 Prevalence of AF in four natural history studies.

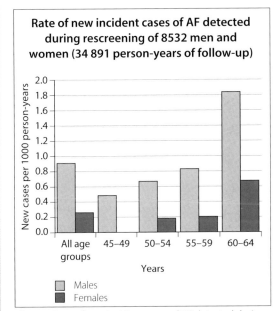

Fig. 1.3 Rate of new incident cases of AF detected during rescreening of 8532 men and women (34 891 person-years of follow-up). Age groups are based on age at baseline. Reproduced with permission from Stewart et al. Heart 2001; 86:516–521.[8]

Age and sex

Incidence of AF increases with increasing age. This has previously been demonstrated in the Framingham Study population, with a prevalence of 0.5% in those aged 50–59, rising to 8.8% of 80–90-year-olds,[10] and has been borne out in other population studies.[4,5,7] The most recent data from the Renfrew-Paisley cohort provides further evidence of the rate of incident cases of AF increasing with age, with a rate of 0.5 male and 0.0 female cases/1000 patient-years in the 45–49-year age group, increasing to 1.8 male and 0.7 female cases/1000 patient- years in those patients aged 60–64 (ages taken at baseline, 20-year follow-up). [8]

Data from the Framingham population also suggests AF is increasing in prevalence (Fig. 1.4).[11] The prevalence in the male Framingham population increased from 3.2% in 1968 to 9.1% in 1989. AF increased as a hospital discharge diagnosis from 30.6/10 000 in 1982, to 59.5/10 000 in 1993. This however could be accounted for by an aging population, increased electrocardiographic surveillance, increases in cardiothoracic surgery or increased myocardial infarction survival, all of which have also occurred over this time.

Although in the general population AF is more common in women than men, the age-adjusted prevalence is higher in men.[4,12] For example, data from Framingham reported the annual incidence of AF in men at 0.9% age 65–74, rising to 1.8% in the 75–84-year-old age group. This rate is much higher than in women, who have average annual incidences of 0.5% and 1.5% for the same age groups.

Race

Although the data on AF in non-white populations are limited, there do seem to be variations in the prevalence of AF in different races. In the Cardiovascular Health Study, 5% of the study population were of Afro-Caribbean origin; in these patients there was noted to be a lower incidence of AF [relative risk (RR) 0.47, 95% confidence interval (CI) 0.22–1.01].[9]

Differences in study design make direct comparisons difficult, but based on population studies there does seem to be a

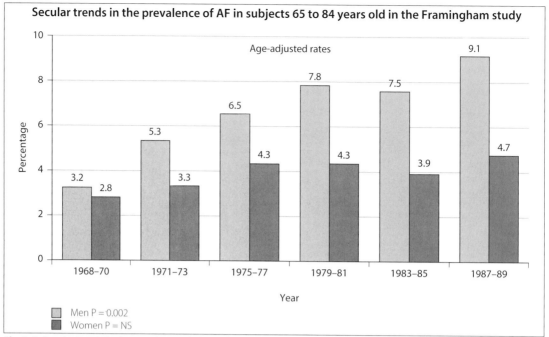

Secular trends in the prevalence of AF in subjects 65 to 84 years old in the Framingham study

Age-adjusted rates

Men P = 0.002
Women P = NS

Fig. 1.4 Secular trends in the prevalence of AF in subjects 65 to 84 years old in the Framingham study. Reproduced with permission from Wolf et al. Am Heart J 1996; 131:790–95.[11]

trend towards a *lower* prevalence of AF in non-white cohorts. One study in India, in which residents of a Himalayan village had one electrocardiogram (ECG), estimated a prevalence of only 0.1%,[13] which is less than the 0.4% prevalence in the general population reported in one USA study who used similar methods.[14] However, only 6% of the Himalayan study population were > 65 years old.

In the west Birmingham AF project, a general practice survey again found a low (0.6%) prevalence of AF reported amongst Indo-Asians aged > 50 years, who comprised 65% of a 25 051 study population.[15] This is in contrast to a survey by Hill et al[16] who reported a prevalence of 3.7% amongst their predominantly Caucasian practice population, although this was looking at > 65-year-olds.[16] A community study in middle-aged to elderly patients in Japan also reported a prevalence of only 1.3%,[17] and in one Thai study the prevalence was only 3.6/1000 population, which again is less than that seen in white population studies.[18]

In hospital based studies there have been comparative findings of the effects of race on prevalence of AF. However, as only an estimated one-third of patients with AF present to hospital,[19] these findings cannot be taken to reflect true prevalence, but trends can be noted. In one survey of acute medical admissions with AF in a city center teaching hospital serving a multiethnic population, the prevalence of AF amongst acute medical admissions was 3.3%.[20] Of the 245 patients with AF, 213 (87%) were white, 10 (4%) were black and 22 (9%) were Indo-Asian. Comparatively, a lower proportion of black and Indo-Asian patients with AF were seen than the proportions in the multiethnic population served by the hospital. In the Northern Manhattan Stroke Study, of those patients presenting with ischemic stroke, AF was more common in whites (29%) than in either black (11%) or Hispanic (11%) patient groups.[21]

These ethnic differences may also reflect the predominant risk factor for the particular ethnic group. For example, hypertension is common amongst Afro-Caribbeans, whilst coronary artery disease is common amongst Indo-Asians in the UK – and not unexpectedly, the commonest etiological factors for AF in Afro-Caribbeans and Indo-Asians are hypertension and ischemic heart disease respectively (Fig. 1.5).[20]

Etiological factors

AF often occurs in association with other cardiovascular disease or recognized risk factors. AF can occur independently in otherwise healthy individuals, in which case it is known as 'lone' AF. A 'strict' definition of lone AF refers to AF in the absence of obvious precipitating factors, in association with a normal ECG (apart from AF), chest X-ray and ECG – it is therefore a

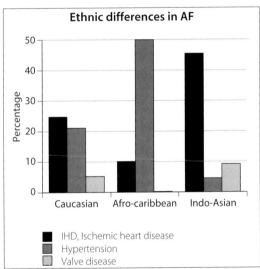

Fig. 1.5 Ethnic differences in the prevalence of atrial fibrillation. Reproduced with permission from Zarifis et al. Br J Clin Pract 1997; 51:91-96.[20]

diagnosis of exclusion. The true prevalence of lone AF varies, and is dependent upon the definition used and population studied. In the Framingham Study, of the 98 patients reported to have developed AF in 1982, 31% had no evidence of cardiovascular disease.[10] However of these patients with 'isolated' AF there were included hypertensive and diabetic patients. In a later report, of the 193 male and 183 female patients in the Framingham population who had developed AF at 30 years follow-up, lone AF occurred in 32 men (16.6%) and 11 women (6%). Again patients with hypertension and diabetes were included in the lone AF group, although the comment is made that the prevalence of either disease in cases compared with controls was not significant (Table 1.1)[22,23]

Cardiovascular risk factors in general are common predisposing conditions seen in association with the development of AF. Hypertension is consistently reported to be associated with an increased risk of developing AF.[9,24,25] Diabetes has also been associated with an increased incidence of AF in some studies.[9,24] In the Framingham population these were the only independent risk factors predictive of AF when adjustments were made for confounding variables. Smoking as a risk factor for AF narrowly failed to reach significance when account was taken of other predisposing factors. Cholesterol levels were not predictive of AF in the Framingham Heart Study and in the Cardiovascular Health Study were associated with reduced risk.

Cardiac disease is also strongly associated with an increased risk of developing AF. Congestive cardiac failure and valvular heart disease have both been

Table 1.1 Prevalence of lone AF from different studies			
Study population	**Age group**	**No. with Lone AF (%)**	**Comorbidity**
Framingham[22]	> 65	11.4	Included hypertension
Mayo clinic[23]	< 60	2.7	No coexisting hypertension

shown to predispose to the development of AF in population studies,[4,24,25] both being associated with a sixfold increase in the Framingham Study. AF is seen as an immediate complication of myocardial infarction (MI), and previous MI is also predictive of AF.[24,25] Although coronary heart disease was noted in about 25% of the men who later developed AF, it was also present in 15% of controls, so this did not reach statistical significance as an independent risk factor in the Framingham cohort.[10]

AF is also seen quite commonly as a complication of both cardiac (33%) and non-cardiac surgery (4% of cases).[26,27] Indeed, AF is the most common arrhythmia seen following cardiac surgery. In the study by Aranki et al[26] looking at the occurrence of AF in patients undergoing coronary artery bypass grafting, of 570 patients studied, 189 developed AF in the postoperative period. Independent predictors of postoperative AF included increasing age [odds ratio (OR)=3 for > 80 years, CI=1.6–5.8, p=0.0007] male sex (OR=1.7, CI=1.1–2.7, p=0.01), hypertension (OR=1.6, CI=1.0–2.3, p=0.03), need for an intraoperative balloon pump (OR=3.5, CI=1.2–10.9, p=0.03), postoperative pneumonia (OR=3.9, CI=1.3–11.5, p=0.01), ventilation for > 24 h (OR=2, CI=1.3–3.2, p=0.003) and return to the intensive care unit (OR=3.2; CI=1.1–8.8, p=0.03).

In a study examining the postoperative course of 4181 patients > 50 years old undergoing non-cardiac surgery, perioperative supraventricular arrhythmias that were persistent or required therapy, occurred in 317 (7.6%) patients. Independent predictors of supraventricular arrhythmia in these patients on multiple regression analysis included: increasing age, male sex, congestive cardiac failure, valvular heart disease, history of asthma, the presence of atrial premature complexes on preoperative ECG, classification III or IV in American Society of Anesthesiologists preoperative assessment and type of procedure (more common in vascular, abdominal and thoracic operations).

Of the other medical conditions commonly associated with AF, lung disease was shown to be an independent risk factor for AF in the Cardiovascular Health Study, but not the Framingham Heart Study.

Hyperthyroidism is also associated with the development of AF.[10] AF occurs in 9–22% of patients with thyrotoxicosis.[28] Signs of hyperthyroidism may be less obvious in the elderly and indeed subclinical hyperthyroidism [indicated by a low thyroid stimulating hormone (TSH), and normal or high Thyroxine (T4) in an asymptomatic patient] has been previously reported with increased frequency in patients with AF.[29]

High alcohol intake or binge drinking is also associated with the development of AF, however in one population study, where the majority of the cohort had only a low to moderate alcohol intake, alcohol consumption was associated with a marginally lower risk of AF.[9] This cohort study, amongst 5201 adults aged > 65 years old followed up for 3 years, found that a low to moderate alcohol intake led to a relative risk reduction in new onset of AF (RR=0.96, CI=0.93–0.99).

Certain ECG features have also been shown to be predictive of AF in several studies.[9,30] Left atrial (LA) size and left ventricular (LV) abnormalities such as reduced ejection fraction and LV hypertrophy have been shown to be independent risk factors for AF. For example, increased LA size was shown to be an independent risk factor for new onset AF in the over 65-year-old Cardiovascular Health Study population (LA size of < 3 cm was given a reference RR of 1, LA size 4.01–5.00 cm conferring an RR of 2.58, CI=1.35–4.94, LA size > 5 cm RR= 4.05, CI=1.96–8.35).[9] In the Framingham population, on multivariate stepwise analysis, increased LA dimension, reduced LV fractional shortening and increased LV wall thickness were all independent predictors for development of non-rheumatic AF.[30]

Prevalence of risk factors for AF often influences the prevalence of AF within a

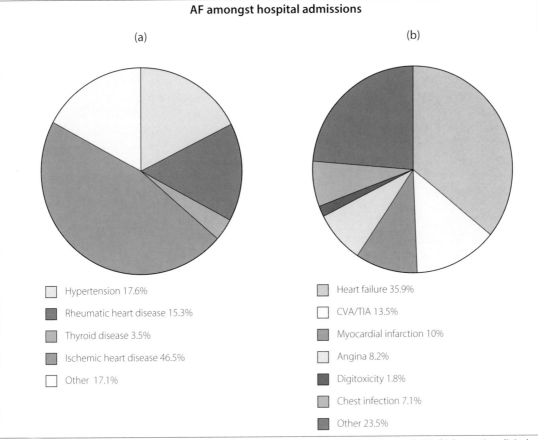

Fig. 1.6 AF among hospital admissions. (a) Etiology of AF amongst acute medial admissions with AF. (b) Presenting clinical features of acute medical admissions with AF. CVA/TIA, cerebrovascular accident/transient ischaemic attack. Reproduced with permission from Lip et al. Br Heart J 1994; 71:92–95.[1]

Key points

Recognized etiological risk factors for AF

Major
- Increasing age
- Hypertension
- Diabetes
- Congestive heart failure
- Valvular heart disease
- Cardiac surgery

Minor
- Hyperthyroidism
- Lung diseases (chronic obstructive pulmonary disease – COPD)
- High alcohol intake

---

population, but also differing risk factors predominate in different populations. For example, in a study in Ethiopia, amongst patients seen in a cardiology clinic for AF, rheumatic heart disease was the commonest predisposing factor,[31] whereas in Western studies hypertension and ischemic heart disease are the commonest causes (Fig. 1.6).[1] Even in a Western population, racial differences in etiology can be observed as demonstrated by one study in the UK where hypertension was the main risk factor in Afro-Caribbean patients with AF, and ischemic heart disease in the Asian population[20] (Table 1.2).[32]

Morbidity and mortality

The potential effects of AF are the result of hemodynamic changes and thromboembolic complications.

Onset of AF can result in a reduction in cardiac output of up to 10–20% regardless

Table 1.2 Stroke risk factors and ethnicity (From Hajat et al[31])

Cerebrovascular	White [n = 995 (79.3%)]	Black [n=203 (16.2%)]	Total [n=1198 (95.5%)]	P
Ischemic heart disease	249 (27.0)	29 (15.5)	278 (25.1)	0.09
Cerebrovascular disease	160 (17.8)	27 (14.6)	187 (17.2)	0.3
Atrial fibrillation	234 (25.0)	13 (6.8)	247 (21.9)	0.001
Hypertension	511 (55.5)	133 (70.7)	644 (58.1)	<0.001
Diabetes mellitus	126 (13.7)	64 (34.0)	190 (17.1)	<0.001
Migraine	72 (8.0)	15 (8.2)	87 (8.1)	0.5
Alcohol	151 (18.0)	18 (10.3)	169)16.7)	<0.001
Smoking	617 (74.3)	87 (51.5)	704 (70.4)	<0.001

Values in parentheses are percentages.

of ventricular rate.[33] Along with fast ventricular rates, this can result in tipping an already compromised ventricle into failure. It has also been suggested that, in a patient with coronary artery disease, sudden increases in ventricular rate associated with uncontrolled AF may precipitate critical cardiac ischemia or even MI. Certainly people with AF do have increased rates of congestive cardiac failure and coronary events, but whether this is cause or effect is uncertain.

AF is associated with a hypercoagulable state,[34] and patients are subsequently at risk of cardiac thromboembolism. Substantial morbidity associated with AF can be related to cerebrovascular events that can occur as a result of this, or intrinsic cerebrovascular atherosclerosis.

AF is an independent risk factor for stroke.[5] Even after adjusting for other stroke risk factors, AF is associated with a rate of stroke approximately five times that of people without AF. Absolute risk for an individual patient, however, increases with age and depends upon the presence of other risk factors such as valvular disease, other cardiovascular disease or cardiac risk factors. Conversely, anticoagulation reduces the risk of stroke in 'at risk' patients with AF.[35] In stroke patients, concurrent AF is associated with greater disability, longer in-hospital patient stay and lower rate of discharge to own home.

AF has also been associated with dementia in the Rotterdam study [odds ratio 2.3 (CI=1.4–3.7)].[36] The same study group found significant positive association between AF and cognitive impairment (OR=1.7, CI=1.2–2.5). A history of stroke in those subjects studied did not account for these associations. Alzheimer disease with cerebrovascular disease was found to be a stronger association than vascular dementia in the Rotterdam study population. Nevertheless the role of silent cerebral infarction, seen with increased frequency in patients with AF,[37] in the pathogenesis of dementia and cognitive impairment in these patients cannot be discounted. Another group examining the cognitive function of 255 hospital inpatients (42 in AF, 213 in sinus rhythm) also found minimental state examinations to be lower in patients with AF compared with those in sinus rhythm, this was retained even after adjustment for other factors associated with mental decline.[38]

Part of the reduction in quality of life due to AF is through the higher incidence of stroke, but there are other factors contributing to impaired functional capacity in these patients. Although some patients with AF are asymptomatic, the majority have some symptoms attributable to the arrhythmia, in the form of palpitations, chest pain, fatigue, dyspnea or dizziness. Initial studies evaluating quality of life in patients with AF indicate a reduced quality of life. The Stroke Prevention in Atrial Fibrillation study investigators aimed to look at functional status in patients with AF using New York Heart Association (NYHA) status, which is an insensitive index, and therefore yielded little result.[39] In a limited study in 69 patients with paroxysmal AF, 47 (68%) of patients thought that having AF interfered with day-to-day life.[40] This was independent of the frequency or duration of their paroxysms of AF. In selected paroxysmal AF patients, particularly those who are very symptomatic or refractory to drug therapy, the approach of AV node ablation and pacemaker insertion has led to an improved quality of life.[41,42]

Patients with AF in association with stroke, MI, heart failure or cardiomyopathy have decreased survival in most studies,[43–46] although some have not shown this (Figs 1.7–1.9).[47–52]

Recent trials have indicated that, even in those AF patients in whom restoration of sinus rhythm is attempted, quality of life, hospitalization rates and long term outcome are not improved.[53,54,55]

Not surprisingly AF is associated with an overall excess mortality. This was independent of associated cardiovascular conditions and risk factors in the Framingham population,[56] being associated with a 1.5–1.9-fold increased mortality risk (Fig. 1.10).

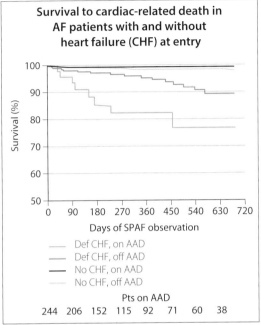

Fig. 1.7 Survival to cardiac-related death in AF patients with and without heart failure (CHF) at entry. SPAF, stroke prevention in atrial fibrillation; CHF, congestive heart failure; AAD, antiarrhythmic drugs. Reproduced with permission from Flaker et al. J Am Coll Cardiol 1992; 20(3):527–532.[51] © 1992 The American College of Cardiology Foundation.

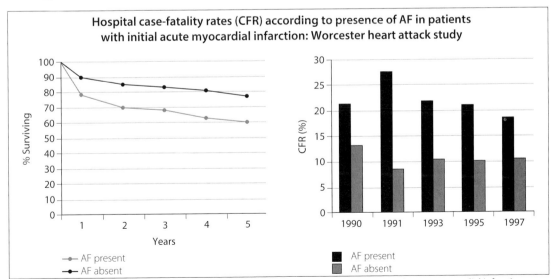

Fig. 1.8 Hospital case-fatality rates (CFR) according to presence of AF in patients with initial acute myocardial infarction: Worcester heart attack study. Reproduced with permission from Goldberg et al. Am Heart J 2002; 143:519–527.[48]

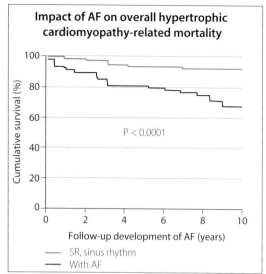

Fig. 1.9 Impact of AF on overall hypertrophic cardiomyopathy-related mortality. Reproduced with permission from Olivotto et al. Circulation 2001; 104:2517–2524.[52]

Key points

Major adverse consequences of AF:

- a 1.5–1.9-fold increase in mortality risk
- a fivefold increase in stroke risk
- a reduced quality of life
- an increased risk of dementia
- an increased burden of health service costs

Costs

As a common arrhythmia and a cause of substantial morbidity and mortality, AF has considerable implications for healthcare expenditure. An estimated 325 000 hospitalizations listed AF as a discharge diagnosis in a report by the American Heart Association [AHA].[57] It has also been reported that healthcare expenditure in the Framingham population was greater in those with AF when compared to those without AF.[58]

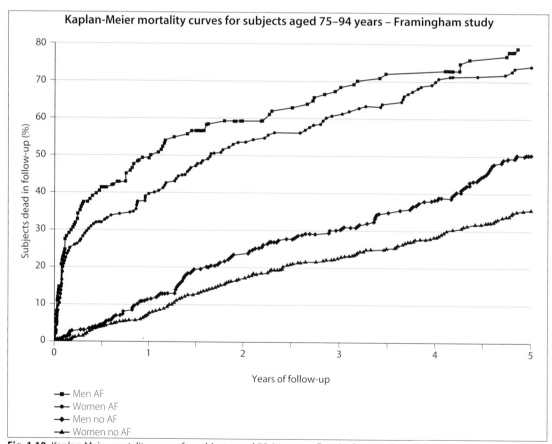

Fig. 1.10 Kaplan-Meier mortality curves for subjects aged 75-94 years – Framingham study.

Because of the increasing use of warfarin in AF patients as stroke prophylaxis, there are considerable increases in demand for anticoagulant services, with increased costs involved in International Normalized Ratio (INR) monitoring and potential bleeding risk. These financial implications should be balanced against the benefits of decreased risk of stroke, which should create healthcare savings in the long term.

Currently, AF is still associated with increased risk of stroke and resultant hospital admissions, readmissions and long-term care impact strongly on the costs associated with this arrhythmia. It has been reported that patients with AF have more severe strokes than stroke patients in sinus rhythm, with survivors having longer hospital stays and increased disability.[43,44] In over 40 years follow-up of the Framingham population, in the 103 patients with AF and stroke, the severity was substantially higher, as was the 30-day mortality (25% in those with AF, compared to 14% in non-AF patients); these differences were still evident at 1 year post stroke, with AF patients also noted to have poorer survival, more recurrences and lower Barthel index scores.[43] In the Copenhagen Stroke Study, for patients with AF, mortality rate was increased 1.7-fold. AF patients also had longer hospital stays compared with those stroke patients in sinus rhythm (50 days vs 40 days, $p < 0.001$), and a lower discharge rate to their own home.[44]

Patients with AF associated with acute MI also have delayed hospital discharge. In the GUSTO-I trial, investigators report a significantly longer inpatient stay in those MI patients with AF, compared to those in sinus rhythm (13 ± 11 days vs 10 ± 9 days, $p=0.0001$).[45]

Postoperative AF also has significant costs, associated with the prolonged hospital stay and treatment of both AF and its complications.[26,27] In the study by Aranki et al[26] after cardiac surgery, for patients who developed postoperative AF the length of hospital stay was reported at

15.3 ± 28.6 days for patients with AF, compared with 9.3 ± 19.6 days for those patients without. Adjusted lengthening of hospital stay attributable to AF being estimated at 4.9 days, translating to increased costs in the region of > $10 000. For non-cardiac operations results were similar, with those patients who developed perioperative arrhythmias staying about 2.5 (CI 1.9–3.1) days longer than the average hospital stay of 8.1 ± 7.8 days. This equates to a 33% increase in inpatient time, with the associated costs this entails.[27]

More recent advances in investigation and treatment of AF, with the use of electrophysiological studies, ablation therapy and atrial cardioversion devices all look set to increase expenditure in the future as their use becomes more commonplace. As the population ages, the prevalence of AF is likely to increase, causing an increasing public health problem. Prevention of AF and treatment of patients with AF and associated cardiovascular disease should reduce mortality and morbidity, particularly associated with stroke, as well as reducing healthcare costs.

OTHER SUPRAVENTRICULAR ARRHYTHMIAS

There are considerably less epidemiological data on supraventricular tachycardias (SVTs) other than AF. A considerable number of supraventricular arrhythmias are asymptomatic. In a study by Page et al[59] monitoring patients with symptomatic supraventricular tachycardias with ambulatory ECG and patient event-recording simultaneously, asymptomatic AF occurred significantly more frequently than symptomatic AF episodes, and asymptomatic SVTs also occurred with notable frequency (Fig. 1.11).[59] This indicates that undetected arrhythmias will underestimate the frequency with which they occur in the general population.

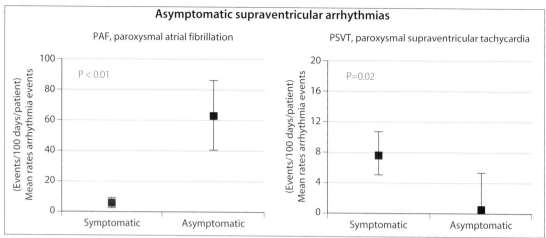

Fig. 1.11 Symptomatic and asymptomatic events in paroxysmal atrial fibrillation (PAF) and paroxysmal supraventricular tachycardia (PSVT). Reproduced with permission from Page et al. Circulation 1994; 89:224–227.[59]

For example, atrial flutter is less common than AF (see Fig. 1.1). The incidence of Wolff-Parkinson-White syndrome in the general population is reported to be 0.1–3% depending on the population studied.[60] One US study reporting on all paroxysmal supraventricular tachycardias in the general population estimated their prevalence at 2.25/1000 persons, and an incidence of 35/100 000 person-years.[61] With an estimate of 89 000 new cases/year, and an estimated 570 000 people with SVT in the USA, this study outlines the common nature of this problem.

VENTRICULAR ARRHYTHMIAS

Key points

Ventricular tachycardia (VT)

- major cause of sudden cardiac death (SCD)
- true incidence unknown, but possibly rising
- coronary artery disease (CAD) and congestive heart failure (CHF) are major risk factors
- most types of VT are definitely malignant

Sudden cardiac death

By their very nature, ventricular arrhythmias, being short lived and life threatening have somewhat unreliable data on their actual rate of occurrence.

Most sudden cardiac deaths (SCDs) are usually caused by acute fatal arrhythmias [ventricular tachycardia (VT) or fibrillation (VF)],[62] and therefore epidemiological data on ventricular arrhythmias is mostly extrapolated from data on sudden cardiac death.

It has been estimated that there are 300 000 SCDs per annum in the USA. Based on the available figures, this makes the overall incidence in the region of 0.1–0.2%/year in the adult population.[63] However this may be an underestimate because figures for out-of-hospital cardiac arrest and sudden death are difficult to ascertain accurately.

From the Framingham data, sudden cardiac death caused 46% of the cardiac mortality in men and 34% mortality in women over a 26-year follow-up,[64] indicating a trend towards an excess mortality in males. The incidence of SCD increases with age[64] and with certain high risk groups, such as those with heart failure (Fig. 1.12).[60]

It should be pointed out that much of the epidemiological data on SCD has been obtained from predominantly white populations. World Health Organization (WHO) data reports the incidence of SCD in industrial populations to vary between

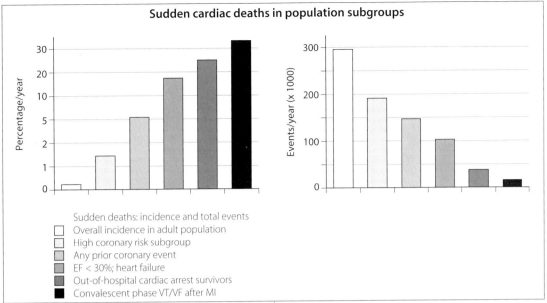

Fig. 1.12 Sudden cardiac deaths in population subgroups. EF, ejection fraction; MI, myocardial infarction; VF, ventricular fibrillation; VT, ventricular tachycardia. Reproduced with permission from Myerberg et al. Circulation 1992; 85(supp I):I2–I10.[63]

19 and 159/100 000 inhabitants/year among men age 35–64 indicating there may be some ethnic variation in incidence.[65]

Other risk factors can be identified for SCD.[63] The most common condition found in association with SCD is ischemic heart disease, although other heart diseases are also associated with an increased risk.

Conditions associated with an increased risk of sudden cardiac death

- Ischemic heart disease

- Cardiomyopathies
  –Hypertrophic cardiomyopathy
  –Idiopathic dilated cardiomyopathy
  –Arrhythmogenic right ventricular dysplasia

- Valvular heart disease
  –Aortic stenosis
  –Mitral valve prolapse

- Electrophysiological abnormalities
  –Wolff-Parkinson-White syndrome
  –Long QT syndrome
  –Conduction system abnormalities
  –Brugada syndrome

- Congenital heart disease

High coronary risk patients without a prior event are estimated to have an annual risk of SCD of 1–2%. Risk of SCD increases in: patients with any prior coronary event (5%), heart failure patients (20%), out-of-hospital cardiac arrest survivors (25–30%) and those with post-MI VT/VF (> 30%). For these patients, the time that they are most at risk of SCD is within the first 6–18 months following an index event.[63,66]

Independent risk factors for SCD differ between males and females. For men, these are in common with cardiac risk factors in general. Cigarette smoking, high body mass index, glucose intolerance, LV hypertrophy, raised cholesterol, and raised systolic blood pressure have all been identified as independent risk factors. In women smoking, LV hypertrophy, raised cholesterol, and raised systolic blood pressure are also risk factors for SCD, along with non-specific ECG changes and low hemoglobin.[67] Parental sudden death has also been identified as a risk factor for sudden death.[68]

As well as being responsible for SCD, ventricular arrhythmias can present asymptomatically, or with symptoms associated with hemodynamic compromise such as palpitations, chest pain, lightheadedness or syncope. Certainly, the different ventricular arrhythmias are associated with differing etiologies and clinical outcomes.

Polymorphic ventricular tachycardia (torsade de pointes)

Polymorphic ventricular tachycardia is traditionally associated with prolongation of the QT interval. This can be congenital, associated with electrolyte imbalance, specific drugs, or with autonomic abnormalities (also see Ch. 13 'Proarrhythmia').

Causes of torsade de pointes

- Congenital prolonged QT syndrome (e.g. Romano Ward syndrome, Jervell-Lange-Nielsen syndrome)

- Electrolyte abnormalities (e.g. hypokalemia, hypocalcemia, hypomagnesemia)

- Drugs
  -tricyclic antidepressants
  -macrolide antibiotics (erythromycin)
  -antifungals (ketaconazole)
  -antihistamines (terfenadine, astemizole)
  -antiarrhythmics (amiodarone, propafenone)

- Stroke

- Anorexia nervosa, etc.

Ventricular tachycardia

Of the patients treated for recurrent symptomatic VT, over 50% have ischemic heart disease. VT has also been associated with dilated cardiomyopathy, hypertrophic cardiomyopathy, right ventricular dysplasia, primary electrical disease, mitral valve prolapse, valvular heart disease, and congenital heart disease.

VT can be catagorized into non-sustained (NSVT) or sustained VT, both of which have different prognostic implications. The occurrence of non-sustained and sustained VT in the acute phase of MI has been estimated to be in the region of 35%.[69]

NSVT is the term used to describe VT that persists for an undefined period (usually more than four beats and less than 30 s) that resolves without intervention. NSVT occurs post-MI in 5–10% of infarct survivors and the prognostic implications are debatable. In contrast, non-sustained VT in the presence of heart failure is quite common, with an estimated prevalence of 35%, and is usually asymptomatic – but in this setting NSVT is associated with an adverse prognosis. NSVT can also occur in normal individuals, but its true prevalence is not known. One cohort study of 24 h ECG recordings in 50 'healthy' medical students with no known heart disease documented the arrhythmia in one individual.[70] The prognosis associated with NSVT in subjects with no structural heart disease is not known.

Sustained VT refers to ventricular tachycardia greater than 30 s in duration or requiring intervention to terminate the arrhythmia. Sustained VT again is seen most commonly in association with ischemic heart disease. Information from follow-up in the GISSI-3 trial, estimated the incidence of late sustained VT (after 48 h, but by 6 weeks) to be about 1%.[71] In comparison with NSVT, sustained VT has a much worse prognosis associated with its presence (Fig. 1.13).[72] Sustained VT can be regarded as stable, when the patient is not hemodynamically compromised and relatively symptom free, or unstable in the presence of serious symptoms and cardiovascular collapse. Some studies had suggested that stable VT was associated with a low risk of sudden death.[73] However, more studies have suggested that both stable and unstable sustained VT are associated with increased risk of sudden death.[74,75] More recently, data from the antiarrhythmics versus implantable

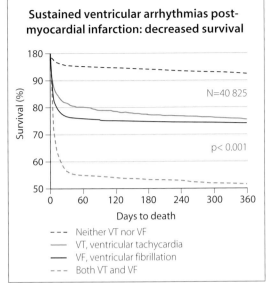

Sustained ventricular arrhythmias post-myocardial infarction: decreased survival

N=40 825

p< 0.001

--- Neither VT nor VF
— VT, ventricular tachycardia
— VF, ventricular fibrillation
--- Both VT and VF

Fig. 1.13 Sustained ventricular arrhythmias post-myocardial infarction: decreased survival. Reproduced with permission from Newby et al. Circulation 1998; 98:2567–2573.[72]

defibrillators (AVID) registry, suggested that stable VT patients may even have a higher mortality than those with unstable sustained VT.[76] The mortality in 440 patients with stable VT was 33.6% compared with the 27.6% mortality observed in unstable sustained VT patients (RR=1.22, p=0.07). Authors therefore

suggesting that the use of implantable cardioverter-defibrillator (ICD) devices may be warranted in stable as well as unstable VT patients to reduce mortality in the future (Fig. 1.14).[77]

Ventricular fibrillation

VF is often preceded by a period of organized VT.[78] Cardiac ischemia is again the most common cause. VF has been estimated to complicate 4.7% of acute MIs[79] with the highest incidence within the 1st hour (Fig. 1.15).[80] VF invariably results in loss of cardiac output, cardiac arrest resulting in death unless promptly treated.

Morbidity and mortality

Looking at inpatient data probably gives us the best picture of mortality and morbidity associated with the various ventricular arrhythmias, although it must be noted that this is often in the context of acute MI.

VF is most often witnessed in the post-MI setting. One study has reported the in-hospital case mortality to be 44%, which is significantly greater than the 5% mortality seen in patients with no VF

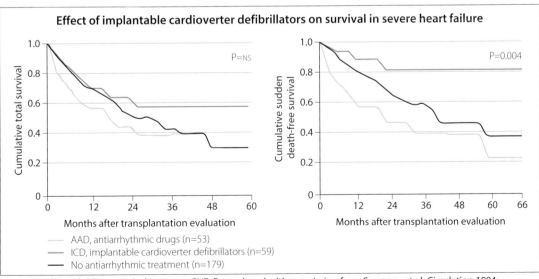

Effect of implantable cardioverter defibrillators on survival in severe heart failure

P=NS

P=0.004

--- AAD, antiarrhythmic drugs (n=53)
— ICD, implantable cardioverter defibrillators (n=59)
— No antiarrhythmic treatment (n=179)

Fig. 1.14 Effect of ICD on survival in severe CHF. Reproduced with permission from Sweeney et al. Circulation 1994; 89(4):1851–1858.[77]

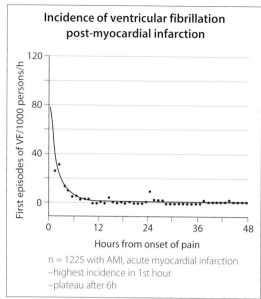

Incidence of ventricular fibrillation post-myocardial infarction

n = 1225 with AMI, acute myocardial infarction
–highest incidence in 1st hour
–plateau after 6h

Fig. 1.15 Incidence of ventricular fibrillation post-myocardial infarction. Reproduced with permission from Sayer et al. Heart 2000;84(3):258–261.[80]

post-MI.[79] This study, which was a retrospective data collection from MI patients admitted 1975–1997, did however show a trend towards decreasing mortality with time, presumably due to increasing surveillance and treatment of post-MI patients.

Post-MI VT is associated with an excess of LV failure, AF/flutter, asystole, and VF in the first 48 h. Patients with VT post-MI, therefore have a more complicated post-MI course, and an increased mortality. In the GISSI-3 study population death rates were found to be 35% at 6 weeks for those with late sustained VT compared with 5% for those without, making late sustained VT a strong independent predictor of mortality post-MI (hazard ratio=6.13, 95% CI=4.56–8.25).[71] In another study looking at the prevalence of NSVT post-MI, by Holter monitoring amongst 325 infarct survivors, only 9% had NSVT shortly following MI. Over a follow-up period of 30 months, 25 of the 325 patients reached the primary endpoint of death, VF or sustained VT.[81] NSVT in the post infarct period carried a relative risk of 2.6 for these primary endpoints, but its predictive value was found to be less than infarct-related artery patency, left ventricular ejection fraction (LVEF) or impaired autonomic tone.

Another study investigating out-of-hospital VT cardiac arrests found monomorphic VT to be more common than polymorphic VT, occurring in 62% of the 190 patients included.[82] The type of VT was not predictive of outcome, with similar rates of successful resuscitation and eventual hospital discharge seen for both groups. Prolonged QTc was predictive of poor outcome in this study. The overall rate of hospital discharge was 28.4%.

VF is the commonest arrhythmia causing cardiac arrest.[83] In Sweden, a survey of out-of-hospital cardiac arrests showed that VF was the arrhythmia on the first ECG recording in 43% of cases,[84] and the authors estimated the incidence of VF at the time of time of cardiac arrest to be in the region of 60–70%, based on these figures. Overall survival for those patients found in VF in this study was 9.5%, which was higher than other rhythms together (where survival was only 1.6%).

Overall, the survival of pre-hospital cardiac arrest patients is best in those patients with VT, intermediate in those with VF and poor in those with bradycardia or asystole.[83]

Costs

There is substantial cost in human lives from ventricular arrhythmias, with survival to hospital discharge for out-of-hospital cardiac arrest estimated at only 2–25%.[85] With this high mortality there is a need for improvement, and minor benefits in survival have been seen where there has been use of automatic external defibrillators as treatment.[86] For the application of prophylactic measures such as ICDs or ablation, the difficulty lies in costs (in terms of both interventional and monetary value) versus benefits. The overall risk of death due to ventricular arrhythmias in the population as a whole is low, therefore prophylactic treatment has

Table 1.3 ICD cost effectiveness	
Treatment of hypertension	$23 200
Heart transplantation	$26 900
Estrogen replacement	$32 900
Neonatal intensive care	$5500–38 800
Renal dialysis	$58 000
Coronary artery bypass	$7200–44 200
ICD*	$7500

*Transvenous/pectoral/increased longevity.
ICD, implantable cardioverter defibrillator

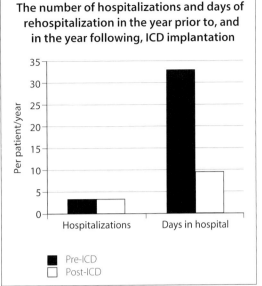

The number of hospitalizations and days of rehospitalization in the year prior to, and in the year following, ICD implantation

Fig. 1.16 The number of hospitalizations and days of rehospitalization in the year prior to, and in the year following, ICD implantation. ICD, implantable cardioverter defibrillator. Reproduced with permission from Valenti et al. Eur Heart J 1996; 17(10):1565–1571.[90] © 1996 The European Society of Cardiology.

centered around high risk groups. With evidence from AVID, Cardiac Arrest Study, Hamburg (CASH), Canadian Implantable Defibrillator Study (CIDS) secondary prevention trials (in patients with previous VF or sustained VT), Multicenter Automatic Defibrillator Implantation Trial (MADIT), Multicenter Unsustained Tachycardia Trial (MUSTT) and numerous ongoing trials (in patients at high risk of VT), demonstrating the survival benefit of ICDs, the treatment of these patients is going to confer high economic and health service costs.[87–89] This is perhaps balanced by reduced hospitalization of these patients and could even be cost effective in direct comparison with other therapies for other conditions (Table 1.3) (Fig. 1.16).[90]

It should however be borne in mind that the majority of fatalities from ventricular arrhythmias occur during the primary event and that this approach does not address primary prevention in the general population.

References

1. Lip GYH, Tean KN, Dunn FG. Treatment of atrial fibrillation in a district general hospital. Br Heart J 1994; 71:92–95.
2. Bialy D, Lehmann MH, Schumacher DN, et al. Hospitalisation for arrhythmias in the United States: Importance of atrial fibrillation. J Am Coll Cardiol 1992; 19:41A.
3. Feinberg WM, Blackshear JL, Laupacis A, et al. Prevalence, age and gender of patients with atrial fibrillation: analysis and implications. Arch Intern Med 1995; 155:469–473.
4. Furberg CD, Psaty BM, Manolio TA, et al for the CHS Collaborative Research Group. Prevalence of atrial fibrillation in elderly subjects (the Cardiovascular Health Study).Am J Cardiol 1994; 74:236–241.
5. Wolf PA, Abbott RD, Kannel WB. Atrial fibrillation as an independent risk factor for stroke: The Framingham Study. Stroke 1991; 22:983–988.
6. Phillips SJ, Whisnant JP, O'Fallon WM, et al. Prevalence of cardiovascular disease and diabetes mellitus in residents of Rochester, Minnesota. Mayo Clin Proc 1990; 65:344–359.
7. Lake FR, Cullen KJ, de Klerk NH, et al. Atrial fibrillation and mortality in an elderly population. Aust NZ J Med 1989; 19:321–326.
8. Stewart S, Hart CL, Hole DJ, et al. Population prevalence, incidence, and predictors of atrial fibrillation in the Renfrew/Paisley study. Heart 2001; 86:516–521.
9. Psaty BM, Manolio TA, Kuller LH, et al. Incidence of and risk factors for atrial fibrillation in older adults. Circulation 1997; 96:2455–2461.
10. Kannel WB, Abbot RD, Savage DD, et al. Epidemiological features of chronic atrial fibrillation. The Framingham Study. N Engl J Med 1982; 306:1018–1022.
11. Wolf PA, Benjamin EJ, Belanger AJ, et al. Secular trends in the prevalence of atrial fibrillation: The Framingham Study. Am Heart J 1996; 131:790–795.
12. Kannel WB, Abbot RD, Savage DD, et al. Coronary heart disease and atrial fibrillation: The Framingham study. Am Heart J 1983; 106:389–396.

13. Kaushal SS, Dasgupta DJ, Prashar BS, et al. Electrocardiographic manifestations of healthy residents of a tribal Himalayan village. J Assoc Phys India. 1995;43:15–16.

14. Ostranderld JR, Brandt RL, Kjelsberg MO, et al. Electrocardiographic findings amongst the adult population of a total natural community, Tecumseh, Michigan. Circulation 1965; 31:888–898.

15. Lip GYH, Bawden L, Hodson R, et al. Atrial fibrillation amongst the indo-asian general practice population: The West Birmingham Atrial Fibrillation Project. Int J Cardiol 1998; 65:187–192.

16. Hill JD, Mottram EM, Killeen PD. Study of the prevalence of atrial fibrillation in general practice patients over 65 years of age. J R Coll Gen Pract 1987; 37:172–173.

17. Nakayama T, Date C, Yokoyama T, et al. A 15.5-year follow-up study of stroke in a Japanese provincial city. Stroke 1997;28:45–52.

18. Kiatchoosakan S, Pachirat O, Chirawatkul A, et al. Prevalence of cardiac arrhythmias in Thai Community. J Med Assoc Thailand 1999; 82:727 (Abstract).

19. Lip GYH, Golding DG, Nazir M, et al. A survey of atrial fibrillation in general practice: The West Birmingham Atrial Fibrillation Project. British Journal of General Practice 1997; 47:285–289.

20. Zarifis J, Beevers DG, Lip GYH. Acute admissions with atrial fibrillation in a British multiracial hospital population. Br J Clin Pract 1997; 51:91–96.

21. Sacco RL, Kargman DE, Zamanillo MC. Race-ethnic differences in stroke risk factors amongst hospitalised patients with cerebral infarction: the Northern Manhattan Stroke Study. Neurology. 1995; 45:659–663.

22. Brand FN, Abbot RD, Kannel WB, et al. Characteristics and prognosis of lone atrial fibrillation: 30 year follow up in the Framingham Study. JAMA 1985; 254:3449–3453.

23. Kopecky SL, Gersh BJ, McGoon MD, et al. The natural history of lone atrial fibrillation population-based study over three decades. N Engl J Med 1987; 317: 669-674

24. Benjamin EJ, Levy D, Vaziri SM, et al. Independent risk factors for atrial fibrillation in a population-based cohort: The Framingham Heart Study. JAMA 1994; 271:840–844

25. Krahn AD, Manfreda J, Tate RB, et al. The natural history of atrial fibrillation: incidence, risk factors and prognosis in the Manitoba Follow-up study. Am J Med 1995; 98:476–484.

26. Aranki SF, Shaw DP, Adams DH, et al. Predictors of atrial fibrillation after coronary artery surgery: current trends and impact on hospital resources. Circulation 1996; 94:390–397.

27. Polanczyk CA, Golman L, Marcantonio ER, et al. Supraventricular arrhythmia in patients having noncardiac surgery: clinical correlates and effect on length of stay. Ann Intern Med 1998; 129:279–285.

28. Woeber KA. Thyrotoxicosis and the heart. N Engl J Med 1992; 327:94–98.

29. Forfar JC, Miller HC, Toft AD. Occult thyrotoxicosis: a correctable cause of 'idiopathic' atrial fibrillation. Am J Cardiol 1979; 44:9–12.

30. Vaziri SM, Larson MG, Benjamin EJ, et al. Echocardiographic predictors of nonrheumatic atrial fibrillation: The Framingham Study. Circulation 1994; 89:724–730.

31. Hajat C, Dundas R, Stewart JA, et al. Cerebrovascular risk factors and stroke subtypes: differences between ethnic groups. Stroke 2001; 32(1):37–42.

32. Maru M. Atrial fibrillation and embolic complications. East Afr Med J 1997; 74:3–5.

33. Clark DM, Plumb VJ, Epstein AE, et al. Haemodynamic effects of an irregular sequence of ventricular cycle lengths during atrial fibrillation. J Am Coll Cardiol 1997; 30:1039–1045.

34. Lip GH. Does atrial fibrillation confer a hypercoagulable state? Lancet 1995; 346:1313–1314.

35. Atrial Fibrillation Investigators: Risk factors for stroke and efficacy of antithrombotic therapy in atrial fibrillation. Arch Intern Med 1994; 154:1449–1457.

36. Ott AO, Breteler MMB, de Bruyne MC, et al. Atrial fibrillation and dementia in a population-based study: The Rotterdam Study. Stroke 1997; 28:316–321.

37. Ezekowitz MD, James KE, Nazarian SM, et al. Silent cerebral infarction in patients with nonrheumatic atrial fibrillation. Circulation 1995; 92;2178–2182.

38. Sabatini T, Frisoni GB, Barbisoni P, et al. Atrial fibrillation and cognitive disorders in older people. J Am Geriatr Soc 2000; 48(4):387–390.

39. Ganiats TG, Browner DK, Dittrich HC. Comparison of quality of wellbeing scale and NYHA functional status classification in patients with atrial fibrillation. Am Heart J 1998; 135;819-24.

40. Hamer ME, Blumenthal JA, McCarthy EA, et al. Quality of life assessment in patients with paroxysmal atrial fibrillation or paroxysmal supraventricular tachycardia. Am J Cardiol 1994; 74:826–829.

41. Brignole M, Gianfranchi L, Menozzi C, et al. Assessment of atrioventricular junction ablation and DDDR mode-switching pacemaker versus pharmacological treatment in patients with severely symptomatic paroxysmal atrial fibrillation. A randomised controlled study. Circulation 1997; 96:2617–2624.

42. Marshall HJ, Harris ZI, Griffith MJ, et al. Atrioventricular nodal ablation and implantation of mode-switching dual chamber pacemakers: effective treatment for drug refractory paroxysmal atrial fibrillation. Heart 1998; 79:543–547.

43. Lin HJ, Wolf PA, Kelly-Haynes M, et al. Stroke severity in atrial fibrillation: the Framingham Study. Stroke 1996; 27:1760–1764.

44. Jorgensen HS, Nakayama H, Reith J, et al. Acute stroke with atrial fibrillation. The Copenhagen Study. Stroke 1996; 10:1765–1769.

45. Crenshaw BS, Ward SR, Granger CB, et al for the GUSTO I Trial investigators. Atrial fibrillation in the setting of acute myocardial infarction: the GUSTO-I experience. J Am Coll Cardiol 1997; 30:406–413.

46. Dries DL, Exner DV, Gersh BJ, et al. Atrial fibrillation is associated with an increased risk for mortality and heart failure progression in patients with asymptomatic and symptomatic left ventricular systolic dysfunction: a retrospective analysis of the SOLVD trials. J Am Coll Cardiol 1998; 32:695–703.

47. Censori B, Camerlingo M, Casto L, et al. Prognostic factors in first-ever stroke in the carotid artery territory seen within 6 hours after onset. Stroke 1993; 24:532–535.

48. Goldberg RJ, Yarzebski J, Lessard D, et al. Recent trends in the incidence rates of and death rates from atrial fibrillation complicating initial acute myocardial infarction: a community-wide perspective. Am Heart J 2002;143(3):519–527.

49. Behar S, Tanne D, Zion M, et al. Incidence and prognostic significance of chronic atrial fibrillation among 5839 consecutive patients with acute myocardial infarction. Am J Cardiol 1992; 70:816–818.

50. Carson PE, Johnson GR, Dunkman WB, et al for the V-HeFT VA cooperative studies group. The influence of atrial fibrillation on prognosis in mild to moderate heart failure: the V-HeFT studies. Circulation 1993;87(suppl VI):VI-102–VI-110.

51. Flaker GC, Blackshear JL, McBride R, et al. Antiarrhythmic drug therapy and cardiac mortality in atrial fibrillation. The Stroke Prevention in Atrial Fibrillation Investigators. J Am Coll Cardiol 1992; 20(3):527–532.

52. Olivotto I, Cecchi F, Casey SA, et al. Impact of atrial fibrillation on the clinical course of hypertrophic cardiomyopathy. Circulation 2001; 104(21):2517–2524.

53. Wyse DG, Waldo AL, DiMarco JP, et al. The Atrial Fibrillation Follow-up Investigation of Rhythm Management (AFFIRM) Investigators. A comparison of rate control and rhythm control in patients with atrial fibrillation. N Engl J Med 2002; 347(23):1825–1833.

54. Van Gelder IC, Hagens VE, Bosker HA, et al. Rate Control Versus Electrical Cardioversion for Persistent Atrial Fibrillation Study Group. A comparison of rate control and rhythm control in patients with recurrent persistent atrial fibrillation. N Engl J Med 2002; 347(23):1834–1840.

55. Hohnloser SH, Kuck K, Lilienthal J. Rhythm or rate control in atrial fibrillation-pharmacological intervention in atrial fibrillation: a randomised trial. Lancet 2000; 356:1789–1794.

56. Benjamin EJ, Wolf PA, D'Agostino RB, et al. Impact of atrial fibrillation on the risk of death: The Framingham Heart Study. Circulation 1998; 98:946–952.

57. American Heart Association. Heart and stroke statistical update. Dallas: American Heart Association; 1999.

58. Wolf PA, Mitchell JB, Baker CS, et al. Impact of atrial fibrillation on mortality, stroke and medical costs. Arch Intern Med 1998; 158:229–234.

59. Page RL, Wilkinson WE, Clair WK, et al. Asymptomatic arrhythmias in patients with symptomatic paroxysmal atrial fibrillation and paroxysmal supraventricular tachycardia. Circulation 1994; 89(1):224–227.

60. Rosner MH. Electrocardiography in the patient with Wolff-Parkinson-White syndrome: Diagnostic and therapeutic issues. Am J Emerg Med 1999; 17:705–714.

61. Orejarena LA, Vidaillet H Jr, DeStefano F, et al. Paroxysmal supraventricular tachycardia in the general population. J Am Coll Cardiol 1998; 31:150–157.

62. Myerberg RJ, Castellanos A. Cardiac arrest and sudden cardiac death. In: Branwald E, ed. Heart disease: a textbook of cardiovascular medicine. 5th edn. New York: WB Saunders; 1997:742–779.

63. Myerberg RJ, Kessler KM, Castellanos A. Sudden cardiac death: structure, function and time-dependence of risk. Circulation 1992; 85 (supp I): I-2–I-10.

64. Kannel WB, Thomas HE. Sudden coronary death: the Framingham study. Ann NY Acad Sci 1982; 382:3–21.

65. World Health Organisation. Technical Report 726. Sudden Cardiac Death. Basel: WHO; 1985:3–26.

66. Furukawa T, Rozanski JJ, Nogami A, et al. Time dependence risk of and predictors for cardiac arrest in survivors of out of hospital cardiac arrest with chronic coronary artery disease. Circulation 1989; 80:599–608.

67. Cupples LA, Gagnon DR, Kannel WB. Long and short-term risk of sudden coronary death. Circulation 1992; 85(suppl I):11–18.

68. Jouven X, Desnos M, Guerot C, et al. Predicting sudden cardiac death in the population: the Paris Prospective Study I. Circulation 1999; 99:1978–1983.

69. Campbell RWF, Murray A, Julian DG. Ventricular arrhythmias in the first 12 hours post myocardial infarction: natural history study. Br Heart J 1981; 46:351–357.

70. Brodsky M, Wu D, Denes P, Kanakis C, Rosen KM. Arrhythmias documented by 24-hour continuous ECG monitoring in 50 male medical students without apparent heart disease. Am J Cardiol 1977; 39:390–395.

71. Volpi A, Cavalli A, Turato R, et al. Incidence and short-term prognosis of late sustained ventricular tachycardia after myocardial infarction: results of the Gruppo Italiano per lo Studio della Sopravivvenza nell'Infarcto Miocardico (GISSI-3) Data Base. Am Heart J 2001; 142(1):87–92.

72. Newby KH, Thompson T, Stebbins A, et al. Sustained ventricular arrhythmias in patients receiving thrombolytic therapy: incidence and outcomes. Circulation 1998; 98:2567–2573.

73. Sarter BH, Finkle GK, Gerszen, et al. What is the risk of sudden cardiac death in patients presenting with haemodynamically stable sustained ventricular tachycardia after myocardial infarction. J Am Coll Cardiol 1996; 28:122–129.

74. Olsen PJ, Woefel A, Simpson RJ, et al. Stratification of sudden death risk in patients receiving long-term amiodarone treatment for sustained ventricular tachycardia or ventricular fibrillation. Am J Cardiol 1993; 71:823–826.

75. Bocker D, Block M, Isbruch F, et al. Benefits of treatment with implantable cardioverter defibrillators in patients with stable ventricular cardiac arrhythmia without cardiac arrest. Br Heart J 1995; 73:158–163.

76. Raitt MH, Renfroe EG, Epstein AE, et al. Stable ventricular tachycardia is not a benign rhythm. Insights from the Antiarrhythmics Versus Implantable Defibrillators (AVID) registry. Circulation 2001; 103:244–252.

77. Sweeney MO, Ruskin JN. Mortality benefits and the implantable cardioverter-defibrillator. Circulation 1994; 89(4):1851–1858. Review.

78. Bayes de Luna A, Coumel P, Leclercq JF. Ambulatory sudden cardiac death: mechanisms of production of fatal arrhythmia on the basis of data from 157 cases. Am Heart J 1989; 117:310–318.

79. Thompson CA, Yarzebski J, Goldberg RJ, et al. Changes over time in case-fatality rates of primary ventricular fibrillation complicating acute myocardial infarction: perspectives from the Worcester Heart Attack Study. Am Heart J 2000; 139:1014–1021.

80. Sayer JW, Archbold RA, Wilkinson P, et al. Prognostic implications of ventricular fibrillation in acute myocardial infarction: new strategies required for further mortality reduction. Heart 2000; 84(3):258–261.

81. Hohnloser SH, Klingenheben T, Zabel M, et al. Prevalence, characteristics and prognostic value during long-term follow up of nonsustained ventricular tachycardia after myocardial infarction in the thrombolytic era. J Am Coll Cardiol 1999; 33:1895–1902.

82. Brady WJ, Debehnke DJ, Laundrie D. Prevalence, theraputic response, and outcome of ventricular tachycardia in the out-of-hospital setting: a comparison of monomorphic ventricular tachycardia, polymorphic ventricular tachycardia, and torsades de pointes. Acad Emerg Med 1999; 6:609–617.

83. Myerberg RJ. Frequency of sudden cardiac death and profiles of risk. Cardiology 1987; 74(supp 2):2–9.

84. Holmberg M, Holmberg S, Herlitz J. Incidence duration and survival of ventricular fibrillation in out-of-hospital cardiac arrest patients in Sweden. Resuscitation 2000; 44:7–17.

85. Eisenberg MS, Horwood BT, Cummins RO, et al. Cardiac arrest and resuscitation: a tale of 29 cities. Ann Emerg Med 1990;19:179–186.

86. Weaver WD, Hill D, Fahrenbruch CE, et al. Use of the automatic external defibrillator in the management of out-of-hospital cardiac arrest. N Engl J Med 1988; 319:661–666

87. Connolly SJ, Hallstrom AP, Cappato R, et al. Meta-analysis of the implantable cardioverter defibrillator secondary prevention trials. AVID, CASH and CIDS studies. Eur Heart J 2000; 21:2071–2078.

88. Moss AJ. Background, outcome, and clinical implications of the Multicenter Automatic Defibrillator Implantation Trial (MADIT). Am J Cardiol 1997;80: 28F-32F

89. Pathmanathan RK, Lau EW, Cooper J, et al. Potential impact of antiarrhythmic drugs versus implantable defibrillators on the management of ventricular arrhythmias: the Midlands trial of empirical amiodarone versus electrophysiologically guided intervention and cardioverter implant registry data. Heart 1998; 80:68–70.

90. Valenti R, Schlapfer J, Fromer M, et al. Impact of the implantable cardioverter-defibrillator on rehospitalizations. Eur Heart J 1996; 17(10):1565–1571.

PATHOPHYSIOLOGY AND ELECTROPHYSIOLOGY

CHAPTER 2

Atrial physiology

Dwayne S G Conway MRCP
City Hospital, Birmingham, UK

Gregory Y H Lip MD FRCP DFM FACC FESC
City Hospital, Birmingham, UK

Understanding normal atrial structure and function helps to explain the consequences of atrial contraction failure, atrial dilatation and arrhythmogenesis

Introduction

Atrial arrhythmias, in particular atrial fibrillation (AF), are the most commonly encountered arrhythmias in routine clinical practice. Whilst this may in part be due to the high early mortality associated with ventricular arrhythmias, atrial arrhythmias may themselves confer significant morbidity and mortality. Indeed, AF carries a risk of stroke approximately fivefold greater than that of patients in sinus rhythm, which is further increased with advancing age and in the presence of certain concomitant diseases, becoming the single commonest cause of stroke in the 80–89-year-old age group.[1] Furthermore, atrial arrhythmias (including AF) may lead to abnormal intracardiac hemodynamics resulting in symptoms of palpitations, dyspnea, fatigue or syncope. The symptoms, morbidity and mortality associated with atrial arrhythmias may be explained by considering the structure, function and physiology of the atria in normal and abnormal conditions.

THE HEALTHY ATRIA: SINUS RHYTHM

Key points
Important physiological atrial functions
● Receiving chamber for venous return
● Booster pump for ventricular stroke volume
● Manometer for ventricular filling via atrial wall stretch
● Impulse generator and heart rate regulator
● Blood volume controller via ANP (in LAA)

In addition to their role as blood-receiving chambers from the pulmonary veins and caval system, the atria contribute to cardiac output via atrial systole, increasing the preload of the ventricles immediately prior to ventricular systole. Atrial systole is regulated by the sinoatrial (SA) node, which initiates a wave of depolarization

spreading across both atria and stimulating contraction of the atrial myocytes. The SA node is a spindle-shaped structure lying less than 1 mm below the epicardial surface at the junction of the superior vena cava and the right atrium, consisting of a fibrous tissue and cellular matrix. The location of the SA node – and subsequent wave of depolarization – accounts for the positive deflection of the 'p' wave in lateral, inferior and anterior (except V_1) leads of the electrocardiogram (ECG) during atrial depolarization. In normal circumstances, the wave of depolarization spreads into the ventricles via the atrioventricular node and the His-Purkinje system, allowing synchrony between atrial and ventricular systolic cycles.

However, atrial systole is not the sole mechanism of ventricular filling. Shortly prior to atrial systole, during left ventricular diastole and relaxation, ventricular pressure falls to a lower level than atrial pressure, causing the atrioventricular (mitral and tricuspid) valves to open, thus allowing 'passive' ventricular filling. The pressure changes within the atria during the cardiac cycle may be assessed by cardiac catheter studies, using pulmonary capillary wedge pressure as a surrogate of left atrial pressure. In addition, the two phases of ventricular filling can be easily visualized by pulse wave spectral Doppler imaging of the mitral valve inflow (Fig. 2.1) and the atria are also easily visualized by two-dimensional or m-mode transthoracic echocardiography, allowing assessment of atrial dimension. Thus echocardiography has become an invaluable non-invasive tool in the assessment of atrial anatomy and hemodynamic function in vivo.

Not all anatomical structures of the atria are clearly seen on transthoracic studies, however; the left and right atrial appendages are seen much more clearly by transesophageal echocardiography (TEE) due to their anatomical location and the proximity of the TEE probe (within the esophagus) to the left atrium. Both the right and left atrial appendages are blind-ending

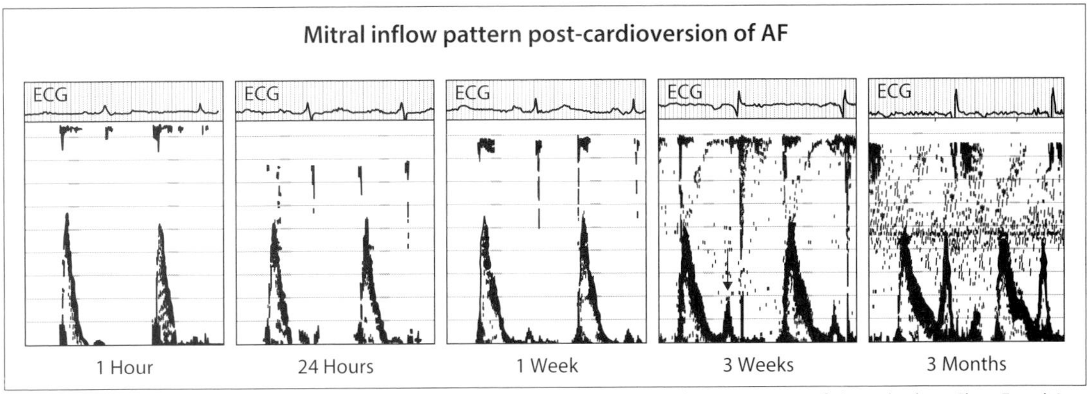

Mitral inflow pattern post-cardioversion of AF

ECG	ECG	ECG	ECG	ECG
1 Hour	24 Hours	1 Week	3 Weeks	3 Months

Fig. 2.1 Spectral Doppler of mitral inflow pattern post-cardioversion of AF and maintenance of sinus rhythm. Clear E and A waves are present at 3 months.

structures and trabeculated (with parallel pectinate muscles), allowing differentiation from the 'bodies' of the right and left atria. Compared with the right atrial appendage, which is broad and triangular, the left atrial appendage (LAA) is longer with a narrower 'neck', increasing the potential for blood-pool stasis within this blind-ending structure (Fig. 2.2). As a consequence, the LAA is the commonest site of intra-atrial thrombus formation in disease states such as AF and (to a lesser extent) mitral stenosis,[2] and both increased LAA size and reduced LAA flow velocity appear to be associated with an increased risk of LAA thrombus in AF and sinus rhythm.[3] In normal circumstances, however, there is a biphasic (or, at slow heart rates, quadriphasic) pattern of blood flow within the LAA,[4] reducing stasis and visible via TEE with pulse wave Doppler (Fig. 2.3). The initial emptying flow from the LAA occurs during ventricular diastole and corresponds with passive left ventricular filling, perhaps due in part to the expanding left ventricle exerting external pressure on the LAA, but mainly related to transmitral blood flow. This is followed by a brief period of LAA filling; both of these phases occur at low flow velocities and may be absent at faster heart rates. The second, more rapid phase of LAA emptying occurs with atrial systole, and appears to be due to active contraction of the LAA. The second (fast) phase of LAA filling follows during ventricular systole, a combination

effect of rising left atrial pressures, elastic recoil of the LAA and increased room for expansion of the LAA within the pericardium (due to the contracting ventricle).

Beyond the contributory role of the atria in cardiac output, they act as vital sensors of blood volume and pressure. Relative to the ventricles, the walls of the atria are thin and pliable, and are thus able stretch in response to increases in blood volume and pressure. Indeed, the LAA may be more distensible still than the left atrium itself, acting as a vital reservoir and pressure sensor in states of increased left atrial pressure and volume overload.[5] The extent of atrial stretch influences several important physiological mechanisms: neuronally-mediated increases in heart rate (with an afferent vagal pathway and an efferent sympathetic pathway) and renin activity,[6] suppression of vasopressin release (promoting diuresis)[7] and secretion of atrial natriuretic peptide (ANP) (further promoting diuresis and sodium wasting). Notably, the atrial appendages contain about 30% of all cardiac ANP and selective dilatation of the atrial appendages in laboratory dogs has been shown to promote diuresis and sodium excretion.[8] Furthermore, removal of the atrial appendages at the time of cardiac surgery has been shown to lead to an impaired release of ANP and inappropriate fluid retention,[9] emphasizing the importance of the atrial appendages in ANP release. In

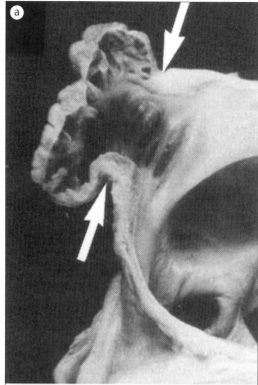

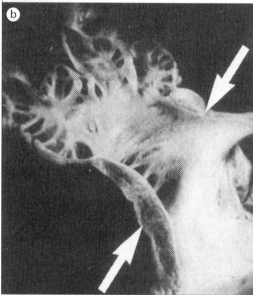

Fig. 2.2 Pathological specimens of the LAA. (a) Bilobed appendage, seen in approximately half of autopsies. (b) Multi-lobed appendage, found in 25% of autopsies. Reproduced with permission from Hart RG, Halperin JL. Atrial fibrillation and stroke: concepts and controversies. Stroke 2001; 32:803–808.

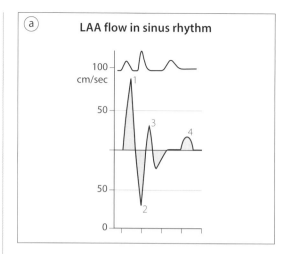

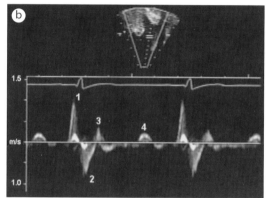

Fig. 2.3 (a) Diagram of LAA flow in sinus rhythm. (b) Pulsed-Doppler tracing of LAA flow in sinus rhythm. 1, LAA contraction; 2, LAA filling; 3, systolic reflection waves (positive and negative); 4, early diastolic LAA outflow. Reproduced with permission from Agmon Y, Khandheria BK, Gentile F, et al. Echocardiographic assessment of the left atrial appendage. J Am Coll Cardiol 1999; 34(7):1867–1877. © 1999 The American College of Cardiology Foundation.

addition to the above homeostatic physiological response mechanisms, an increased atrial size has been shown to be associated with an increased risk of AF,[10] and an increased risk of thromboembolic complications of this condition,[11] although the latter may be due to an association with other prothrombotic conditions such as hypertension.

Due to the multiple roles of the atria and atrial appendages (as receiving chambers for venous return, capacitance vessels in states of increased atrial pressures, sensors of atrial volume and stretch, potential sites of thrombosis and regulators of heart rate, stroke volume and circulating blood volume), any atrial arrhythmia represents a change from the 'healthy' state and may be either a precipitant or a consequence of changes in the anatomical, physiological or hemodynamic state of the atria, in addition to a precipitant or consequence of disorders anatomically remote from the atria.

ATRIAL FIBRILLATION

The term 'atrial fibrillation' describes the chaotic electrical activity resulting from the integration of several coexisting re-entrant wavefronts continuously sweeping around the atria. The electrophysiological mechanisms of AF will be discussed in detail in Chapter 3, but it appears that the persistence of AF is often related to increased atrial size, allowing a critical mass of anatomical substrate for the persistence of the disorganized electrical wavefronts. Atrial hypertrophy and dilatation are thus risk factors for the initiation and permanence of AF, and AF may therefore be subsequent to conditions which increase left atrial 'workload' (such as hypertension, left ventricular hypertrophy and left ventricular dysfunction). However, AF may also occur as a response to a hyperadrenergic state (such as infection or exercise), thyrotoxicosis or an alcoholic 'binge', suggesting the relationship between AF and anatomical and physiological changes in the atria is not simply a function of left atrial size. Indeed, of all the atrial arrhythmias, AF carries the worst long-term prognosis and it is thus not surprising that AF is associated with a multitude of changes in atrial anatomy and physiology.

Atrial anatomy and atrial fibrillation

Left atrial enlargement is a common finding in AF. Many conditions predisposing to AF are known to have effects on the left atrium, which are likely to be contributory to the initiation and maintenance of AF. However, there is evidence that chronic AF itself can lead to progressive left atrial dilatation,[12] with left atrial enlargement related to the duration of AF, and indeed that the process is reversible with cardioversion and long-term maintenance of sinus rhythm.[13] An association between increased LAA size and AF has also been observed in postmortem[14] and TEE[3] studies.

Left atrial dilatation reduces the probability of successful cardioversion and maintenance of sinus rhythm.[15] Furthermore, left atrial dilatation promotes blood-pool stasis within the left atrium, which can be visualized on TEE as spontaneous echo contrast (SEC) (a swirling, smoke-like pattern) (Fig. 2.4) or reduced left atrial appendage flow velocities measured by pulse wave Doppler (Fig. 2.5), and may thus increase the risk of intra-atrial thrombogenesis.[3,16] Indeed, the first Stroke Prevention in Atrial Fibrillation (SPAF) study reported that an increased left atrial size corrected for body surface area was an independent predictor for stroke,[17] although a more recent meta-analysis of three trials suggested that isolated left atrial dilatation per se was not an independent risk factor, when all other clinical variables are accounted for.[18] However, the association between left atrial size and

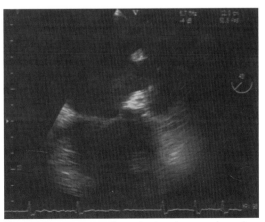

Fig. 2.4 Spontaneous echocontrast on transesophageal echocardiography.

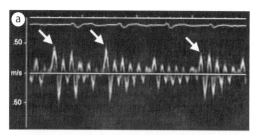

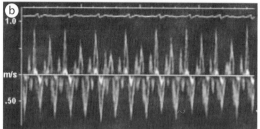

Fig. 2.5 (a) Pulsed-Doppler tracing of LAA flow in AF. Note the rapid fibrillatory flow waves, which are of higher velocity during ventricular diastole than systole. (b) Pulsed-Doppler tracing of LAA flow in AFL (with a 2:1 ventricular response). Flutter flow waves are, in general, slower and of higher velocity than fibrillatory flow waves. Reproduced with permission from Agmon Y, Khandheria BK, Gentile F, et al. Echocardiographic assessment of the left atrial appendage. J Am Coll Cardiol 1999; 34(7):1867–1877. © 1999 The American College of Cardiology Foundation.

thromboembolic risk may still represent a possible pathological mechanism, and an increased LAA size has also been shown to associate with LAA stasis and an increased risk of LAA thrombosis.[3]

Atrial histology and atrial fibrillation

Key points

Atrial histology and hemodynamics in AF

- Atrial wall fibrosis
- Structural changes in atrial myocytes
- Inflammatory cell infiltration
- Endothelial abnormality on scanning electron microscopy
- Atrial contraction failure
- Atrial stasis and dilatation
- Atrial mechanical remodeling ('stunning')

Despite the link between left atrial size and AF, it is seldom possible to identify the exact mechanisms predisposing to AF, as the condition may occur in patients with normal atrial size or apparently free of coexisting disease. However, patchy areas of fibrotic change have been described on histological examination of atrial tissue from patients with AF.[19] These fibrotic changes may be due to inflammatory or degenerative processes, but it is difficult to establish whether these areas predispose to AF (perhaps acting as excitable foci or affecting atrial refractoriness), whether they are themselves a consequence of AF, or whether they may merely be innocent associations of coexisting disease. Atrial fibrosis appears to be inducible in a canine heart failure model of AF, but does not resolve after termination of the arrhythmia.[20] It has been demonstrated in goat models that sustained AF itself leads to a change in structure of atrial myocytes.[21] Myocytes increased in size (up to 195%), with a reduction in myofibrils, accumulation of glycogen, alterations in mitochondrial structure, fragmentation of sarcoplasmic reticulum and dispersion of nuclear chromatin. However, there were few signs of cellular degeneration and the interstitial space remained unaltered, suggesting a different pathological process to the fibrosis seen in human AF atrial tissue. Nonetheless, these myocyte changes may account for the delay in return of atrial systole that occurs after successful cardioversion of AF. In a separate study, Frustaci and colleagues[22] noted that atrial biopsies from patients with lone AF demonstrated different patterns of histological change: two cases had atrial myocyte hypertrophy with vacuolar degeneration and fibrillolysis (similar to the observations in the goat model), eight had lymphomononuclear infiltrates with myocyte necrosis (suggestive of localized inflammation) and two had non-specific fibrotic change only. It is therefore possible that localized inflammatory and degenerative change may predispose to at least two-thirds of apparent lone AF. In support of the inflammatory hypothesis, increased circulating levels of C-reactive protein (CRP) have been described in AF.[23]

Inflammatory molecules such as CRP have been implicated in the prothrombotic mechanisms behind coronary atherothrombosis,[24] but their role in the prothrombotic state of AF remains unclear.

Hemodynamic aspects of atrial fibrillation

The presence of AF confers an alteration in hemodynamic state via two mechanisms: the loss of atrial systole and the irregular, fast ventricular response. Atrial systole is lost as a result of both the chaotic electrical activity itself and the resulting myopathic changes to the atrial myocytes. Thus AF leads to a fall in stroke volume, varying from about 10% in normal individuals to over a third in the elderly (who are particularly reliant on the contribution of atrial systole due to a reduction in left ventricular compliance and reduced passive left ventricular filling). The reduction in stroke volume in AF is most marked at higher heart rates due to reduced left ventricular filling time. Furthermore, if the heart rate in AF remains uncontrolled it may lead to cellular changes in the left ventricular myocardium, which promote left ventricular dilatation and systolic dysfunction, so-called 'tachycardia-induced cardiomyopathy'.

In addition to a reduction in cardiac output, these mechanisms are also responsible for intra-atrial blood stasis and an increase in left atrial pressure, which can lead to atrial 'stretch' (causing an increase in ANP production) and increased pulmonary venous pressure. The hemodynamic changes in AF account for much of the symptoms and clinical manifestations of AF, namely palpitations, reduced exercise tolerance and dyspnea. Indeed, AF may commonly be associated with reduced left ventricular function: in addition to tachycardia-induced cardiomyopathy following AF, this association may be due to pre-existing left ventricular dysfunction resulting in an increase in left atrial pressure and size and precipitating AF. Following myocardial infarction, the development of new AF is a poor prognostic sign.[25]

The adverse hemodynamic effects of AF may be successfully abolished with the return and maintenance of sinus rhythm. Cardioversion has been shown to confer a significant improvement in left ventricular ejection fraction and exercise capacity among patients with AF[26,27] and for these reasons has long been a goal in the treatment of AF. However, there are no prospective randomized controlled trials demonstrating a reduction in mortality rate by cardioversion of AF, and the potential benefits of a 'rhythm-control' versus 'rate-control' approach may be offset by the unfavorable side-effect profile of many 'rhythm-control' drugs and by the increase in hospital admissions which has also been described using this approach.[26] Furthermore, cardioversion and maintenance of sinus rhythm may be difficult to achieve for many AF patients in clinical practice, and the results of several prospective randomized controlled trials (PIAF, AFFIRM and RACE) have consistently shown no overall benefit in the 'rhythm control' approach over rate control and anticoagulation.[26,28,29]

Thrombogenesis and stroke

Thrombogenesis and Virchow's triad in AF

- Left atrial stasis (in LAA)
- 'Rough' endothelium on scanning electron microscopy
- A prothrombotic state is definitely present (increased platelet activation, increased D-dimer and von Willebrand factor)

AF is an important risk factor for stroke, conferring an increase in risk approximately five times that of the general population.[30] However, this risk depends upon the presence or absence of certain additional risk factors. For example, the risk is 18 times greater in the presence of rheumatic heart disease, but even in non-valvular AF, other factors (including advancing age, hypertension, diabetes, left ventricular dysfunction or hypertrophy, or previous thromboembolism) may lead to an increased risk.

Thrombus is usually formed within the left atrial appendage prior to subsequent embolism.[2] The precise mechanisms predisposing to thrombus formation and embolization are unclear, but abnormalities in blood flow within the left atrium and its appendage are understood to be of importance. The loss of atrial systole in AF results in increased stasis of blood within the left atrium. The irregular, fast ventricular response also reduces effective left ventricular filling and promotes left atrial stasis. Left atrial stasis may be visualized on TEE as SEC. This phenomenon occurs due to increased interaction between erythrocytes and fibrinogen molecules in states of reduced blood flow, increasing echocardiographic 'backscatter',[31] and has been shown to independently predict an increased risk of thromboembolism.[32] Further studies have demonstrated reduced flow velocities in the LAA in AF, with a change in Doppler waveform, and these changes have also been associated with presence of LAA thrombus (which may be present in as many as 15% of patients presenting with recent-onset AF), SEC and increased risk of subsequent thromboembolism.[33] While mitral stenosis further reduces effective transit of blood from the left atrium to the left ventricle (thus increasing thromboembolic risk), mitral regurgitation may reduce thromboembolic risk by a 'stirring' effect of the regurgitant jet in the left atrium, thus reducing stasis.

The importance of abnormal hemodynamics in thrombus formation is better understood than mechanisms of subsequent embolism. However, the transition from AF to sinus rhythm (in paroxysmal AF or following cardioversion) appears to be a particular time of increased risk, with an approximately 7% risk of thromboembolism associated with direct

current (DC) cardioversion if anticoagulation is not used. This may be due to the return of left atrial systole leading to embolization of preformed thrombus, but there is often a period of atrial 'stunning' following cardioversion (which may last up to 3 weeks) whereby the left atrial contractile function initially *decreases* prior to return of atrial systole.[13] Furthermore, there is still a risk of thromboembolism in the period following cardioversion even in those in whom pre-existing thrombus has been excluded by TEE,[34] adding weight to the theory that there may be an increased propensity to thrombus *formation* immediately postcardioversion, rather than simply an increase in embolism.

The term 'atrial stunning' is perhaps a misnomer: the phenomenon has been described in both electrical and pharmacological cardioversion of AF (but is not seen in cardioversion of ventricular arrhythmias) and varies according to the duration of prior AF, suggesting it is related to electrophysiological and cellular changes caused by the AF itself, rather than the effect of cardioversion.

There is also a clustering of thromboembolic events around the time of onset of AF, and after the transition from paroxysmal to chronic AF, suggesting a change in rhythm does play a role in thromboembolism, although the relative contribution to thrombogenesis versus embolism is unclear. However, the size and mobility of LAA thrombus are known determinants of embolic risk, which is increased if the thrombus exceeds 1.5 cm diameter or appears pedunculated and mobile.[35]

Despite the above evidence, blood flow abnormalities alone may not be sufficient to induce left atrial thrombus formation. Indeed, the thromboembolic risk in patients with 'lone' AF is relatively low, despite the loss of atrial systole. Virchow's triad theory of thrombogenesis postulates that abnormal vessel wall and intravascular constituents are also needed for thrombus formation, in addition to blood flow abnormalities. On a macroscopic level, an increased left atrial size might be considered evidence of abnormal vessel wall, and has been shown to predict subsequent thromboembolism in AF, although this association may simply be a reflection of comorbidity such as hypertension.[18] Left atrial (and/or left atrial appendage) enlargement has also been associated with the presence of SEC and intra-atrial thrombus.[31]

However, there is further evidence of abnormal 'vessel wall' in AF at microscopic and molecular levels. Masawa et al[36] described 'rough endocardium', a macroscopically wrinkled appearance due to edematous and fibrous thickening, with small areas of endothelial denudation and thrombotic aggregation visible by scanning electron microscopy in necropsy specimens of left atrial tissue from patients with AF and cerebral embolism. They also noted a significantly higher proportion of these features among these cases than among cases with cerebral embolism that had been in sinus rhythm. In another necropsy study, Shirani et al[37] described a significantly higher prevalence of LAA endocardial fibroelastosis in AF than in sinus rhythm. Furthermore, increased endocardial expression of von Willebrand factor (vWf) has been described in patients with 'overloaded' atrial appendages with a correlation between endocardial vWf expression and adherent platelet thrombus,[38] and raised plasma levels of vWf have been shown to associate with ultrastructural changes in the atrial appendage endocardium of patients with mitral valve disease (Fig. 2.6).[39] Many of the patients in the latter two studies were in AF, although the studies were not sufficiently powered to detect whether AF itself contributes to these changes. However, these studies demonstrate evidence of endocardial abnormalities in patients with (or at high risk of) AF, which might provide a substrate for thrombus adhesion.

The final part of Virchow's triad, namely abnormal procoagulant blood constituents, have also been described in

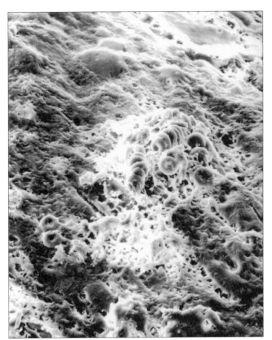

Fig. 2.6 Severely damaged left atrial appendage endocardial surface with thrombotic mass in a patient with atrial fibrillation and mitral valve disease. Reproduced with permission from Goldsmith I, Kumar P, Carter P, et al. Atrial endocardial changes in mitral valve disease: A scanning electron microscopy study. Am Heart J 2000; 140(5): 777–784.

AF, suggesting that AF represents a truly hypercoagulable state (Fig. 2.7).[40] Kumagai and colleagues[41] described increased fibrin D-dimer (an index of fibrin turnover or 'hypercoagulability') in chronic AF compared to healthy controls in sinus rhythm, a finding subsequently confirmed by Lip et al.[42] Furthermore, successful cardioversion to sinus rhythm appears to reduce levels of fibrin D-dimer,[43] suggesting that the presence of AF itself may be driving the increased hemostatic state. Further evidence of increased thrombogenesis in AF has been described, using prothrombin fragment 1+2 (F1+2)[44,45] fibrinopeptide A[46–49] and thrombin–antithrombin III (TAT) complex[50] as indices, and there is evidence that full-dose warfarin treatment may 'normalize' levels of fibrin D-dimer[42] and F1+2.[51] Furthermore, Feinberg et al[52] found an association between high levels of F1+2 and cardioembolic events in AF, although this

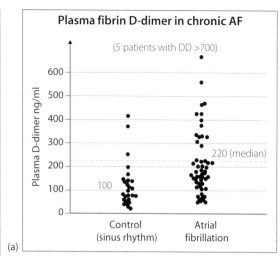

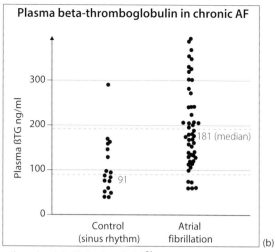

Fig. 2.7 (a) Plasma fibrin D-dimer in chronic AF. (b) Plasma beta-thromboglobulin in chronic AF.[54]

relationship disappeared after adjustment for age. However, whilst these studies use markers of increased fibrin turnover to demonstrate evidence of an ongoing hypercoagulable state in AF, the markers are not themselves *promoters* of coagulation and thus may not strictly fulfil Virchow's triad.

In simple terms, the known intravascular promoters of thrombus formation are platelets and the proteins of the coagulation 'cascade', via their interaction with each other and the vascular endothelium. Evidence supporting increased platelet activation in AF has been provided by numerous studies[53–56] (Table 2.1),[31,52–54,56–62] but there are some conflicting studies,[63,64] which may reflect the variety of available methods with which to assess platelet function without an obvious 'gold standard'.[65] Whilst the majority of the evidence suggests platelet activation may be increased in AF, the evidence that this relates to the increased thrombotic risk in AF is conflicting. Although Heppel[58] found an independent association between raised levels of the platelet marker beta-thromboglobulin and intra-atrial thrombus on TEE, a much larger study[52] found no association between plasma levels of beta-thromboglobulin and subsequent thromboembolic events among participants in the SPAF III trial.

Furthermore, plasma levels of soluble P-selectin were unrelated to estimated stroke risk among patients from SPAF III,[59] despite associations between soluble P-selectin level and atherothrombotic risk factors such as smoking and peripheral vascular disease in these patients. The importance of platelet activation in AF is therefore uncertain.

In addition to increased markers of platelet activation, Gustafsson et al[53] demonstrated increased plasma fibrinogen, fibrin D-dimer and vWf in AF, which has since been confirmed by Lip et al[42] and Li-Saw-Hee et al.[66] vWf may be a particularly important procoagulant factor, due to its ability to interact with platelets and factor VIII[67] as an index of endothelial damage or dysfunction (due to increased release of vWf from endothelial cells[68]) and as an established marker of poor prognosis in cardiovascular disease.[69] Indeed, Lip et al[42] found a significant positive correlation between plasma levels of fibrin D-dimer and vWf (in keeping with the role of this molecule or the endothelium in thrombogenesis) and Heppel et al,[58] in addition to their findings for beta-thromboglubulin, found raised levels of vWf to be predictive of the presence of left atrial appendage thrombus seen on TEE in AF patients. Among 1321 participants in the SPAF III trial, plasma vWf level was

Table 2.1 The prothrombotic state of atrial fibrillation: a summary of key studies of platelet activation in AF

Author	Year	No of AF cases included in study	Study Findings	Comment
Yamauchi[56]	1986	99	Raised plasma levels of BTG and PF4 in AF	The first case-control study to describe evidence of platelet activation in AF
Gustafsson[53]	1990	40	Raised plasma levels of BTG and PF4 in AF. Levels among AF cases with or without recent stroke were higher than levels among both healthy controls and stroke patients in sinus rhythm	Further evidence of platelet activation in AF
Black[31]	1993	135	The presence of SEC visible on TEE was not associated with increased BTG in AF	A large TEE study. SEC (a risk factor for thromboembolism in AF) not apparently linked to platelet activation
Lip[54]	1996	51	Raised BTG levels in AF are reduced by full-dose warfarin, not aspirin-based therapy	Evidence that full-dose warfarin may lead to greater reductions in platelet activation in AF than aspirin-based prophylaxis
Pongratz[57]	1997	60	Raised BTG and sP-sel among AF patients with stroke or LA thrombus compared to both healthy controls and AF without thromboembolism	Evidence suggesting platelet activation is associated with embolic or 'pre-embolic' status in AF
Heppel[58]	1997	109	BTG and PF4 higher among AF cases with LA thrombus than AF cases without. Raised BTG levels independently associated with LA thrombus	Another large TEE study. Suggests an association does exist between platelet activation and LA thrombosis in AF
Feinberg[52]	1999	1338	No relationship between plasma levels of BTG and subsequent stroke risk	Large prospective substudy among participants in the SPAF III trial. No apparent link between platelet activation and subsequent stroke incidence in AF. However, **all** participants in SPAF III received antithrombotic therapy (warfarin or aspirin-based)
Conway[59]	2002	1321	No relationship between recognised risk factors for stroke in AF (apart from diabetes) and plasma sP-sel	Further sub-studies from among the SPAF III cohort. Despite using an alternative platelet marker to BTG, once again no evidence of a link between platelet activation and stroke. However, **all** participants in SPAF III received antithrombotic therapy (warfarin or aspirin-based)
Conway[60]	2002	994	Plasma sP-sel levels not associated with subsequent stroke	

Table 2.1 *cont'd*

Author	Year	No of AF cases included in study	Study Findings	Comment
Kamath[61]	2002	238	Raised BTG and GpV among AF patients on no antithrombotic therapy, but no evidence of enhanced platelet aggregation using ex vivo methods. No effect of warfarin or aspirin on indices of platelet function	Although some evidence for platelet activation, overall a conflicting picture with no apparent effect of antithrombotic therapy. Authors suggest that platelet function may not be important in determining thrombogenesis in AF
Conway[62]	2003	162	No difference in plasma sP-sel between AF and matched controls	A substudy of the Rotterdam Study (a large community-based study of an elderly population) – No evidence of platelet activation in AF

Despite suggestions of increased platelet activation in AF in earlier studies, such findings are not confirmed by more recent studies (often with larger sample sizes and more rigorous statistical method). Furthermore, although platelet activation appears enhanced among AF cases with LA thrombus or previous embolism, large prospective studies have failed to confirm that this translates into increased stroke risk. Platelet activation is notoriously difficult to assess accurately and therefore, although a role for platelets in AF-related stroke remains unproven, it cannot be completely excluded.

BTG, beta-thromboglobulin; PF4, platelet factor 4; TEE, transesophageal echocardiography; SEC, spontaneous echocontrast; SPAF III, the third Stroke Prevention in Atrial Fibrillation trial; sP-sel, soluble P-selectin; GpV, glycoprotein V.

associated with the presence of four stroke risk factors independently of each other (heart failure, previous stroke, increasing age and diabetes) and with overall estimated stroke risk.[59] Follow-up data from this study suggests raised plasma vWf levels may be predictive of subsequent cardiovascular events, independently of known clinical risk factors.[60]

Conversely, despite having been shown to be both an independent predictor for stroke among the general population in the Edinburgh Artery Study[70] and an associate of left atrial SEC in the setting of AF,[16,31] elevated plasma fibrinogen (the immediate precursor to insoluble fibrin in the coagulation cascade) did not predict thromboembolic events in a study of 621 participants in the SPAF III trial.[52]

Plasma levels of other prothrombotic molecules (including tissue factor[71]) are also raised in AF and abnormalities of

fibrinolytic pathways (raised levels of plasminogen activator inhibitor-1) have been described,[72] but their relationship to stroke risk and other clinical factors has not been fully explored. Factor V Leiden was not linked to thromboembolic events in SPAF III.[52]

Despite the evidence for abnormal hemostatic factors in AF, AF itself is an extremely heterogeneous condition, often reflecting additional (often undiagnosed) underlying cardiovascular pathologies that might themselves account for the abnormalities seen. Although some studies examining hemostatic markers in AF have attempted to adjust for these potential confounders, the numbers of cases in these studies were small and often compared to healthy controls, making adjustment difficult. In a large epidemiological study from the Framingham offspring population,[73] raised levels of hemostatic markers among AF cases compared to the general population became non-significant when additional cardiovascular pathologies were accounted for. However, numbers of AF cases in the study were still relatively small (n=47) and, in view of the independent association observed between levels of vWf and AF in the Rotterdam Study,[62] the presence of a true relationship between AF itself and hemostatic markers is not in doubt. The association with some hemostatic markers and risk factors would nevertheless seem consistent with the variable risk of stroke and thromboembolic events in AF (dependent on the presence of such additional conditions).

It has been suggested that circulating levels of certain hemostatic markers in AF may be altered by exercise[74] and may not reflect intra-atrial levels,[75] but the evidence for these suggestions is not supported by all studies.[76] Furthermore, there does not appear to be significant circadian or diurnal variation in levels of hemostatic markers in AF,[66] suggesting a persistently hypercoagulable state in AF, detectable by measurement of markers from peripheral venous blood. Nonetheless, the relationships between hemostatic markers (including vWf), AF, cardiovascular comorbidity and the risk of subsequent stroke need further evaluation to determine which factors are related to AF per se, which are related to co-morbidities and which might determine cardiovascular risk in AF.

A summary of the main studies of procoagulant intravascular abnormalities in AF is shown in Table 2.2.[31,41–43,52,53,58–60,62,71,73,,77,78]

Additional intravascular effects of atrial fibrillation

The physiological effects of AF extend beyond alterations in hemostasis, yet even these other physiological factors could have implications for thrombogenesis, stroke and cardiovascular morbidity. AF has been shown to lead to an increased secretion of ANP, with plasma levels noticeably higher during episodes of AF than during sinus rhythm in patients with paroxysmal AF,[79] and rapidly decreased by successful direct-current cardioversion.[80–82] The increase in ANP during AF may be due to the electrophysiological changes of the atrial myocytes, or simply reflect an increase in intra-atrial pressure. ANP may be responsible for the increase in hematocrit that has been observed in AF (and paroxysms of AF),[63,75] and this in turn may be partly responsible for the presence of SEC in AF, due to increased interaction between erythrocytes and fibrinogen.[31] Whether hemoconcentration due to ANP might also increase interaction between platelets, endothelium and molecules of the coagulation cascade is unclear. In addition to these effects, a reduction in circulating volume due to ANP might exacerbate the fall in cardiac output due to the loss of atrial systole and exacerbate symptoms of fatigue, presyncope or malaise.

Interestingly, whilst the short-term effect of AF appears to be an increase in ANP secretion (which may be due to increased atrial pressures or an increase in heart rate), the presence of chronic AF appears to lead to a reduction in ANP production due to degenerative change in the atria.[83] Indeed, a low ANP is associated with an increased probability of recurrent AF following successful cardioversion, perhaps reflecting the degree of atrial degeneration.[84] Paradoxically, a *high* brain natriuretic peptide (BNP) level is associated with an increased probability of recurrent AF following successful cardioversion,[84] although as BNP is predominantly secreted by the ventricles this is most likely to reflect impaired left ventricular function (which is itself known to reduce the chance of successful cardioversion and maintenance of sinus rhythm, presumably due to increased atrial workload).

Other important physiological changes which have been described in AF include an increase in Big endothelin-1[85] and a decrease in nitric oxide activity,[86] both of which may reflect dysfunctional

Table 2.2 The prothrombotic state of atrial fibrillation: a summary of key studies of pro-coagulant factors in AF

Author	Year	No of AF cases included in study	Study Findings	Comment
Kumagai[41]	1990	73	Raised levels of fibrin D-dimer in AF	The first case-control study to describe a prothrombotic state in AF
Gustafsson[53]	1990	40	Raised plasma levels of fibrin D-dimer, fibrinogen and vWf in AF	Further evidence of a prothrombotic state in AF
Black[31]	1993	135	Raised fibrinogen and haematocrit associated with SEC in AF	Evidence of rheological abnormalities associated with SEC. Rheological disturbances may underlie the increased thrombotic risk associated with SEC
Lip[42, 43]	1995 & 1996	87	Raised plasma levels of fibrin D-dimer, fibrinogen and vWf in AF. A correlation between D-dimer and vWf. D-dimer levels reduced both by warfarin therapy and cardioversion to sinus rhythm	Evidence that the prothrombotic state in AF may be modified by antithrombotic therapy or reversion to sinus rhythm. Also, a suggested association between endothelial dysfunction (vWf) and the prothrombotic state (D-dimer) in AF
Heppel[58]	1997	109	Plasma vWf independently associated with presence of LA thrombus on TEE	Suggests an association between endothelial dysfunction (vWf) and LA thrombosis in AF
Feinberg[52]	1999	1338	No relationship between plasma levels of fibrinogen or prothrombin fragment F1+2 and subsequent stroke risk	Large prospective sub-study among participants in the SPAF III trial – Failed to identify a marker capable of predicting stroke in AF. However, **all** participants in SPAF III received antithrombotic therapy (warfarin or aspirin-based)
Li-Saw-Hee[77]	2000	61	Raised fibrin D-dimer, fibrinogen and vWf in AF not affected by low-dose warfarin or aspirin (alone or combination)	In accordance with clinical trial observations, no significant effect on indices of the prothrombotic state is seen with 'low-dose' warfarin regimens
Li-Saw-Hee[78]	2001	69	Fibrinogen and vWf levels related to subtype of AF. Levels in *permanent* and *paroxysmal* AF significantly higher than controls, but no difference between *persistent* AF and controls	Suggests that the prothrombotic state might be associated with the 'permanence' or 'burden' of AF

Table 2.2 *cont'd*

Author	Year	No of AF cases included in study	Study Findings	Comment
Feng[73]	2001	47	No significant difference in levels of fibrinogen, vWf or PAI-1 between AF cases and matched population controls	Data from the Framingham offspring population. Despite a huge sample population, the relatively small number of AF cases may have led to an underestimation of relationships between AF and the prothrombotic state
Conway[62]	2003	162	No difference in plasma fibrinogen levels between AF and matched controls, but an independent association between AF and vWf levels in women	A substudy of the Rotterdam Study (a large community-based study of an elderly population). Despite failing to prove a link with fibrinogen levels, there appeared to be a definite association between AF and vWf levels *among women* not explained by other clinical factors. The study raises the possibility of gender differences in the prothrombotic mechanisms of AF, and confirms a link between AF and endothelial dysfunction (vWf)
Chung[71]	2002	25	Raised plasma levels of VEGF and tissue factor TF in AF. A strong correlation between VEGF and TF.	Evidence of another potential mechanism of thrombosis in AF, via TF-mediated coagulation pathway. Also, evidence that angiogenic factors may be raised in AF and may relate to the prothrombotic state
Conway[59]	2002	1321	Plasma levels of vWf rise in relation to estimated stroke risk using clinical criteria. Heart failure, age, prior stroke, diabetes and body mass index are independent associates of vWf in AF	Further sub-studies from among the SPAF III cohort. Finally, proof that an index of the prothrombotic state (vWf) is clearly linked both to clinical risk factors and *independently* to subsequent stroke.
Conway[60]	2002	994	Plasma vWf levels independently predict stroke and cardiovascular mortality/morbidity in AF, after adjusting for clinical factors	Endothelial dysfunction or vWf itself may be implicated in mechanisms of stroke in AF. Note: **all** participants in SPAF III received antithrombotic therapy (warfarin or aspirin-based)

Clear evidence exists for a prothrombotic state in AF, which may be modified by warfarin therapy or cardioversion, while aspirin or low-dose warfarin appear less effective. Abnormalities of rheology (fibrinogen, haematocrit), vascular wall (vWf, VEGF) and coagulation factors (TF) exist in AF, fulfilling Virchow's triad for thrombogenesis. Perhaps most notable of these factors, vWf is associated with several stroke risk factors and is independently predictive of LA thrombus and future stroke. Links with other pathological processes (angiogenesis, inflammation) may exist, and ongoing studies continue to unravel the complexities of the prothrombotic state of AF. It is hoped that this greater understanding may eventually identify potential therapeutic targets and aid risk stratification in AF.

vWf, von Willebrand factor; TEE, transesophageal echocardiography; SEC, spontaneous echocontrast; SPAF III, the third Stroke Prevention in Atrial Fibrillation trial; PAI-1, plasminogen activator inhibitor type-1; VEGF, vascular endothelial growth factor; TF, tissue factor.

endothelium and play a role in inappropriate vasomotor responses. Low nitrate activity may also be associated with an increase in platelet activation, through reduced platelet cGMP.[86] More recently still, raised circulating levels of CRP[23] and vascular endothelial growth factor (VEGF)[71] have been described in AF, suggesting involvement of inflammatory and angiogenic processes in the condition. Inflammatory molecules including CRP have been linked to thrombogenesis in other cardiovascular conditions,[24] and VEGF levels correlate strongly with levels of tissue factor (an important molecule in the coagulation cascade) in AF,[71] suggesting each of these processes may be involved in thrombogenesis in AF.

ATRIAL FLUTTER

Echocardiographic studies of atrial flutter have revealed visible atrial contractions occurring with each flutter wave, although the atrial contraction sequence is reversed compared to sinus rhythm, with left preceding right atrial contraction.[87] Furthermore, the rapid atrial rate of atrial flutter is not compatible with a sustained 1:1 conduction to the ventricles; thus, in the usual setting of 2:1 or 3:1 conduction block at the AV node, atrioventricular synchrony is lost in atrial flutter. As a consequence atrial pressures may rise and lead to a similar hemodynamic profile as seen in AF, and ANP is similarly elevated in atrial flutter as in AF.[79] Furthermore, the risk factors for development and persistence of atrial flutter are in essence the same as for AF, including an increased left atrial size[88] although the electrophysiological properties of the atria in flutter and AF are quite different (see Ch. 3).

For the above reasons, atrial flutter is often regarded as a single entity with AF in epidemiological studies, thus the precise risk of LAA thrombus formation and stroke in atrial flutter per se is unclear. There is inconsistency between TEE studies regarding the prevalence of LAA thrombus

and SEC in atrial flutter.[89,90] Indeed, atrial flutter commonly coexists with paroxysms of AF (so-called 'flutter-fibrillation') and there is evidence that these features are more frequent among patients with known episodes of AF than those with 'pure' atrial flutter.[91] The presence of atrial contraction in atrial flutter would be expected to reduce left atrial stasis compared to AF, and higher LAA flow velocities are seen in atrial flutter compared to AF,[91] thus thromboembolic risk might be expected to be lower in 'pure' flutter. However, there are to date no studies examining plasma markers of hemostasis and thrombosis in atrial flutter per se.[92] Overall, due to the increased risk of thromboembolism and the difficulty in differentiating cases of 'pure' flutter from 'flutter-fibrillation', it is sensible clinical practice to apply the same criteria for thromboprophylaxis as in AF, until more evidence of a reduced risk in atrial flutter is available from large-scale epidemiological studies.

ATRIOVENTRICULAR RE-ENTRANT TACHYCARDIAS AND ATRIOVENTRICULAR NODAL RE-ENTRANT TACHYCARDIAS

Atrioventricular re-entrant tachycardias (AVRTs) and atrioventricular nodal re-entrant tachycardias (AVNRTs) are both caused by the presence of abnormal re-entrant circuits between atria and ventricles or within the AV node itself. These re-entrant circuits are discussed in detail in Chapter 3. Both AVRTs and AVNRTs result in a change from the normal sequence of atrial and ventricular depolarization and contraction. However, the degree of hemodynamic change may depend on the size of the re-entrant circuit, with the smaller circuit of AVNRTs increasing the likelihood of simultaneous atrial and ventricular contraction, resulting in 'cannon A waves' in the jugular venous pressure waveform.[93] Both types of arrhythmia lead to an increase in atrial pressure with resultant secretion of ANP, but this effect is more pronounced in AVNRTs than AVRTs.[94] Both types of arrhythmia are frequently accompanied by the symptom of polyuria (again, more commonly in AVNRTs), which is likely to be due both to the increase in ANP and a reduction in Vasopressin, leading to an increase in renal prostaglandin E2.[95] However, the increase in ANP in these arrhythmias is paralleled by an increase in plasma endothelin, which has antagonistic actions to ANP.[96] Despite the rise in endothelin these mechanisms induce diuresis and natriuresis and reduce circulating volume, which together with the loss of AV synchrony leads to a fall in cardiac output and relative hypotension, leading to symptoms of syncope, presyncope and malaise. Patients also experience palpitations due to the rapid ventricular response and vigorous neck pulsations, especially in AVNRTs (due to cannon A waves).

There are few studies of hemostatic factors in AVRTs or AVNRTs, although patients with paroxysmal AVRTs or AVNRTs appear to have similar levels of fibrin D-dimer and fibrinogen to healthy controls in sinus rhythm.[97] This finding is in keeping with epidemiological evidence, which does not show an increased risk of stroke in these conditions.

SINUS TACHYCARDIA

Whilst AF may be the most common sustained cardiac arrhythmia, perhaps the most commonly observed short-term change from 'normal sinus rhythm' is sinus tachycardia, representing simply an increase in the heart rate above the expected 'normal' range of 60–100 beats per minute (bpm). It is usually seen as a normal physiological response to exercise or high adrenergic states such as emotional stress and, as such, will usually resolve gradually once the stimulus is removed. In the rare case of a persistent sinus tachycardia, an underlying cause (such as an undiagnosed infection or endocrine abnormality) should be sought. Sinus tachycardia rarely, if ever, represents the presence of organic heart disease and, as the synchrony between atria and ventricles is maintained, it rarely causes significant hemodynamic disturbance (although may lead to a fall in systemic blood pressure at very fast rates, due to reduced LV filling time) and is not associated with an increased thromboembolic risk. Nonetheless, the symptoms of palpitations from sinus tachycardia, especially if persistent, may be sufficiently unpleasant for the patient to seek medical advice.

SINUS BRADYCARDIA

As in the case of sinus tachycardia, sinus bradycardia most commonly represents an appropriate physiological response (e.g. high 'vagal tone' among young fit athletes). Once more, due to the maintenance of atrio-ventricular synchrony, there is minimal hemodynamic disturbance unless heart rates fall sufficiently low to result in a significant fall in cardiac output (which may result in dyspnoea, or syncope as an early sign of systemic hypoperfusion), and there is no evidence for a change in thromboembolic risk. In the case of symptomatic sinus bradycardia, underlying causes should be sought (medications and hypothyroidism are common causes when a 'normal' physiological response is unlikely). Cardiac disease is uncommon, although calcific degeneration of the SA node among the elderly or the presence of ischemic heart disease (usually of the right coronary system) may occasionally lead to sinus bradycardia.

SUMMARY

Atrial arrhythmias are associated with a wide variety of changes from the 'normal' atrial anatomy and physiology of sinus rhythm. An understanding of the abnormalities of atrial anatomy and physiology associated with atrial arrhythmias helps to reveal the mechanisms behind the significant morbidity and mortality that may be a consequence of these conditions. Atrial fibrillation, in keeping with the prognostic importance of this arrhythmia, is associated with the greatest degree of variation from 'normal' atrial anatomy and physiology, and these abnormalities are linked to both the hemodynamic and thromboembolic consequences of AF. As our understanding of these abnormal physiological mechanisms improves, we may identify new therapeutic targets for treating the causes, consequences and symptoms of atrial arrhythmias.

References

1. Wolf PA, Abbott RD, Kannel WB. Atrial fibrillation as an independent risk factor for stroke: the Framingham Study. Stroke 1991; 22(8):983–988.
2. Blackshear JL, Odell JA. Appendage obliteration to reduce stroke in cardiac surgical patients with atrial fibrillation. Ann Thorac Surg 1996; 61(2):755–759.
3. Pollick C, Taylor D. Assessment of left atrial appendage function by transesophageal echocardiography. Implications for the development of thrombus. Circulation 1991; 84(1):223–231.
4. Jue J, Winslow T, Fazio G, et al. Pulsed Doppler characterization of left atrial appendage flow. J Am Soc Echocardiogr 1993; 6(3 Pt 1):237–244.
5. Davis CA III, Rembert JC, Greenfield JC Jr. Compliance of left atrium with and without left atrium appendage. Am J Physiol 1990; 259(4 Pt 2):H1006–H1008.
6. Annat G, Grandjean B, Vincent M, et al. Effects of right atrial stretch on plasma renin activity. Arch Int Physiol Biochim 1976; 84(2):311–315.
7. Grindstaff RR, Cunningham JT. Cardiovascular regulation of vasopressin neurons in the supraoptic nucleus. Exp Neurol 2001; 171(2):219–226.
8. Kappagoda CT, Linden RJ, Snow HM. The effect of distending the atrial appendages on urine flow in the dog. J Physiol 1972; 227(1):233–242.
9. Omari BO, Nelson RJ, Robertson JM. Effect of right atrial appendectomy on the release of atrial natriuretic hormone. J Thorac Cardiovasc Surg 1991; 102(2):272–279.
10. Vaziri SM, Larson MG, Benjamin EJ, et al. Echocardiographic predictors of nonrheumatic atrial fibrillation. The Framingham Heart Study. Circulation 1994; 89(2):724–730.
11. Benjamin EJ, D'Agostino RB, Belanger AJ, et al. Left atrial size and the risk of stroke and death. The Framingham Heart Study. Circulation 1995; 92(4):835–841.
12. Sanfilippo AJ, Abascal VM, Sheehan M, et al. Atrial enlargement as a consequence of atrial fibrillation. A prospective echocardiographic study. Circulation 1990; 82(3):792–797.
13. Manning WJ, Leeman DE, Gotch PJ, et al. Pulsed Doppler evaluation of atrial mechanical function after electrical cardioversion of atrial fibrillation. J Am Coll Cardiol 1989; 13(3):617–623.
14. Ernst G, Stollberger C, Abzieher F, et al. Morphology of the left atrial appendage. Anat Rec 1995; 242(4):553–561.
15. Hoglund C, Rosenhamer G. Echocardiographic left atrial dimension as a predictor of maintaining sinus rhythm after conversion of atrial fibrillation. Acta Med Scand 1985; 217(4):411–415.
16. Asinger RW, Koehler J, Pearce LA, et al. Pathophysiologic correlates of thromboembolism in nonvalvular atrial fibrillation: II. Dense spontaneous echocardiographic contrast (The Stroke Prevention in Atrial Fibrillation [SPAF-III] study). J Am Soc Echocardiogr 1999; 12(12):1088–1096.
17. The Stroke Prevention in Atrial Fibrillation Investigators. Predictors of thromboembolism in atrial fibrillation: II. Echocardiographic features of patients at risk. Ann Intern Med 1992; 116(1):6–12.
18. Echocardiographic predictors of stroke in patients with atrial fibrillation: a prospective study of 1066 patients from 3 clinical trials. Arch Intern Med 1998; 158(12):1316–1320.
19. Unverferth DV, Fertel RH, Unverferth BJ, et al. Atrial fibrillation in mitral stenosis: histologic, hemodynamic and metabolic factors. Int J Cardiol 1984; 5(2):143–154.
20. Shinagawa K, Shi YF, Tardif JC, et al. Dynamic nature of atrial fibrillation substrate during development and reversal of heart failure in dogs. Circulation 2002; 105(22):2672–2678.
21. Ausma J, Wijffels M, Thone F, et al. Structural changes of atrial myocardium due to sustained atrial fibrillation in the goat. Circulation 1997; 96(9):3157–3163.
22. Frustaci A, Chimenti C, Bellocci F, et al. Histological substrate of atrial biopsies in patients with lone atrial fibrillation. Circulation 1997; 96(4):1180–1184.
23. Chung MK, Martin DO, Sprecher D, et al. C-reactive protein elevation in patients with atrial arrhythmias: inflammatory mechanisms and persistence of atrial fibrillation. Circulation 2001; 104(24):2886–2891.
24. Lagrand WK, Visser CA, Hermens WT, et al. C-reactive protein as a cardiovascular risk factor: more than an epiphenomenon? Circulation 1999; 100(1):96–102.
25. Pizzetti F, Turazza FM, Franzosi MG, et al. Incidence and prognostic significance of atrial fibrillation in acute myocardial infarction: the GISSI-3 data. Heart 2001; 86(5):527–532.

26. Hohnloser SH, Kuck KH, Lilienthal J. Rhythm or rate control in atrial fibrillation—Pharmacological Intervention in Atrial Fibrillation (PIAF): a randomised trial. Lancet 2000; 356(9244):1789–1794.

27. Kieny JR, Sacrez A, Facello A, et al. Increase in radionuclide left ventricular ejection fraction after cardioversion of chronic atrial fibrillation in idiopathic dilated cardiomyopathy. Eur Heart J 1992; 13(9):1290–1295.

28. AFFIRM Investigators. Survival in patients presenting with atrial fibrillation: the Atrial Fibrillation Follow-up Investigation of Rhythm Management (AFFIRM) study. N Engl J Med 2002;347:1825–1833.

29. Van Gelder IC, Hagens VE, Bosker HA, et al. A comparison of rate control and rhythm control in patients with recurrent persistent atrial fibrillation. N Engl J Med 2002; 347:1834–1840.

30. Wolf PA, Dawber TR, Thomas HE, et al. Epidemiologic assessment of chronic atrial fibrillation and risk of stroke: the Framingham study. Neurology 1978; 28(10):973–977.

31. Black IW, Chesterman CN, Hopkins AP, et al. Hematologic correlates of left atrial spontaneous echo contrast and thromboembolism in nonvalvular atrial fibrillation. J Am Coll Cardiol 1993; 21(2):451–457.

32. The Stroke Prevention in Atrial Fibrillation Investigators Committee on Echocardiography Transesophageal echocardiographic correlates of thromboembolism in high-risk patients with nonvalvular atrial fibrillation. Ann Intern Med 1998; 128(8):639–647.

33. Goldman ME, Pearce LA, Hart RG, et al. Pathophysiologic correlates of thromboembolism in nonvalvular atrial fibrillation: I. Reduced flow velocity in the left atrial appendage (The Stroke Prevention in Atrial Fibrillation [SPAF-III] study). J Am Soc Echocardiogr 1999; 12(12):1080–1087.

34. Klein AL, Grimm RA, Murray RD, et al. Use of transesophageal echocardiography to guide cardioversion in patients with atrial fibrillation. N Engl J Med 2001; 344(19):1411–1420.

35. Leung DY, Davidson PM, Cranney GB, et al. Thromboembolic risks of left atrial thrombus detected by transesophageal echocardiogram. Am J Cardiol 1997; 79(5):626–629.

36. Masawa N, Yoshida Y, Yamada T, et al. Diagnosis of cardiac thrombosis in patients with atrial fibrillation in the absence of macroscopically visible thrombi. Virchows Arch A Pathol Anat Histopathol 1993; 422(1):67–71.

37. Shirani J, Alaeddini J. Structural remodeling of the left atrial appendage in patients with chronic non-valvular atrial fibrillation: Implications for thrombus formation, systemic embolism, and assessment by transesophageal echocardiography. Cardiovasc Pathol 2000; 9(2):95–101.

38. Fukuchi M, Watanabe J, Kumagai K, et al. Increased von Willebrand factor in the endocardium as a local predisposing factor for thrombogenesis in overloaded human atrial appendage. J Am Coll Cardiol 2001; 37(5):1436–1442.

39. Goldsmith I, Kumar P, Carter P, et al. Atrial endocardial changes in mitral valve disease: a scanning electron microscopy study. Am Heart J 2000; 140(5):777–784.

40. Lip GYH. Does atrial fibrillation confer a hypercoagulable state? Lancet 1995; 346:1313–1314.

41. Kumagai K, Fukunami M, Ohmori M, et al. Increased intracardiovascular clotting in patients with chronic atrial fibrillation. J Am Coll Cardiol 1990; 16(2):377–380.

42. Lip GY, Lowe GD, Rumley A, et al. Increased markers of thrombogenesis in chronic atrial fibrillation: effects of warfarin treatment. Br Heart J 1995; 73(6):527–533.

43. Lip GY, Rumley A, Dunn FG, et al. Plasma fibrinogen and fibrin D-dimer in patients with atrial fibrillation: effects of cardioversion to sinus rhythm. Int J Cardiol 1995; 51(3):245–51.

44. Topcuoglu MA, Haydari D, Ozturk S, et al. Plasma levels of coagulation and fibrinolysis markers in acute ischemic stroke patients with lone atrial fibrillation. Neurol Sci 2000; 21(4):235–240.

45. Tsai LM, Chen JH, Tsao CJ. Relation of left atrial spontaneous echo contrast with prethrombotic state in atrial fibrillation associated with systemic hypertension, idiopathic dilated cardiomyopathy, or no identifiable cause (lone). Am J Cardiol 1998; 81(10):1249–1252.

46. Giansante C, Fiotti N, Miccio M, et al. Coagulation indicators in patients with paroxysmal atrial fibrillation: effects of electric and pharmacologic cardioversion. Am Heart J 2000; 140(3):423–429.

47. Kahn SR, Solymoss S, Flegel KM. Nonvalvular atrial fibrillation: evidence for a prothrombotic state. CMAJ 1997; 157(6):673–681.

48. Uno M, Tsuji H, Sawada S, et al. Fibrinopeptide A (FPA) levels in atrial fibrillation and the effects of heparin administration. Jpn Circ J 1988; 52(1):9–12.

49. Yamamoto K, Ikeda U, Fukazawa H, et al. Effects of aspirin on status of thrombin generation in atrial fibrillation. Am J Cardiol 1996; 77(7):528–530.

50. Iga K, Izumi C, Inoko M, et al. Increased thrombin-antithrombin III complex during an episode of paroxysmal atrial fibrillation. Int J Cardiol 1998; 66(2):153–156.

51. Kistler JP, Singer DE, Millenson MM, et al. Effect of low-intensity warfarin anticoagulation on level of activity of the hemostatic system in patients with atrial fibrillation. BAATAF Investigators. Stroke 1993; 24(9):1360–1365.

52. Feinberg WM, Pearce LA, Hart RG, et al. Markers of thrombin and platelet activity in patients with atrial fibrillation: correlation with stroke among 1531 participants in the stroke prevention in atrial fibrillation III study. Stroke 1999; 30(12):2547–2553.

53. Gustafsson C, Blomback M, Britton M, et al. Coagulation factors and the increased risk of stroke in nonvalvular atrial fibrillation. Stroke 1990; 21(1):47–51.

54. Lip GY, Lip PL, Zarifis J, et al. Fibrin D-dimer and beta-thromboglobulin as markers of thrombogenesis and platelet activation in atrial fibrillation. Effects of introducing ultra-low-dose warfarin and aspirin. Circulation 1996; 94(3):425–431.

55. Minamino T, Kitakaze M, Sanada S, et al. Increased expression of P-selectin on platelets is a risk factor for silent cerebral infarction in patients with atrial fibrillation: role of nitric oxide. Circulation 1998; 98(17):1721–1727.

56. Yamauchi K, Furui H, Taniguchi N, et al. Plasma beta-thromboglobulin and platelet factor 4 concentrations in patients with atrial fibrillation. Jpn Heart J 1986; 27(4):481–487.

57. Pongratz G, Brandt-Pohlmann M, Henneke KH, et al. Platelet activation in embolic and preembolic status of patients with non-rheumatic atrial fibrillation. Chest 1997; 111(4):929–933.

58. Heppell RM, Berkin KE, McLenachan JM, et al. Haemostatic and haemodynamic abnormalities associated with left atrial thrombosis in non-rheumatic atrial fibrillation. Heart 1997; 77(5):407–411.

59. Conway DS, Pearce LA, Chin BSP, et al. Plasma von Willebrand factor and soluble P-selectin as indices of endothelial damage and platelet activation in 1321 patients with non-valvular atrial fibrillation: relationship to stroke risk factors. Circulation 2002; 106(15):1962–1967.

60. Conway DSG, Pearce LA, Chin BSP, et al. High plasma von Willebrand factor levels predict future stroke, myocardial infarction and vascular death in 994 patients with atrial fibrillation. Eur Heart J 2002; 23(suppl):239 (abstract 1292)

61. Kamath S, Blann AD, Chin BS, et al. A study of platelet activation in atrial fibrillation and the effects of antithrombotic therapy. Eur Heart J 2002; 23(22):1788–1795.

62. Conway DS, Heeringa J, Van Der Kuip DA, et al. Atrial fibrillation and the prothrombotic state in the elderly: the Rotterdam study. Stroke 2003; 34(2):413–417.

63. Sohara H, Miyahara K. Effect of atrial fibrillation on the fibrino-coagulation system—study in patients with paroxysmal atrial fibrillation. Jpn Circ J 1994; 58(11):821–826.

64. Nagao T, Hamamoto M, Kanda A, et al. Platelet activation is not involved in acceleration of the coagulation system in acute cardioembolic stroke with nonvalvular atrial fibrillation. Stroke 1995; 26(8):1365–1368.

65. Kamath S, Blann AD, Lip GY. Platelets and atrial fibrillation. Eur Heart J 2001; 22(24):2233–2242.

66. Li-Saw-Hee FL, Blann AD, Lip GY. A cross-sectional and diurnal study of thrombogenesis among patients with chronic atrial fibrillation. J Am Coll Cardiol 2000; 35(7):1926–1931.

67. Denis CV. Molecular and cellular biology of von Willebrand factor. Int J Hematol 2002; 75(1):3–8.

68. Blann A, Seigneur M. Soluble markers of endothelial cell function. Clin Hemorheol Microcirc 1997 Jan-Feb;17(1):3–11

69. Jansson JH, Nilsson TK, Johnson O. von Willebrand factor in plasma: a novel risk factor for recurrent myocardial infarction and death. Br Heart J 1991; 66(5):351–355.

70. Smith FB, Lee AJ, Fowkes FG, et al. Hemostatic factors as predictors of ischemic heart disease and stroke in the Edinburgh Artery Study. Arterioscler Thromb Vasc Biol 1997; 17(11):3321–3325.

71. Chung NA, Belgore F, Li-Saw-Hee FL, et al. Is the hypercoagulable state in atrial fibrillation mediated by vascular endothelial growth factor? Stroke 2002; 33(9):2187–2191.

72. Roldan V, Marin F, Marco P, et al. Anticoagulant therapy modifies fibrinolytic dysfunction in chronic atrial fibrillation. Haemostasis 2000; 30(4):219–224.

73. Feng D, D'Agostino RB, Silbershatz H, et al. Hemostatic state and atrial fibrillation (the Framingham Offspring Study). Am J Cardiol 2001; 87(2):168–171.

74. Furui H, Taniguchi N, Yamauchi K, et al. Effects of treadmill exercise on platelet function, blood coagulability and fibrinolytic activity in patients with atrial fibrillation. Jpn Heart J 1987; 28(2):177–184.

75. Peverill RE, Harper RW, Smolich JJ. Inverse relation of haematocrit to cardiac index in mitral stenosis and atrial fibrillation. Int J Cardiol 1999; 71(2):149–155.

76. Li-Saw-Hee FL, Blann AD, Goldsmith I, et al. Indexes of hypercoagulability measured in peripheral blood reflect levels in intracardiac blood in patients with atrial fibrillation secondary to mitral stenosis. Am J Cardiol 1999; 83(8):1206–1209.

77. Li-Saw-Hee FL, Blann AD, Lip GY. Effects of low-dose warfarin, aspirin–warfarin combination therapy, and dose-adjusted warfarin on thrombogenesis in chronic atrial fibrillation. Stroke 2000; 31(4):828–833.

78. Li-Saw-Hee FL, Blann AD, Gurney D, et al. Plasma von Willebrand factor, fibrinogen and soluble P-selectin levels in paroxysmal, persistent and permanent atrial fibrillation. Effects of cardioversion and return of left atrial function. Eur Heart J 2001; 22(18):1741–1747.

79. Nilsson G, Pettersson A, Hedner J, et al. Increased plasma levels of atrial natriuretic peptide (ANP) in patients with paroxysmal supraventricular tachyarrhythmias. Acta Med Scand 1987; 221(1):15–21.

80. Petersen P, Kastrup J, Vilhelmsen R, et al. Atrial natriuretic peptide in atrial fibrillation before and after electrical cardioversion therapy. Eur Heart J 1988; 9(6):639–641.

81. Arakawa M, Miwa H, Noda T, et al. Alternations in atrial natriuretic peptide release after DC cardioversion of non-valvular chronic atrial fibrillation. Eur Heart J 1995; 16(7):977–985.

82. Fujiwara H, Ishikura F, Nagata S, et al. Plasma atrial natriuretic peptide response to direct current cardioversion of atrial fibrillation in patients with mitral stenosis. J Am Coll Cardiol 1993; 22(2):575–580.

83. Yoshihara F, Nishikimi T, Sasako Y, et al. Plasma atrial natriuretic peptide concentration inversely correlates with left atrial collagen volume fraction in patients with atrial fibrillation: plasma ANP as a possible biochemical marker to predict the outcome of the maze procedure. J Am Coll Cardiol 2002; 39(2):288–294.

84. Mabuchi N, Tsutamoto T, Maeda K, et al. Plasma cardiac natriuretic peptides as biochemical markers of recurrence of atrial fibrillation in patients with mild congestive heart failure. Jpn Circ J 2000; 64(10):765–771.

85. Masson S, Gorini M, Salio M, et al. Clinical correlates of elevated plasma natriuretic peptides and Big endothelin-1 in a population of ambulatory patients with heart failure. A substudy of the Italian Network on Congestive Heart Failure (IN-CHF) registry. IN-CHF Investigators. Ital Heart J 2000; 1(4):282–288.

86. Minamino T, Kitakaze M, Sato H, et al. Plasma levels of nitrite/nitrate and platelet cGMP levels are decreased in patients with atrial fibrillation. Arterioscler Thromb Vasc Biol 1997; 17(11):3191–3195.

87. Fujii J, Foster JR, Mills PG, et al. Dual echocardiographic determination of atrial contraction sequence in atrial flutter and other related atrial arrhythmias. Circulation 1978; 58(2):314–321

88. Pozen RG, Pastoriza J, Rozanski JJ, et al. Determinants of recurrent atrial flutter after cardioversion. Br Heart J 1983; 50(1):92–96.

89. Bikkina M, Alpert MA, Mulekar M, et al. Prevalence of intraatrial thrombus in patients with atrial flutter. Am J Cardiol 1995; 76(3):186–189.

90. Corrado G, Sgalambro A, Mantero A, et al. Thromboembolic risk in atrial flutter. The FLASIEC (Flutter Atriale Societa Italiana di Ecografia Cardiovascolare) multicentre study. Eur Heart J 2001; 22(12):1042–1051.

91. Santiago D, Warshofsky M, Li Mandri G, et al. Left atrial appendage function and thrombus formation in atrial fibrillation-flutter: a transesophageal echocardiographic study. J Am Coll Cardiol 1994; 24(1):159–164.

92. Lip GY, Kamath S. Thromboprophylaxis for atrial flutter. Eur Heart J 2001;22(12):984–987.

93. De Vecchis R, Zarrelli V, Imperatore A, et al. [Differences in the symptomatology of paroxysmal supraventricular tachycardias in relation to the different sites of localization of the arrhythmic reentry circuit. Clinical picture, semiologic and genetic aspects] Diversita di sintomatologia nelle tachicardie parossistiche sopraventricolari (TPSR) correlata alla differente localizzazione del circuito aritmico di rientro. Analisi del quadro clinico e considerazioni semeiogenetiche. Minerva Cardioangiol 1993; 41(1-2):1–16.

94. Abe H, Nagatomo T, Kobayashi H, et al. Neurohumoral and hemodynamic mechanisms of diuresis during atrioventricular nodal reentrant tachycardia. Pacing Clin Electrophysiol 1997; 20(11):2783–2788.

95. Fujii T, Kojima S, Imanishi M, et al. Different mechanisms of polyuria and natriuresis associated with paroxysmal supraventricular tachycardia. Am J Cardiol 1991; 68(4):343–348.

96. Li C, Tian R, Zhu L, et al. Changes of plasma endothelin and atrial natriuretic peptide during the onset and after termination of paroxysmal supraventricular tachycardia. Chin Med Sci J 1995; 10(3):161–164.

97. Lip GY, Lowe GD, Rumley A, et al. Fibrinogen and fibrin D-dimer levels in paroxysmal atrial fibrillation: evidence for intermediate elevated levels of intravascular thrombogenesis. Am Heart J 1996; 131(4):724–730.

CHAPTER 3

Electro-physiology for clinicians: pathophysio-logical aspects

Ernest W Lau MD MA MRCP
University of Ottawa Heart Institute, Ottawa, Canada

Gregory Y H Lip MD FRCP DFM FACC FESC
City Hospital, Birmingham, UK

The basis for clinical arrhythmias is cellular electrophysiological disturbances leading to abnormal impulse generation and conduction or both

Introduction

The management of arrhythmias has been greatly transformed in the last three decades due to major developments in both cellular and clinical electrophysiology. These developments have led to a better understanding of the genesis of arrhythmias, and hence a more logical approach to their management. This chapter will examine the mechanisms of arrhythmias, with a view to providing an adequate theoretical basis for understanding and planning the practical management of these conditions.

The mechanisms of arrhythmias can be divided into three main categories:

1. abnormalities in impulse initiation–
2. abnormalities in impulse conduction;
3. simultaneous abnormalities in impulse initiation and conduction (see Table 3.1).[1]

The electrophysiological mechanisms of arrhythmias impart properties that help with their identification and management clinically (Table 3.2). However, before the mechanisms of arrhythmias can be studied, some knowledge of how the cardiac impulse is normally generated and conducted within the heart is necessary.

Table 3.1 Mechanisms and examples of arrhythmias

Mechanisms	Examples
Abnormalities in impulse initiation	
Automaticity	
normal pacemaker	Sick sinus syndrome
	Inappropriate sinus tachycardia
	Sinus arrhythmia
ectopic pacemakers	Atrial tachycardia
	Junctional ectopic (His bundle) tachycardia
abnormal automaticity	Accelerated idioventricular rhythm
Triggered activity	
Early afterdepolarization (EAD)	Torsades de pointes (initiation)
Delayed afterdepolarization (DAD)	Digitalis-toxicity related arrhythmias
	Right ventricular outflow tract tachycardia
Abnormal impulse conduction	
Conduction block	Sinus node dysfunction
	AV node block
Ordered re-entry	Sinus node re-entrant tachycardia
	Atrial flutter
	Atrial tachycardia
	AV nodal re-entrant tachycardia
	AV re-entrant tachycardia
	Most ventricular tachycardia
	Bundle branch re-entrant tachycardia
Random re-entry	Atrial fibrillation
	Torsades de pointes (perpetuation)
	Ventricular fibrillation
Reflection	No known clinical example
Simultaneous abnormalities in impulse initiation and conduction	
Parasystole	Sinus rhythm with complete heart block and an infranodal escape rhythm
	Frequent ventricular or atrial ectopic beats

AV, atrioventricular

Table 3.2 Correlation between electrophysiological mechanisms and clinical characteristics of arrhythmias

Mechanism	Onset	Offset	Effect of pacing
Normal automaticity – normal pacemaker	Gradual	Gradual	Suppresses but does not initiate
Normal automaticity – ectopic pacemaker	Gradual	Gradual	Suppresses but does not initiate
Abnormal automaticity	Abrupt	Abrupt	Does not suppress or initiate
Early afterdepolarization	Preceding brady-cardia or short-long-short sequence	Abrupt	Suppresses onset, but does not initiate or terminate
Delayed afterdepolarization	Often initial warm-up	Often terminal slow-down	Can initiate and occasionally terminate
Ordered re-entry	Abrupt (within 1 beat); might be initiated by ≥ 1 ectopic beats	Usually abrupt (within 1 beat) but may slow down before spontaneous termination	Initiate, reset, entrain and terminate
Random re-entry	Abrupt	Abrupt	Can initiate, but does not reset, entrain or terminate

NORMAL IMPULSE GENERATION AND CONDUCTION

Normal impulse initiation and conduction

- Sinoatrial node   = The controlling normal pacemaker
- Intra-atrial nodal tracts
- Atrioventricular node (AVN)   With slow conduction
- His bundle
- Left and right bundle branches   With fast conduction
- Purkinje fibers

The heart is served by a specialized conduction system designed to initiate and coordinate the spread of electrical (and hence mechanical) activation throughout the heart (Fig. 3.1). The system comprises the sinoatrial node (SAN), the atrial

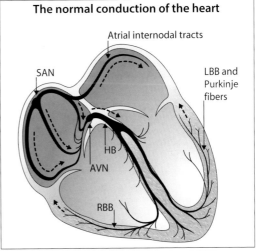

The normal conduction of the heart

Atrial internodal tracts

SAN

LBB and Purkinje fibers

HB

AVN

RBB

Fig. 3.1 The normal conduction of the heart. SAN, sinoatrial node; AVN, atrioventricular node; HB, His bundle; LBB, left bundle branch; RBB, right bundle branch.

internodal tracts, the atrioventricular node (AVN), the His bundle, the left and right bundle branches, and the Purkinje fibers.

The cells in the specialized conduction system are different from the ordinary atrial and ventricular myocardial cells in manifesting automaticity, i.e. they are intrinsically capable of spontaneously discharging and hence generating a cardiac rhythm. The means by which spontaneous discharge happens is through the development of a 'pacemaker' potential during phase 4 of the action potential; when the pacemaker potential reaches the depolarization threshold, an action potential results (Fig. 3.2). The pacemaker potential in the SAN and AVN cells is mediated by a fall in potassium conductance and a rise in calcium conductance, even though a rise in sodium conductance also plays a minor role.[2]

The rate at which a pacemaker cell discharges is governed by three factors:

1. the maximum resting membrane potential;
2. the threshold potential; and
3. the slope of the depolarization potential.

Usually, the SAN, with the highest intrinsic rate (60–100/min) dominates other subsidiary latent pacemakers at the AVN and His bundle (intrinsic rates 40–60/min) and the bundle branches (intrinsic rate 20–40/min) through overdrive suppression.[3] However, the latent pacemakers can occasionally escape from the control of the SAN and dominate the cardiac rhythm.

From the usual pacemaker in the SAN, the cardiac impulse is conducted to the rest of the heart via a specialized conduction system of cardiac cells (Fig. 3.1). From the SAN situated at the junction between the superior vena cava and the right atrium, the cardiac impulse is conducted via the atrial myocardium to the AVN. Specialized atrial internodal tracts speed up conduction within the atria, enhancing the synchrony of contraction.

The AVN, situated on the right atrial side of the interatrial septum, normally provides the only electrical connection between the atria and ventricles through the insulating fibrous atrioventricular ring. Conduction through the AVN is slow (0.05 m/s) compared with the atrial or ventricular muscle (0.5 m/s), introducing a delay of 0.1–0.2 s (normally) between the onset of atrial and ventricular systole. The delay ensures atrial contraction is finished before ventricular contraction begins, and hence adequate diastolic ventricular filling for effective systolic contraction.

From the AVN, the cardiac impulse is conducted down the His bundle and the left and right bundle branches in the interventricular septum at the speed of 1 m/s to reach the Purkinje fibers, which ramify throughout the ventricular myocardium. Conduction through the Purkinje fibers is very fast at 5 m/s, ensuring that all parts of both ventricles are excited and hence contract almost simultaneously.

A consequence of the rapid, nearly simultaneous activation of the extensive balk of ventricular myocardium is the narrowness of the QRS complex on the surface electrocardiogram (ECG) (normally ≤ 120 ms). This fact is clinically important for two reasons. First, it provides an important clue to the mechanism of an arrhythmia. When the QRS complex of a rhythm is broad (> 140 ms), activation of

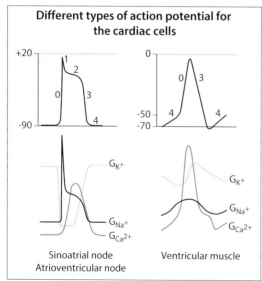

Fig. 3.2 Different types of action potential for the cardiac cells.

the ventricular myocardium is slow, which can be only due to either defects within the His-Purkinje system (i.e. aberrant conduction) or activation of the ventricular myocardium through some less efficient means other than the specialized Purkinje fibers (e.g. an accessory pathway or the ordinary ventricular myocardium).[4–6] Second, when the QRS complex is broad, ventricular contraction is less synchronized and hence less effective, which might contribute or lead to the development of cardiac failure and affect the long-term prognosis.[7–11] In this light, cardiac resynchronization therapy through biventricular pacing may improve the hemodynamic and clinical performance of patients with heart failure and broadened QRS complexes, a hypothesis which is supported by the results from randomized clinical trials.[12–17]

Apart from its intrinsic properties, the electrical and mechanical activities of the heart are also modulated by external influences, especially from the autonomic nervous system.

Key points
Importance of QRS width

- Narrow QRS (≤ 0.12 s):   Fast (and mostly normal) myocardial activation
- Broad QRS (> 0.14 s):   Slow and ineffective myocardial activation

ABNORMALITIES IN IMPULSE INITIATION

Abnormalities in impulse initiation can be by either automaticity or triggered activity. The crucial difference between the two lies in the mechanism of action potential generation. As mentioned above, automaticity means generation of an action potential through spontaneous depolarization during phase 4. In contrast, triggered activity depends on afterdepolarizations, or oscillations in membrane potential that follow the upstroke of an action potential, which can sometimes reach the depolarization threshold for the generation of another action potential.[18] Thus, whereas automaticity can occur in the absence of any recent electrical activity, triggered activity must be immediately preceded by a cardiac impulse.

Automaticity

Automaticity takes place normally in the SAN and other parts of the specialized conduction system of the heart, but can also take place abnormally in other cardiac cells in certain situations.

Normal pacemaker

The normal pacemaker of the heart is the SAN. In certain situations, the sinus rate can become either too slow (e.g. sick sinus syndrome, during a vasovagal attack) or too fast (the syndrome of inappropriate sinus tachycardia) than is physiologically 'appropriate'. There will be a certain level of arbitrariness in deciding what is a physiologically 'appropriate' sinus rate for a patient. For example, a sinus rate of 120/min will be appropriate for someone during agitation, exertion or even in septic shock but not at rest. On the other hand, a sinus rate of 40/min might be appropriate for a young trained athlete with no symptoms but not an 80-year-old person complaining of lethargy and dyspnea. When the sinus rate is inappropriately high at rest or increases disproportionately with minimal exertion in the absence of reversible factors (e.g. hyperthyroidism, fever or orthostatic hypotension), the diagnosis will be the syndrome of inappropriate sinus tachycardia.[19] Conversely, when the sinus rate is inappropriately slow in the absence of reversible factors (e.g. hypothyroidism, beta-blockade), the diagnosis will be sick sinus syndrome.[20,21] However, the sick sinus syndrome often also reflects defects in other parts of the specialized conduction system, as the latent pacemakers in the AVN, His bundle or bundle branches fail to speed up sufficiently to provide an adequate escape rhythm heart rate. Finally, when the vagal tone is high, as can be the case among the young, marked beat-to-beat variation in the sinus rate can result. This form of sinus arrhythmia is physiological and of no clinical significance.

Clinically, the hallmarks of automatic arrhythmias of the SAN are that they are of gradual onset and offset, and can be suppressed but not initiated by pacing (Table 3.2).

Key points		
Arrhythmia mechanisms		
● Abnormal automaticity:		Often in ischemia with partial depolarization
● Triggered activity		
● Early afterdepolarization		(EAD) in bradycardia Long QT
● Delayed afterdepolarization		(DAD) in tachycardia

Ectopic pacemakers

A latent ectopic pacemaker can dominate the cardiac rhythm if:

1. the intrinsic rate of the SAN falls below that of the latent pacemaker;
2. the intrinsic rate of the latent pacemaker rises above that of the SAN; or
3. the impulse from the SAN is prevented from reaching (hence suppressing) the latent pacemaker due to conduction block.

The first scenario happens in the sick sinus syndrome. The second scenario happens in certain cases of atrial tachycardia[22] and junctional ectopic (His bundle) tachycardia.[23,24] Junctional ectopic tachycardia is a rare form of tachycardia most common among infants and children, especially postoperatively after surgery for congenital heart disease.[25,26] The third scenario happens due to simultaneous

abnormalities in impulse initiation and conduction and will be discussed later.

Like automatic arrhythmias of the SAN, arrhythmias due to normal automaticity in ectopic foci tend to be of gradual onset and offset and can be suppressed but not initiated by pacing (Table 3.2).

Abnormal automaticity

The atrial and ventricular myocardial cells, which are outside the specialized conduction system of the heart and hence not latent pacemakers, can sometimes acquire automaticity. A common setting in which this happens is ischemia-induced myocardial injury. In such a situation, the myocardial cell loses its ability to maintain the normal resting membrane potential (−90 to −80mV) and becomes partially depolarized (−65 to −30mV). This partial depolarization leads to further spontaneous depolarization and eventually the initiation of a full-blown potential. But for abnormal automaticity to manifest, the abnormal automatic focus needs to discharge at a rate faster than the normal pacemaker of the heart, the SAN. Abnormal automaticity in Purkinje cells in the ischemic region is believed to underlie the phenomenon of accelerated idioventricular rhythm, which occasionally accompanies a myocardial infarction, especially during reperfusion, be it by thrombolysis or coronary angioplasty (Fig. 3.3).[27–30]

Like normal automaticity, abnormal automaticity cannot be initiated by pacing (Table 3.2). However, unlike normal automaticity, abnormal automaticity tends to be of abrupt onset and offset and is not amenable to overdrive suppression. The latter features set abnormal automaticity apart from normal automaticity.

Triggered activity

Triggered activity can be due to either early afterdepolarization (EAD), which occurs during the repolarization of action potential (Fig. 3.4a) or delayed

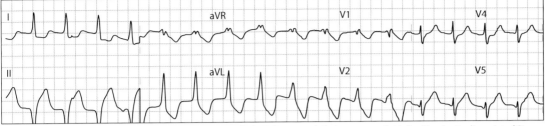

Fig. 3.3 Accelerated idioventricular rhythm after thrombolysis for acute inferior myocardial infarction (note dissociated P waves).

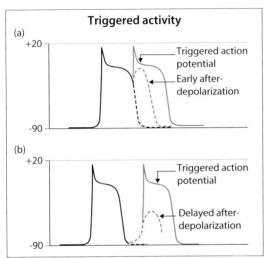

Fig. 3.4 Triggered activity.

afterdepolarization, which occurs when repolarization is complete or nearly complete (Fig. 3.4b).

Early afterdepolarization

EAD occurs during the plateau phase (phase 2) or early repolarization (phase 3) of the action potential (Fig. 3.4a). EAD is favoured by prolongation of the action potential and delay in repolarization.[31] Clinically, this manifests as lengthening of the QT interval on the ECG, giving rise to the so-called 'long QT syndromes'.[32–34] The long QT syndromes (LQTS) can be either congenital or acquired, and are clinically important for their association with a specific form of polymorphic ventricular tachycardia called torsades de pointes (TdP),[31] a term coined by Dessertenne to describe an undulating ECG pattern of periodically changing axis and morphology of the QRS complex that seems to twist around an imaginary baseline.[35] TdP can cause syncope or even sudden cardiac death.[36] But whereas EAD may provide the trigger, other factors (mainly spatial dispersion of repolarization) will also need to be present for the activation generated by EAD to propagate and perpetuate, in order that TdP can develop.[37]

As the duration of the action potential is positively correlated with the preceding cycle length,[38] EAD commonly starts immediately after a long preceding RR interval. This occurs in the presence of either a general bradycardia or a long compensatory pause after an ectopic beat (Table 3.2). The former gives rise to the clinical syndrome of bradycardia-dependent TdP.[39,40] The latter gives rise to the classical short-long-short sequence which occasionally immediately precedes the onset of TdP.[41–43]

TdP is typically of abrupt onset and offset (Table 3.2). As EAD is favored by a long preceding cycle length, pacing at a more rapid rate is frequently successful in suppressing EAD and the onset of TdP.[44–46] [47–49] However, once started, TdP cannot be reset or terminated by pacing (Table 3.2).

Delayed after depolarization

Delayed afterdepolarization (DAD) is favored by intracellular calcium overloading and is believed to be due to a transient inward current activated by abnormalities in the release and sequestration of calcium ions by the sarcoplasmic reticulum.[50,51] The potential generated by DAD may not reach the depolarization threshold and hence not lead to the generation of an action potential. The successful generation of an action potential by DAD is favored by adrenergic stimulation and a reduction in the preceding cycle length (or an increase in the heart rate).[52,53] Hence commonly, arrhythmias initiated by DAD happens when the intracellular calcium level is high (e.g. digitalis exposure), or when adrenergic stimulation and heart rate are elevated (e.g. during physical exertion).[54,55] The clinical arrhythmias attributable to DAD include those associated with digitalis toxicity[56] and right ventricular outflow tract tachycardia.[57]

Arrhythmias due to DAD often show initial warm-up and terminal slow-down, and can be induced by pacing, especially in the presence of an isoproterenol infusion.[58,59] Occasionally, arrhythmias due to DAD terminate after pacing, but only after a few extra beats (Table 3.2).

Components of a re-entrant circuit

- An electrically inert center (may be an anatomical obstacle)
- A slow conduction zone is critical
- Differential refractoriness creates a unidirectional block

ABNORMALITIES IN IMPULSE CONDUCTION

Abnormality in impulse conduction means slowed conduction or conduction block. There are several possible mechanisms by which conductional abnormalities may occur, including:

1. the cardiac tissue is dead (i.e. scar tissue);
2. the cardiac tissue is still refractory after the passage of a recent depolarization;
3. the cardiac tissue is hyperdepolarized to a lower than normal resting potential (e.g. as a result of ischemia, electrolyte disturbance or drugs);
4. the propagating activation wavefront is not strong enough to excite the cardiac tissue, which is fully excitable (i.e. decremental conduction and block).

Conduction block

The impulse from the SAN may fail to reach and activate the ventricular myocardium due to conduction block in either the AVN or the exit from the SAN to the atrial myocardium (exit block). The relief from overdrive suppression allows the more slowly discharging and usually dormant automatic foci in the His bundle, bundle branches or Purkinje fibers to exert themselves and take control of the cardiac rhythm. The resulting escape rhythm can have a narrow QRS complex if the dominating ectopic focus is in the AVN or the His bundle, or a broad QRS complex if the dominant ectopic focus is situated in the bundle branches or Purkinje fibers. Whatever the seat of ectopic focus, the escape rhythm is invariably slower than is normal (i.e. bradycardia) and often does not speed up adequately in response to physiological demands such as exertion. Regardless of the site of conduction block, the resulting condition can usually be satisfactorily treated with permanent pacemaker implantation.

Ordered re-entry

Ordered re-entry,[60] or classical re-entry as described by Mines,[61] is responsible for the majority of regular tachycardias clinically observed.[62] It was with remarkable foresight that Mines first proposed such a mechanism back in 1914 using isolated strips of cardiac muscle cut into rings,[61] even though it took more than six decades for technology to catch up and allow in vivo demonstration of the operation of this mechanism in human clinical tachycardias.[63–65]

The pre-requisites for an ordered re-entrant circuit are:

1. a central area of electrical inertia;
2. differential refractoriness in the two limbs of a re-entrant circuit; and
3. a slow conduction zone (Fig. 3.5).

A central area of electrical inertia provides a focus for the activation wavefront to circle around (Fig. 3.5a). Differential refractoriness in the two limbs

of the circuit allows the establishment of a unidirectional block in response to the tachycardia trigger, which usually takes the form of one or more premature beats, and the initiation of re-entry (Fig. 3.5b). In order that re-entry be perpetuated, the circulating activation wavefront must not encounter any refractory tissue in the circuit. This requires the cycle length (the time for the activation wavefront to circle once) to be longer than the refractory period at any point and the presence of an excitable gap in the circuit (Fig. 3.5c).

In the human heart, the crucial condition for re-entry perpetuation, namely, the existence of an excitable gap in the circuit, will usually not be fulfilled unless a slow conduction zone exists in the circuit to prolong the cycle length (Fig. 3.5d). Using the action potential duration as a surrogate for the effective refractory period, the wavelength and hence minimum size of a re-entrant circuit which can be sustained in different parts of the heart can be estimated by the product of the local conduction velocity and action potential duration (Table 3.3).[66] As should be evident from Table 3.3, most parts of the human heart (with the exception of the AVN) will not be physically large enough to contain a re-entrant circuit without the existence of a slow conduction zone. In actual fact, the slow conduction zone is the most critical component of the re-entrant circuit and may even be considered as the circuit itself, insofar as ablation of the slow zone will abolish the circuit whereas ablation elsewhere in the circuit will merely modify but not destroy it (Fig. 3.6).[67] Figure 3.6 also highlights the fact that only the slow conduction zone may be anatomically well-defined and other parts are more variable, giving rise to a 'figure of eight' form of re-entry.[68]

The presence of an excitable gap within the re-entrant circuit is important electrophysiologically, for it provides a window for engaging the re-entrant circuit and modifying the associated tachycardia through pacing (Fig. 3.7). In fact, such an ability is regarded as a hallmark of

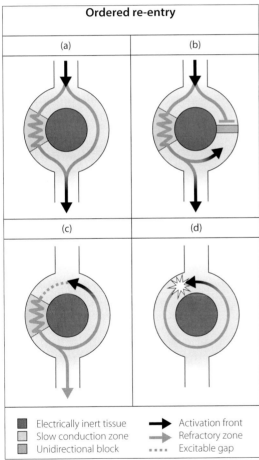

Ordered re-entry

| (a) | (b) |
| (c) | (d) |

Legend:
- ■ Electrically inert tissue
- □ Slow conduction zone
- ■ Unidirectional block
- ➜ Activation front
- ➜ Refractory zone
- ···· Excitable gap

Fig. 3.5 Ordered re-entry. (a) Normal conduction. (b) Initiation of re-entry by a critically timed premature impulse encounters unidirectional block in one limb but not the other of the re-entrant circuit due to differential refractoriness. (c) Perpetuation of re-entry relies on the presence of an 'excitable gap' of tissue, which in turn relies on a slow zone of conduction. (d) In the absence of an excitable gap, the activation wavefront encounters refractory tissue and re-entry is terminated.

Table 3.3 Abilities of different parts of the heart in sustaining a re-entrant circuit

Site	Conduction velocity (cm/s)	Action potential duration (s)	Minimum size of a re-entry circuit (cm)
Atria	50	0.2	10
Atrioventricular node	5	0.2	1
Ventricle	50	0.3	15
His bundle and its bundle branches	100	0.3	30
Purkinje fibers	500	0.4	200

(Based on figures taken from Bray et al 66)

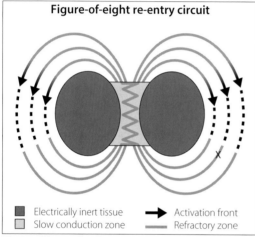

Figure-of-eight re-entry circuit

- ■ Electrically inert tissue
- □ Slow conduction zone
- → Activation front
- ▬ Refractory zone

Fig. 3.6 'Figure-of-eight' re-entry circuit. Ablation at point X in the re-entrant circuit will modify the circuit (and the consequent tachycardia) but not abolish it, whereas ablation within the slow conduction zone will destroy the circuit and abolish all arrhythmias dependent on it.

re-entry.[1] When a premature extra stimulus S_1 enters the re-entrant circuit through the excitable gap, it generates an orthodromic (in the same direction as the circulating wavefront) and an antidromic (opposite in direction to the circulating wavefront) wavefronts (Fig. 3.7a). The antidromic wavefront from S_1 inevitably collides with the circulating wavefront and is extinguished (Fig. 3.7a, c). If the orthodromic wavefront from S_1 does not encounter any refractory tissue created by the preceding circulating wavefront, it will circle around the re-entrant circuit,

'resetting' the tachycardia by bringing the next beat forward in time (Fig. 3.7a,c). If the tachycardia is continuously reset to a faster rate (shorter cycle length) by pacing, entrainment of the re-entrant circuit has occurred.[65,67,69] However, if an extra stimulus S_2 is so premature that its orthodromic wavefront encounters refractory tissue, then the tachycardia will be terminated (Fig. 3.7b,c). In order that this is possible, it is necessary that the refractory period be non-uniform in the re-entrant circuit – for the orthodromic wavefront from S_2 to reach the refractory tail left by the preceding circulating wavefront, the part of the re-entrant circuit immediately leading to the collision site must be non-refractory and able to conduct. In the simple model depicted in Figure 3.7(c), the slow conduction zone is presumed to have a longer refractory period than the rest of the circuit and contains the site where the orthodromic wavefront of S_2 encounters refractory tissue. If refractory period is uniform in the re-entrant circuit, then theoretically re-entry can never be terminated by an extra stimulus, no matter how premature it is (Fig. 3.7d). Another theoretical possibility for the orthodromic wavefront of a premature extra stimulus to be extinguished is for it to travel faster than the circulating wavefront, so that it can catch up with refractory tissue (Fig. 3.7e). However, this is highly unlikely as

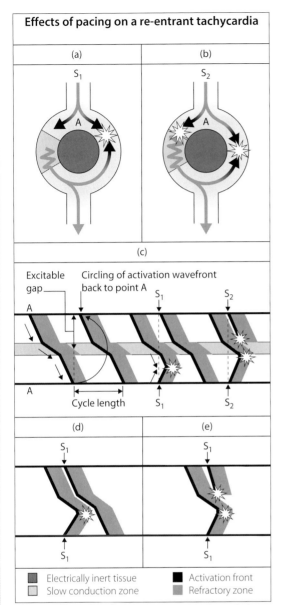

Effects of pacing on a re-entrant tachycardia

(a) (b)

S₁ S₂

A A

(c)

Excitable gap

Circling of activation wavefront back to point A

A

S₁ S₂

A

Cycle length S₁ S₂

(d) (e)

S₁ S₁

S₁ S₁

| ■ Electrically inert tissue | ■ Activation front |
| □ Slow conduction zone | ■ Refractory zone |

Fig. 3.7 Effects of pacing on a re-entrant tachycardia (see text for details)

myocardial tissues tend to conduct either more slowly or at the same speed as the interval between successive stimuli decreases (i.e. 'decremental' conduction).[70] The presence of an excitable gap makes it possible to induce, terminate, reset (i.e. advance the next tachycardia cycle without altering the cycle length)[71,72] or entrain (i.e. continuously reset the tachycardia to a faster than intrinsic rate)[65,69,73] a re-entrant tachycardia through pacing, which serves

as a hallmark of ordered re-entry (Table 3.2).

The key components of a re-entrant circuit (a central area of electrical inertia, a unidirectional block and a slow conduction zone) can occur by both anatomical and functional mechanisms. The central region of electrical inertia may be provided by anatomical barriers (e.g. scar tissue, the tricuspid annulus) or functional in nature (due to refractoriness). Unidirectional block and slow conduction may be caused by physiological (e.g. in the AVN, or when activation traverses across rather than along a cardiac cell – i.e. anisotropy[74] or pathological regional heterogeneity (e.g. due to fibrous tissue intermingling with live cardiac cells after a myocardial infarction, or disorganized muscle fibers as in hypertrophic cardiomyopathy) in excitability, refractoriness and conduction velocity.

Ordered re-entry imparts some properties common to all arrhythmias by this mechanism (Table 3.2). First, as the activation wavefront of the arrhythmia must traverse the same circuit path, whence electrical excitation spreads to other parts of the heart, in exactly the same way over and over again, the activation pattern of the heart, be it recorded endocardially with electrodes during electrophysiology study or on the surface ECG, will stay constant from beat to beat, i.e. a regular tachycardia. By definition, if a tachycardia is irregular, the arrhythmia cannot be due to ordered re-entry. (In reality, minor variations in the cycle length, QRS axis or morphology can be demonstrated to exist when measured accurately with the aid of high-resolution electronic equipment during electrophysiology study, but such minor variations are not usually discernible by the naked human eye or even when measured out with a ruler or a pair of callipers on the ECG.) Second, the tachycardia is usually initiated by one or a few premature beats (mirroring the process illustrated in Fig. 3.5b) (Fig. 3.8) and may also be terminated or reset (i.e. brought forward

Initiation of an ordered re-entrant tachycardia by a single premature beat (*)

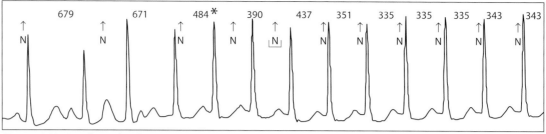

| 679 | | 671 | | 484 * | | 390 | | 437 | 351 | 335 | 335 | 335 | 343 | 343 |

Fig. 3.8 Initiation of an ordered re-entrant tachycardia by a single premature beat (*).

temporally) by a premature beat (mirroring the processes illustrated in Fig. 3.7). This feature is particular useful in diagnosing tachycardias recorded on Holter monitoring. Third, a re-entrant circuit is either on-going or not; hence tachycardias due to ordered re-entry are typically of very abrupt onset and offset (i.e. within one beat), even though occasionally the tachycardia may gradually slow down prior to spontaneous termination.

The clinically important arrhythmias due to re-entry include atrioventricular re-entrant tachycardia (AVRT), atrioventricular nodal re-entrant tachycardia (AVNRT), some cases of atrial tachycardia, atrial flutter and regular monomorphic ventricular tachycardia (VT) (Table 3.1). Less common arrhythmias due to re-entry are sinus nodal re-entrant tachycardia (SNRT).[75] The re-entrant circuits can either be large and anatomically definable (i.e. macro re-entrant), as are the cases of AVRT and atrial flutter, or minute (i.e. micro re-entrant), as are most cases of regular monomorphic VT.

Key points

Features of ordered re-entry

- An excitable gap must be present to perpetuate the arrhythmia
- Pacing modifies the spontaneous tachycardia
- Entrainment by continuous resetting the tachycardia is typical
- The tachycardia is always regular and usually initiated by an extrasystole

Random re-entry

Random re-entry,[60] or leading-circle re-entry,[76] serves as an alternative to ordered re-entry. Instead of retracing anatomically the same circuit path repeatedly, the activation wavefront opportunistically excites whatever adjacent tissue that is excitable. In such a situation, the central area of electrical inertia will be functional (i.e. due to refractoriness induced by electrical activation) and hence shift with time. Moreover, there will not be an excitable gap, which prevents external interaction with the circuit through pacing (Table 3.2). The absence of an excitable gap also means a random re-entry circuit can be smaller (and with a faster resulting tachycardia) than an ordered re-entry circuit. In fact, the rate of a random re-entry tachycardia is often close to that permitted by the refractory period of the involved cardiac tissue.

The crucial substrate of random re-entry is spatial dispersion in refractoriness, in order that an activation wavefront will always find some adjacent tissue excitable and hence not be extinguished. Because of the 'wandering' nature of the seat of the re-entrant circuit, the electrical activation of the heart, and hence the ECG manifestation, of the resulting arrhythmia will not be constant but changes from beat to beat. Multiple activation wavefronts or excitation wavelets can operate side by side simultaneously, adding to the apparent randomness (or chaos) of the pattern of electrical activation of the heart over time. When random re-entry happens in the atria, as in atrial fibrillation (AF), the electrical activation of the atria is often too fractionated to generate any sizeable atrial signal for the randomness to be appreciated on the surface ECG. However, AF manifests the random nature of atrial activation by the irregular pattern of ventricular response. When random re-entry happens in the ventricles, an irregular pattern of QRS complex timing, morphology and axis on the ECG can be expected. Such a manifestation on the ECG is seen with polymorphic VT and ventricular fibrillation (VF). Both the importance of spatial dispersion in refractoriness and the operation of random re-entry have been experimentally demonstrated in the case of the specific form of polymorphic VT, TdP.[37]

Reflection

Reflection is a special form of re-entry which happens in a linear bundle (down to a single muscle fiber). The two ends of the bundle are separated by one zone of depressed conduction and excitation can oscillate between the two ends through electrotonic activation provided conduction is sufficiently slow in the central zone. Reflection has only been demonstrated in vitro but not in vivo, and no clinical arrhythmia has been associated with this mechanism.[77,78]

ABNORMALITIES IN IMPULSE INITIATION AND CONDUCTION

When a second autonomous rhythm exists simultaneously and operates side by side with normal sinus rhythm, parasystole results. This is possible because the source of the second rhythm, be it caused by automaticity or re-entry, is connected to the rest of the heart by an area of unidirectional block, which protects it from being suppressed or terminated by the sinus rhythm but allows it to intermittently capture other areas of the heart when they are not refractory from the previous sinus impulse.[79–82] In this respect, complete heart block with an ectopic escape rhythm originating from below the AVN in the

Junctional parasystole with dissociated P waves (*) and hypotension recorded during cardiac catheterization

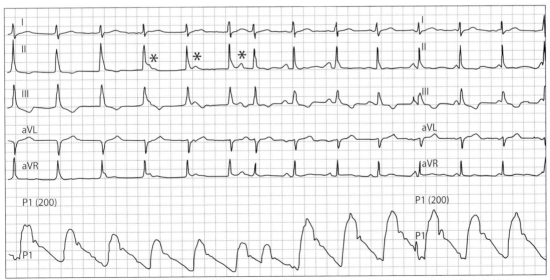

Fig. 3.9 Junctional parasystole with dissociated P waves (*) and hypotension recorded during cardiac catheterization.

presence of non-conducted SAN impulses can be regarded as a special case of parasystole. When frequent atrial or ventricular ectopic beats exist in the presence of an adequate sinus rate, parasystole may also be in operation. An example of junctional parasystole associated with dissociated P waves and hypotension (most probably due to the loss of coordinated atrial transport) recorded during cardiac catheterization is shown in Figure 3.9.

CONCLUSIONS

This chapter links the findings from cellular and clinical electrophysiological studies to the various arrhythmic phenomena observed clinically. Such knowledge should provide a better understanding of the rationale behind different aspects of the practical management of arrhythmias.

References

1. Waldo AL, Wit AL. Mechanisms of cardiac arrhythmias. Lancet 1993; 341:1189–1193.
2. Surawicz B. Automaticity. In: Electrophysiologic basis of ECG and cardiac arrhythmias. Baltimore: Williams & Wilkins; 1995:80–108.
3. Vassalle M. The relationship among cardiac pacemakers: overdrive suppression. Circ Res 1977; 41:269–277.
4. Griffith MJ, Garratt CJ, Mounsey P, et al. Ventricular tachycardia as default diagnosis in broad complex tachycardia. Lancet 1994; 343:386–388.
5. Lau EW, Ng GA, Griffith MJ. Variability in the manifestation of pre-excited atrial fibrillation: its quantification, theoretical origin and diagnostic potential. Ann Noninvasive Electrocardiol 2001; 6:117–122.
6. Lau EW, Pathmanathan RK, Ng GA, et al. Electrocardiographic criteria for diagnosis of irregular broad complex tachycardia with a high sensitivity for pre-excited atrial fibrillation. Pacing Clin Electrophysiol 2000; 23:2040–2045.
7. Wilensky RL, Yudelman P, Cohen AI, et al. Serial electrocardiographic changes in idiopathic dilated cardiomyopathy confirmed at necropsy. Am J Cardiol 1988; 62:276–283.
8. Grines CL, Bashore TM, Boudoulas H, Olson S, et al. Functional abnormalities in isolated left bundle branch block. The effect of interventricular asynchrony. Circulation 1989; 79:845–853.
9. Shamim W, Francis DP, Yousufuddin M, et al. Intraventricular conduction delay: a prognostic marker in chronic heart failure. Int.J Cardiol 1999; 70:171–178.
10. Shamim W, Yousufuddin M, Cicoria M, et al. Incremental changes in QRS duration in serial ECGs over time identify high risk elderly patients with heart failure. Heart 2002; 88:47–51.
11. Xiao HB, Brecker SJ, Gibson DG. Effects of abnormal activation on the time course of the left ventricular pressure pulse in dilated cardiomyopathy. Br Heart J 1992; 68:403–407.
12. Cazeau S, Ritter P, Bakdach S, et al. Four chamber pacing in dilated cardiomyopathy. Pacing Clin Electrophysiol 1994; 17:1974–1979.
13. Nishimura RA, Hayes DL, Holmes DRJ, et al. Mechanism of hemodynamic improvement by dual-chamber pacing for severe left ventricular dysfunction: an acute Doppler and catheterization hemodynamic study. J Am Coll Cardiol 1995; 25:281–288.
14. Leclercq C, Cazeau S, Le BH, et al. Acute hemodynamic effects of biventricular DDD pacing in patients with end-stage heart failure. J Am Coll Cardiol 1998; 32:1825–1831.
15. Kass DA, Chen CH, Talbot MW, et al. Ventricular pacing with premature excitation for treatment of hypertensive-cardiac hypertrophy with cavity-obliteration. Circulation 1999; 100:807–812.
16. Cazeau S, Leclercq C, Lavergne T, et al. Effects of multisite biventricular pacing in patients with heart failure and intraventricular conduction delay. N Engl J Med 2001; 344:873–880.
17. Linde C, Leclercq C, Rex S, et al. Long-term benefits of biventricular pacing in congestive heart failure: results from the MUltisite STimulation in cardiomyopathy (MUSTIC) study. J Am Coll Cardiol 2002; 40:111–118.
18. Cranefield PF. Action potentials, afterpotentials, and arrhythmias. Circ Res 1977; 41:415–423.
19. Krahn AD, Yee R, Klein GJ, et al. Inappropriate sinus tachycardia: evaluation and therapy. J Cardiovasc Electrophysiol 1995; 6:1124–1128.
20. Kaplan BM, Langendorf R, Lev M, et al. Tachycardia-bradycardia syndrome (so-called 'sick sinus syndrome'). Pathology, mechanisms and treatment. Am J Cardiol 1973; 31:497–508.
21. Evans R, Shaw DB. Pathological studies in sinoatrial disorder (sick sinus syndrome). Br Heart J 1977; 39:778–786.
22. Steinbeck G, Hoffman E. 'True' atrial tachycardia. Eur Heart J 1998; 19(suppl E):E10–E12.
23. Wren C. Incessant tachycardias. Eur Heart J 1998; 19 (suppl E):E32–E36.
24. Wren C. Mechanisms of fetal tachycardia. Heart 1998; 79:536–537.
25. Villain E, Vetter VL, Garcia JM, et al. Evolving concepts on the management of congenital junctional ectopic tachycardia. Circulation 1990; 81:1544–1549.

26. Dodge-Khatami A, Miller OI, Anderson RH, et al. Impact of junctional ectopic tachycardia on postoperative morbidity following repair of congenital heart defects. Eur J Cardiothorac Surg 2002; 21:255–259.

27. Rosen MR, Wit AL, Hoffman BF. Electrophysiology and pharmacology of cardiac arrhythmias. VI. Cardiac effects of verapamil. Am Heart J 1975; 89:665–673.

28. Spear JF, Michelson EL, Spielman SR, et al. The origin of ventricular arrhythmias 24 hours following experimental anterior septal coronary artery occlusion. Circulation 1977; 55:844–852.

29. Ferrier GR, Moffat MP, Lukas A. Possible mechanisms of ventricular arrhythmias elicited by ischemia followed by reperfusion. Studies on isolated canine ventricular tissues. Circ Res 1985; 56:184–194.

30. Wehrens XH, Doevendans PA, Ophuis TJ, et al. A comparison of electrocardiographic changes during reperfusion of acute myocardial infarction by thrombolysis or percutaneous transluminal coronary angioplasty. Am Heart J 2000; 139:430–436.

31. El-Sherif N. Early afterdepolarizations and arrhythmogenesis. Experimental and clinical aspects. Arch Mal Couer Vaiss 1991; 84:227–234.

32. Jackman WM, Clark M, Friday KJ, et al. Ventricular tachyarrhythmias in the long QT syndromes. Med Clin North Am 1984; 68:1079–1109.

33. Jackman WM, Friday KJ, Anderson JL, et al. The long QT syndromes: a critical review, new clinical observations and a unifying hypothesis. Prog Cardiovasc Dis 1988; 31:115–172.

34. El-Sherif N, Turitto G. The long QT syndrome and torsade de pointes. Pacing Clin Electrophysiol 1999; 22:91–110.

35. Dessertenne F. La tachycardie ventriculaire a deux foyers opposes variables. Arch Mal Couer Vaiss 1966; 59:263–272.

36. Ben-David J, Zipes DP. Torsades de pointes and proarrhythmia. Lancet 1993; 341:1578–1582.

37. El-Sherif N, Caref EB, Yin H, et al. The electrophysiological mechanism of ventricular arrhythmias in the long QT syndrome. Tridimensional mapping of activation and recovery patterns. Circ Res 1996; 79:474–492.

38. Brorson L, Olsson SB. Right atrial monophasic action potential in healthy males. Studies during spontaneous sinus rhythm and atrial pacing. Acta Med Scand 1976; 199:433–446.

39. Brachmann J, Scherlag BJ, Rosenshtraukh LV, et al. Bradycardia-dependent triggered activity: relevance to drug-induced multiform ventricular tachycardia. Circulation 1983; 68:846–856.

40. Shimizu W, Tanaka K, Suenaga K, et al. Bradycardia-dependent early afterdepolarizations in a patient with QTU prolongation and torsade de pointes in association with marked bradycardia and hypokalemia. Pacing Clin Electrophysiol 1991; 14:1105–1111.

41. Cranefield PF, Aronson RS. Torsade de pointes and other pause-induced ventricular tachycardias: the short-long-short sequence and early afterdepolarizations. Pacing Clin Electrophysiol 1988; 11:670–678.

42. Locati EH, Maison-Blanche P, Dejode P, et al. Spontaneous sequences of onset of torsade de pointes in patients with acquired prolonged repolarization: quantitative analysis of Holter recordings. J Am Coll Cardiol 1995; 25:1564–1575.

43. Vos MA, Gorenek B, Verduyn SC, et al. Observations on the onset of torsade de pointes arrhythmias in the acquired long QT syndrome. Cardiovasc Res 2000; 48:421–429.

44. Crawford MH, Karliner JS, O'Rourke RA, et al. Prolonged Q-T interval syndrome. Successful treatment with combined ventricular pacing and propanolol. Chest 1975; 68:369–371.

45. DiSegni E, Klein HO, David D, et al. Overdrive pacing in quinidine syncope and other long QT-interval syndromes. Arch Intern Med 1980; 140:1036–1040.

46. Wilmer CI, Stein B, Morris DC. Atrioventricular pacemaker placement in Romano-Ward syndrome and recurrent torsades de pointes. Am J Cardiol 1987; 59:171–172.

47. Eldar M, Griffin JC, Abbott JA, et al. Permanent cardiac pacing in patients with the long QT syndrome. J Am Coll Cardiol 1987; 10:600–607.

48. Moss AJ, Liu JE, Gottlieb S, et al. Efficacy of permanent pacing in the management of high-risk patients with long QT syndrome. Circulation 1991; 84:1524–1529.

49. Eldar M, Griffin JC, Van HG, et al. Combined use of beta-adrenergic blocking agents and long-term cardiac pacing for patients with the long QT syndrome. J Am Coll Cardiol 1992; 20:830–837.

50. Ferrier GR, Moe GK. Effect of calcium on acetylstrophanthidin-induced transient depolarizations in canine Purkinje tissue. Circ Res 1973; 33:508–515.

51. Ferrier GR. The effects of tension on acetylstrophanthidin-induced transient depolarizations and aftercontractions in canine myocardial and Purkinje tissues. Circ Res 1976; 38:156–162.

52. El-Sherif N, Gough WB, Zeiler RH, et al. Triggered ventricular rhythms in 1-day-old myocardial infarction in the dog. Circ Res 1983; 52:566–579.

53. Moak JP, Rosen MR. Induction and termination of triggered activity by pacing in isolated canine Purkinje fibers. Circulation 1984; 69:149–162.

54. Wu D, Kou HC, Hung JS. Exercise-triggered paroxysmal ventricular tachycardia. A repetitive rhythmic activity possibly related to afterdepolarization. Ann Intern Med 1981; 95:410–414.

55. Palileo EV, Ashley WW, Swiryn S, et al. Exercise provocable right ventricular outflow tract tachycardia. Am Heart J 1982; 104:185–193.

56. Ferrier GR. Digitalis arrhythmias: role of oscillatory afterpotentials. Prog Cardiovasc Dis 1977; 19:459–474.

57. Griffith MJ, Garratt CJ, Rowland E, et al. Effects of intravenous adenosine on verapamil-sensitive 'idiopathic' ventricular tachycardia. Am J Cardiol 1994; 73:759–764.

58. Buxton AE, Waxman HL, Marchlinski FE, et al. Right ventricular tachycardia: clinical and electrophysiologic characteristics. Circulation 1983; 68:917–927.

59. Buxton AE, Marchlinski FE, Doherty JU, et al. Repetitive, monomorphic ventricular tachycardia: clinical and electrophysiologic characteristics in patients with and patients without organic heart disease. Am J Cardiol 1984; 54:997–1002.

60. Hoffman BF, Rosen MR. Cellular mechanisms for cardiac arrhythmias. Circ Res 1981; 49:1–15.

61. Mines GR. On circulating excitations in heart muscle and their possible relations to tachycardia and fibrillation. Trans R Soc Can Ser 1914; 8:43–52.

62. Wit AL, Cranefield PF. Reentrant excitatiom as a cause of cardiac arrhythmia. Am J Physiol 1978; 235:H1–H17.

63. Okumura K, Henthorn RW, Epstein AE, et al. Further observations on transient entrainment: importance of pacing site and properties of the components of the reentry circuit. Circulation 1985; 72:1293–1307.

64. Almendral JM, Stamato NJ, Rosenthal ME, et al. Resetting response patterns during sustained ventricular tachycardia: relationship to the excitable gap. Circulation 1986; 74:722–730.

65. Waldo AL. Atrial flutter: entrainment characteristics. J Cardiovasc Electrophysiol 1997; 8:337–352.

66. Bray JJ, Cragg PA, MacKnight ADC, et al. Cardiovacular system: introduction and the heart. In: Lecture notes on human physiology. Oxford: Blackwell Science; 1994:367–404.

67. Stevenson WG, Sager PT, Friedman PL. Entrainment techniques for mapping atrial and ventricular tachycardias. J Cardiovas Electrophysiol 1995; 6:201–216.

68. El-Sherif N, Mehra R, Gough WB, et al. Ventricular activation patterns of spontaneous and induced ventricular rhythms in canine one-day-old myocardial infarction. Evidence for focal and reentrant mechanisms. Circ Res 1982; 51:152–166.

69. Waldo AL, Plumb VJ, Arciniegas JG, et al. Transient entrainment and interruption of the atrioventricular bypass pathway type of paroxysmal atrial tachycardia. A model for understanding and identifying reentrant arrhythmias. Circulation 1983; 67:73–83.

70. Josephson ME. Electrophysiological investigation: general concepts. In: Clinical cardiac electrophysiology: techniques and interpretations. Philadelphia: Lea & Febiger; 1992:22–70.

71. Rosenthal ME, Stamato NJ, Almendral JM, et al. Resetting of ventricular tachycardia with electrocardiographic fusion: incidence and significance. Circulation 1988; 77:581–588.

72. Rosenthal ME, Stamato NJ, Almendral JM, et al. Coupling intervals of ventricular extrastimuli causing resetting of sustained ventricular tachycardia secondary to coronary artery disease: relation to subsequent termination. Am J Cardiol 1988; 61:770–774.

73. Brugada P, Wellens HJ. Entrainment as an electrophysiologic phenomenon. J Am Coll Cardiol 1984; 3:451–454.

74. Spach MS, Dolber PC, Heidlage JF. Influence of the passive anisotropic properties on directional differences in propagation following modification of the sodium conductance in human atrial muscle. A model of reentry based on anisotropic discontinuous propagation. Circ Res 1988; 62:811–832.

75. Weisfogel GM, Batsford WP, Paulay KL, et al. Sinus node re-entrant tachycardia in man. Am Heart J 1975; 90:295–304.

76. Allessie MA, Bonke FI, Schopman FJ. Circus movement in rabbit atrial muscle as a mechanism of tachycardia. III. The 'leading circle' concept: a new model of circus movement in cardiac tissue without the involvement of an anatomical obstacle. Circ Res 1977; 41:9–18.

77. Antzelevitch C, Jalife J, Moe GK. Characteristics of reflection as a mechanism of reentrant arrhythmias and its relationship to parasystole. Circulation 1980; 61:182–191.

78. Rozanski GJ, Jalife J, Moe GK. Reflected reentry in nonhomogeneous ventricular muscle as a mechanism of cardiac arrhythmias. Circulation 1984; 69: 163–173.

79. Glass L, Goldberger AL, Belair J. Dynamics of pure parasystole. Am J Physiol. 1986; 251:H841–H847.

80. Kinoshita S. Mechanisms of intermittent ventricular parasystole due to type II second degree entrance block. J Electrocardiol 1983; 16:7–14.

81. Kinoshita S, Nakagawa K, Kato N, et al. Mechanism of supraventricular parasystole. Circulation 1982; 65:208–212.

82. Cohen H, Langendorf R, Pick A. Intermittent parasystole – mechanism of protection. Circulation 1973; 48:761–774.

Electro-physiology: diagnostic aspects

Ernest W Lau MD MA MRCP
University of Ottawa Heart Institute, Ottawa, Canada

Gregory Y H Lip MD FRCP DFM FACC FESC
City Hospital, Birmingham, UK

For the ordinary clinician, the ECG remains the most important diagnostic tool

Introduction

The practical management of arrhythmias, both in terms of diagnosis and treatment, has been transformed in the last three decades by the development of diagnostic and interventional electrophysiology (EP), which centers around two approaches.[1] The first approach involves the temporary percutaneous placement of electrode catheters within the heart for defining the mechanism of an arrhythmia (i.e. an EP study) and possibly destroying it through the delivery of radiofrequency (RF) electrical energy, providing a definitive 'cure' for the arrhythmia at the same sitting as its diagnosis.[2–18] The second approach involves the permanent subcutaneous placement of implantable devices (e.g. loop recorder[19–22] or cardioverter-defibrillator[23–27]) for continuously monitoring the patient's cardiac rhythm and delivering appropriate therapy accordingly (back-up pacing for bradycardia and overdrive pacing or cardioversion/defibrillator for tachycardia).[28] In comparison, the developments in antiarrhythmic drug therapy have been much less spectacular. Rather disappointingly, antiarrhythmic drugs remain unpredictable and often ineffective in suppressing arrhythmias, are poorly tolerated and have many side-effects (some of which are potentially life threatening).[29] With further refinements in mapping[30–36] and ablation technologies,[37–41] the scope of ablation therapy for arrhythmias stands to expand even more.[42–51] Improved battery technology and detection algorithms also mean that implantable devices can be expected to become longer lasting and more reliable in diagnosing and treating arrhythmias in the future.

Even though technological advances have opened up new, exciting opportunities in the management of arrhythmias, they are mainly in the hands of the specialist electrophysiologists. For the ordinary clinician, the electrocardiogram (ECG) remains the most important diagnostic tool, and anti-arrhythmic drugs and pacing (temporary or permanent) the only therapeutic modalities readily available. Thus this chapter will confine itself to the ECG and not the EP diagnosis of arrhythmias, and concentrate on their acute rather than long-term treatment. An account on the theoretical basis of the mechanisms of arrhythmias, which should facilitate the comprehension of this chapter, has been separately provided.

DIAGNOSIS OF BRADYCARDIAS

A simple schema for diagnosing bradycardias by the ECG is shown in Figure 4.1. When P waves are invisible, it is either because the atria are engaged in low-amplitude fibrillatory activities or the sinoatrial node (SAN) is not activating the atria. The former situation occurs in atrial fibrillation (AF). The latter situation occurs when either the SAN is not discharging (i.e. sinus arrest) or the impulse from the SAN is prevented from entering the atria (i.e. exit block). When P waves are visible, the SAN may be going too slow (sinus bradycardia, sick sinus syndrome), or sinus impulses are not being conducted 1:1 to the ventricles (i.e. second or third degree block in the atrioventricular node (AVN)) (Figs 4.2 and 4.3). Most cases of sick sinus syndrome and AVN block occur among the elderly, even though AVN block can also occur either congenitally[52–54] or after cardiac surgery.[55]

ACUTE TREATMENT OF BRADYCARDIAS

The acute management of any form of bradycardia is simple – temporary pacing. When the facilities for temporary pacing are not available, vagolytic agent (e.g. atropine) or sympathomimetic agent (e.g. isoprenaline) can be tried. However, if the bradycardia is well tolerated and

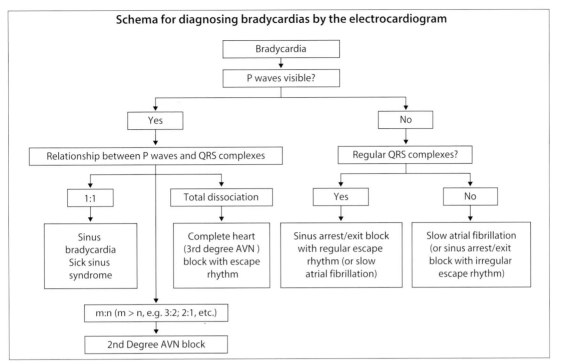

Fig. 4.1 Schema for diagnosing bradycardias by the electrocardiogram. AVN, atrioventricular node.

First degree atrioventricular nodal block with aberrant conduction and intermittent complete heart block with a broad complex escape rhythm

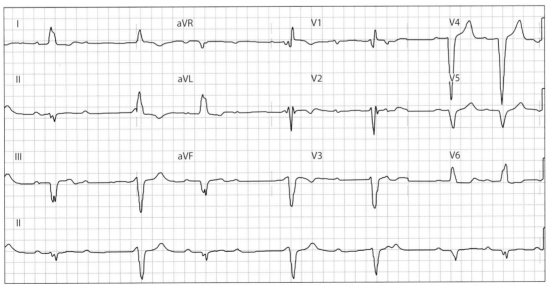

Fig. 4.2 First degree atrioventricular nodal block with aberrant conduction and intermittent complete heart block with a broad complex escape rhythm.

Wenckebach atrioventricular node block

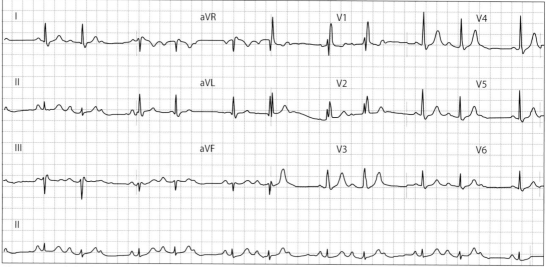

Fig. 4.3 Wenckebach atrioventricular node block.

haemodynamically stable, temporary pacing may not be indicated. The management strategy for such a situation will be to rectify any reversible potential causes of bradycardia (i.e. hypothyroidism, excessive rate-limiting drugs) or proceed direct to permanent pacemaker implantation. Regardless of the exact electrophysiological mechanism, bradycardias can almost always be satisfactorily treated with permanent pacemaker implantation.[56]

Basic tools for arrhythmia diagnosis

- 12-lead surface ECG
- Routine monitor ECG in CCU
- Conventional Holter- or event recording
- A thorough patient history

DIAGNOSIS OF TACHYCARDIAS

Even though an EP study with placement of intracardiac electrodes is often necessary for the exact diagnosis, much information can still be drawn, and many important inferences made, about the mechanism of an arrhythmia from examining the surface ECG. Moreover, for the majority of clinicians who do not specialize in EP or cardiology, the ECG remains the only portal with which they are familiar into the center of an arrhythmia. Apart from the ECG during tachycardia, the ECGs in sinus rhythm and during the initiation and termination of arrhythmia, and the patient's background history (age, gender, past medical history, drug exposure, family history) are also of interest and may provide vital clues.

The ECG diagnosis of tachycardias can be guided by three considerations:

1. width of the QRS complex;
2. regularity of the tachycardia; and
3. nature of atrial activity and its relationship to the QRS complexes.

Width of the QRS complex

The width of the QRS complex allows inference on the mechanism of ventricular activation. The usual narrow QRS complex requires highly synchronized activation of the ventricular myocardium, which can only be achieved when the specialized, rapidly conducting His-Purkinje system (HPS) is used for the activation of the

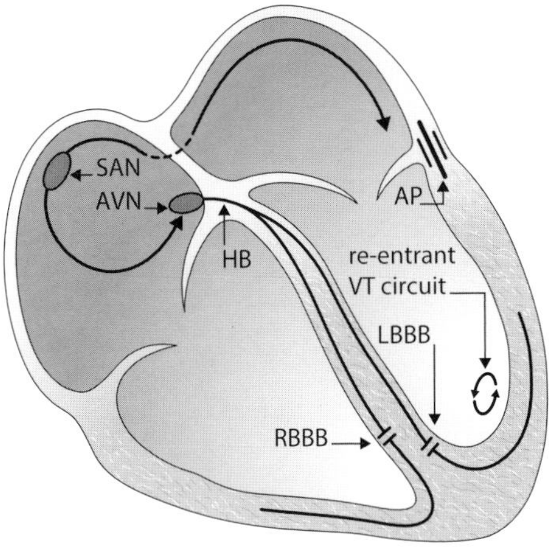

Fig. 4.4 Electrophysiological mechanisms of broad complex tachycardias. AP, accessory pathway; SAN, sinoatrial node; AVN, atrioventricular node; HB, His bundle; LBB, left bundle branch block; RBB, right bundle branch block; VT, ventricular tachycardia.

majority of the ventricular myocardium. When the QRS complex is broad, three explanations are possible: aberrant conduction, pre-excitation or a ventricular origin of the tachycardia (Fig. 4.4).

Aberrant conduction occurs due to bundle branch block (BBB) – when one of the bundle branches is blocked in the antegrade conduction, part of the ventricular myocardium will be activated by slow propagation of electrical activation through the ordinary ventricular myocardium. Aberrant conduction can be pre-existent, rate dependent (i.e. only becomes evident during tachycardia) or due to concealed retrograde penetration of one of the bundle branches during tachycardia.[57]

Pre-excitation occurs when a significant amount of ventricular myocardium is captured by antegrade conduction down one or more accessory pathways.[58] Histologically, an accessory pathway is an area of working myocardial fibers breaching the fibrous, electrically insulating atrioventricular annulus to link up the atrial myocardium with the ventricular myocardium or one of the fascicles of the

HPS.[59–62] An antegradely conducting accessory pathway causes pre-excitation of the part of the ventricular myocardium into which it inserts ahead of other parts of the myocardium by the AVN/HPS, and this manifests as a shortened PR interval. As the ventricular insertion site of an accessory pathway is usually into ordinary working myocardium (close to the base of the heart), spread of excitation to the rest of ventricular myocardium is slow through electrotonic conduction. Thus pre-excitation manifests as an initial slurred upstroke/downstroke (δ wave) to an overall broadened QRS complex on the ECG. These ECG features together with palpitations constitute the Wolff-Parkinson-White syndrome pattern) (Fig. 4.5).[63] It is possible to deduce the anatomical location of an accessory pathway on the basis of the pre-excitation pattern it generates on the ECG.[4,64–67] However, pre-excitation may be inapparent or latent if the accessory pathway is situated in the free wall of the left ventricle, a long way away from the SAN.[68,69] Also, some (concealed) accessory pathways only conduct retrogradely in a ventriculoatrial direction and do not cause pre-excitation at all. Any tachycardia which uses one or more accessory pathway for antegrade conduction to the ventricles (i.e. a pre-excited tachycardia) will have a broad QRS complex.

A ventricular origin of tachycardia applies to ventricular tachycardia (VT) and ventricular fibrillation (VF). In such a situation, similar to the case of pre-excitation, activation of ventricular myocardium is slow through electrotonic conduction and hence not well synchronized, resulting in a broad QRS complex.

At this point, it is worthwhile mentioning the term 'supraventricular tachycardia' (SVT), which is effectively taken to mean a narrow complex tachycardia by most clinicians. However, a narrow complex tachycardia is not necessarily truly 'supraventricular', in the sense of having the entire tachycardia mechanism confined to the atria and the

Manifest pre-excitation

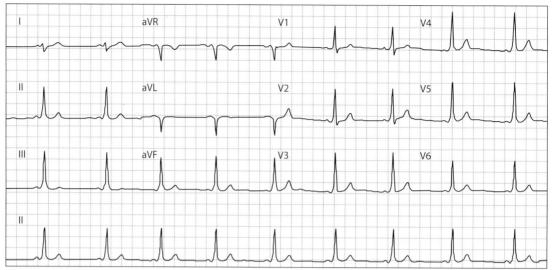

Fig. 4.5 Manifest pre-excitation. Note shortened PR interval, δ wave and broad QRS complex.

AVN independent of the ventricles. A prime example of this apparent contradiction is orthodromic AVRT, for which the ventricles are an integral part of the tachycardia mechanism despite the usually narrow QRS complex (in the absence of aberrant conduction) during tachycardia. A better definition of an SVT is one for which antegrade activation of the ventricles by the HPS is compatible with (but may or may not be necessary for) the maintenance of the tachycardia. In this light, a distinction can be drawn between 'true' SVT, for which participation of the ventricles is not necessary for its perpetuation, and 'pseudo' SVT, for which activation of the ventricles via the HPS is essential for its perpetuation (Table 4.1). Aberrant conduction and pre-excitation will turn any SVT (and otherwise narrow complex tachycardia) into a broad complex tachycardia. However, in the case of a pre-excited tachycardia, the accessory pathway can be either an integral part of the tachycardia mechanism (e.g. antidromic AVRT) or a mere bystander (e.g. atrial tachycardia in the presence of an accessory pathway).

It is not always easy to tell whether a broad QRS complex is due to aberrant conduction, pre-excitation or a ventricular origin. A simple way of distinguishing SVT with aberrant conduction from VT or pre-excited tachycardia is by comparing the QRS morphology pattern during tachycardia with that of typical left bundle branch block (LBBB) or right bundle branch block (RBBB) (Fig. 4.6), but this is by no means fool-proof.[70,71] Certain forms of VT and pre-excited tachycardia can have typical BBB morphology patterns[72] whereas aberrant conduction does not always have the classical BBB morphology patterns.[73] Another approach is to compare the QRS morphology pattern on the ECG during sinus rhythm with that during tachycardia, but this method is again fallible. For example, aberrant conduction and pre-excitation may be only intermittent, rate dependent or latent and not always

Table 4.1 Inferences from nature of atrial signal and its relationship to QRS complexes during a tachycardia

Relationship between atrial signals and QRS complexes	Nature of atrial signal and inferences	Examples
More atrial signals than QRS complexes	Ventricles not needed for perpetuation of tachycardia	'True' SVT: (inappropriate) sinus tachycardia SNRT atrial flutter atrial tachycardia AVNRT – with 2nd degree AVN block
More QRS complexes than atrial signals	Atria not needed for perpetuation of tachycardia atrial signals	VT
Atrial signals ('P' waves) and QRS complexes in 1:1 ratio		
RP interval < PR' interval during a RR' interval (short RP tachycardias)	Antegrade P wave: AVN conduction slow compared with tachycardia rate	(Inappropriate) sinus tachycardia SNRT atrial tachycardia
	Retrograde P wave: retrograde limb of re-entrant circuit conducts faster than antegrade limb	Typical 'slow-fast' AVNRT AVRT with rapidly retrogradely conducting accessory pathway
RP interval > PR' interval during a RR' interval (long RP tachycardias)	Antegrade P wave: AVN conduction fast compared to tachycardia rate	(Inappropriate) sinus tachycardia SNRT atrial tachycardia
	Retrograde P wave: retrograde limb of re-entrant circuit conducts more slowly than antegrade limb	Atypical 'fast-slow' or 'slow-slow' AVNRT AVRT with slowly retrogradely conducting accessory pathway, e.g. PRJT

AVN, atrioventricular node; SVT, supraventricular tachycardia; VT, ventricular tachycardia; SNRT, sinus node re-entrant tachycardia; AVNRT, atrio-ventricular nodal re-entrant tachycardia; AVRT, atrioventricular nodal re-entrant tachycardia; PJRT, permanent junctional re-entrant tachycardia

apparent on the sinus rhythm ECG. (Latent pre-excitation can be unmasked with adenosine.[68,74]) VT can also have a QRS morphology pattern exactly the same as that during sinus rhythm.[75,76]

Regularity of tachycardia

Regularity of tachycardia can be defined in terms of RR interval and QRS morphology/axis.

Irregularity in the RR interval of a cardiac rhythm can be due to:

1. irregularity in atrial impulse generation;
2. inconsistency in AVN conduction of atrial impulses; or
3. a combination of the two.

Irregularity in atrial impulse generation means random re-entry, i.e. AF. Inconsistency in AVN conduction means second degree AVN block, which can produce an irregular ventricular response in spite of regular atrial impulse generation. This is most often evident in the case of atrial flutter with AVN block (e.g. 2:1, 3:1). Inconsistency in AVN

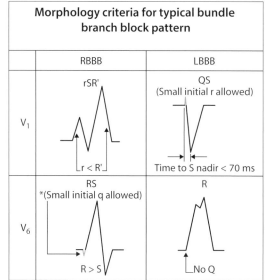

Morphology criteria for typical bundle branch block pattern

	RBBB	LBBB
V₁	rSR' ⎣r < R'⎦	QS (Small initial r allowed) Time to S nadir < 70 ms
V₆	RS *(Small initial q allowed) R > S	R No Q

Fig. 4.6 Morphology criteria for typical bundle branch block pattern. RBBB, right bundle branch block; LBBB, left bundle branch block; *< 2 mm in depth and < 40 ms in width.

conduction is inconsistent with a pseudo SVT (i.e. orthodromic AVRT). Finally, irregularity in atrial impulse generation and inconsistency in AVN conduction can coexist and contribute to the irregularity in RR interval simultaneously, as is most likely the actual case with AF.

Irregularity in QRS morphology/axis signifies variation in the activation pattern of the ventricles, and can be due to:

1. variation in the route(s) of antegrade conduction to the ventricles;
2. variation in the spread of electrical activation within the ventricles; or
3. a combination of the two.

The route(s) of antegrade conduction to the ventricles can vary due to intermittent aberrant conduction, or different beat-to-beat result of the competition between the AVN/HPS and one or more accessory pathway (i.e. pre-excitation) in capturing the ventricular myocardium.[77] The spread of electrical activation within the ventricles can vary greatly from beat-to-beat when it is by random re-entry, as in VF or polymorphic VT. A combination of the two mechanisms happens in the setting of a ventricular arrhythmia (i.e. independent of the atria for maintenance) competing with a supraventricular source of impulses for activation of the ventricular myocardium, as in the case of capture/fusion beats during VT.

A tachycardia regular in both RR interval and QRS morphology/axis is most consistent with ordered re-entry, but is also compatible with enhanced automaticity (normal, ectopic or abnormal) or triggered activity. In reality, minor variations in RR interval and QRS morphology/axis exist even for tachycardias due to such mechanisms when assessed with highly sensitive electronic equipment during EP study, but the fluctuations are usually too minute to be discerned by the naked eye on the ECG so the tachycardias will appear effectively regular. However, any otherwise regular 'true' SVT can be turned irregular by second degree AVN block (e.g. atrial tachycardia with Wenckebach AVN block), intermittent aberrant conduction or variable pre-excitation.

Nature of atrial activity and its relationship to the QRS complex

Atrial activity may not always be evident on the ECG during a tachycardia, but its relationship with the QRS complexes can often shed light on the tachycardia mechanism (Table 4.1).

Atrial activity can be represented by flutter wave, antegrade P wave or retrograde P wave on the ECG, and the three manifestations can be partially distinguished on the basis of the morphology and axis of the atrial signal. Flutter waves are characterized by the classical 'saw-tooth' appearance and should be easy to recognize. An atrial signal is likely to be an antegrade P wave if it is normal in morphology and axis (and similar to that observed during sinus rhythm). However, an atrial signal abnormal in morphology and axis (and different from the P wave in sinus rhythm) can be either a retrograde P wave or an antegrade P wave emanating from an abnormal atrial site (e.g. an ectopic focus situated in the left atrium).

During a tachycardia, atrial signals can either exist in a 1:1 ratio to the QRS complexes or not. When there are more atrial signals than QRS complexes, the ventricles are not needed for maintenance of the tachycardia, i.e. 'true' SVT. When there are more QRS complexes than atrial signals, the atria are not needed for maintenance of the tachycardia, i.e. VT. When atrial signals and QRS complexes exist in a 1:1 ratio, during a tachycardia cycle defined by two consecutive QRS complexes (i.e. an RR' interval), the atrial signal ('P' wave) can be temporally more tightly associated with the preceding QRS complex (i.e. the RP interval < the PR' interval) or the following QRS complex (i.e. the RP interval > the PR' interval). This defines two categories of tachycardias: short RP tachycardias (the RP interval < the PR' interval) and long RP tachycardias (the RP interval > the PR' interval). The relative lengths of the RP and PR' intervals together with the nature of the atrial signal help identify the underlying tachycardia mechanism (Table 4.1). However, in the case of short RP tachycardias, the atrial signal may be obscured by the preceding QRS complex and its existence can only be inferred.

Diagnostic schema for tachycardias

The three considerations mentioned above allow the establishment of a systematic approach to the diagnosis of tachycardias (Table 4.2).

(Inappropriate) sinus tachycardia

Sinus tachycardia is characterized by a P wave of identical morphology and axis as during sinus rhythm. Because the tachycardia is due to automaticity, there is typically a period of warm-up and cool-down at the beginning and end. Sinus tachycardia is inappropriate when the sinus rate is too fast for the physiological condition of the patient.[78]

Sinus node re-entrant tachycardia

Sinus node re-entrant tachycardia (SNRT) again has a P wave of morphology and axis identical to that during sinus rhythm.[79] Because SNRT is due to re-entry, unlike sinus tachycardia, SNRT is typically of abrupt onset and termination. SNRT is amenable to RF ablation.[80]

Atrial tachycardia

Atrial tachycardia is a 'true' SVT (Fig. 4.7) and can be due to either enhanced ectopic automaticity or intra-atrial re-entry. Both mechanisms are often associated with structural heart disease, especially in the way of previous cardiac surgery, as surgical scars can provide the anatomical barriers to conduction needed for re-entry.[13] Atrial tachycardia can be incessant and lead to the development of tachycardiomyopathy which is reversible on treatment.[81–83]

The P wave morphology and axis may point towards the site of an ectopic atrial focus.[84] A positive P wave in lead V_1 suggests a left atrial focus. A positive or biphasic P wave in lead aVL suggests a right atrial focus. The P wave axis, as determined by the polarity of P wave in the inferior leads, helps to distinguish a superiorly situated focus (positive P waves in inferior leads) from an inferiorly situated focus (negative P waves in superior leads) in both the right and left atria.

Atrial fibrillation

AF usually manifests as an irregular narrow complex tachycardia with no distinct atrial activity on the ECG. Occasionally organized atrial activity are discernible in certain leads (especially V_1) and the arrhythmia can be mistaken for

Table 4.2 Schema for diagnosing tachycardias by the electrocardiogram

	Irregular	Regular
Narrow QRS complex ⇒ ventricular activation through the His-Purkinje system	AF 'true' SVT (i.e. does not require ventricles for perpetuation) with variable AVN conduction	<u>Flutter waves</u> atrial flutter <u>Short RP interval</u> inappropriate sinus tachycardia SNRT atrial tachycardia typical AVNRT orthodromic AVRT <u>Long RP interval</u> inappropriate sinus tachycardia SNRT atrial tachycardia permanent junctional re-entrant tachycardia atypical AVNRT <u>Special form of VT</u> fascicular tachycardia
Broad QRS complex ⇒ ventricular activation 1. through the His-Purkinje system with BBB 2. via accessory pathways (pre-excitation) 3. originating from within ventricular myocardium	AF with BBB 'true' SVT with variable AVN conduction and BBB pre-excited AF polymorphic VT/ TdP VF	<u>Typical BBB morphology of QRS</u> any form of SVT with BBB special forms of VT: RVOT tachycardia (LBBB) bundle branch re-entrant tachycardia (LBBB>RBBB) special form of pre-excitation: Mahaim tachycardia (LBBB) <u>Atypical BBB morphology of QRS</u> pre-excitation: antidromic AVRT VT: most cases

AVN, atrioventricular node; BBB, bundle branch block; LBBB, left bundle branch block; RBBB,: right bundle branch block; SVT, supraventricular tachycardia; VT, ventricular tachycardia; AF, atrial fibrillation; SNRT, sinus node re-entrant tachycardia; AVNRT, atrioventricular nodal re-entrant tachycardia; AVRT, atrio-ventricular re-entrant tachycardia; TdP, torsades de pointes; VF, ventricular fibrillation.

atrial flutter or atrial tachycardia (Fig. 4.8). The ECG manifestation of atrial activity during AF is related to the number of wandering wavelets participating in random re-entry: the fewer wavelets are involved, the coarser the AF and vice versa.[85,86]

Pre-excited atrial fibrillation: When AF happens in the presence of pre-excitation, an irregular broad complex tachycardia results. When only one accessory pathway is present, the morphology pattern of the pre-excited QRS complex tends to be constant (Fig. 4.9). But when multiple accessory pathways are present, the morphology pattern of the pre-excited QRS complex can be highly variable due to shifting degrees of fusion between pre-excitation via different accessory pathways (Fig. 4.10).[77]

The major differential diagnosis for pre-excited AF is AF with aberrant conduction. Whereas AF with aberrant conduction is relatively 'benign', pre-excited AF can degenerate into VF, which is believed to be the mechanism of sudden cardiac death in patients with the Wolff-Parkinson-White syndrome.[87,88] Moreover, standard treatments for AF such as verapamil can be highly dangerous for pre-excited AF.[89–92] It is thus important that the

Atrial tachycardia with 2:1 atrioventricular nodal block

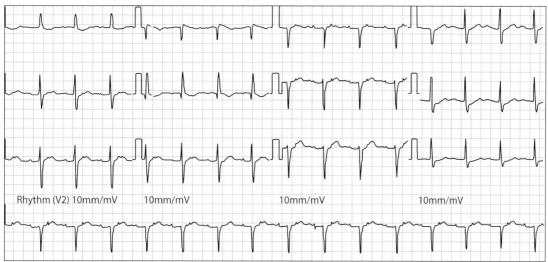

Fig. 4.7 Atrial tachycardia with 2:1 atrioventricular nodal block.

Atrial fibrillation

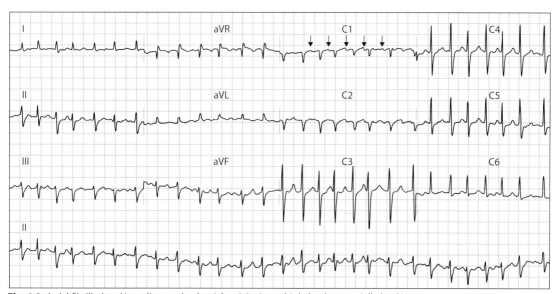

Fig. 4.8 Atrial fibrillation. Note disorganized atrial activity in multiple leads, especially lead V_1.

two conditions can be distinguished, but that should not be difficult as specific diagnostic criteria exist for this purpose.[71,77]

Atrial flutter

Atrial flutter is due to a macroentrant circuit confined to the atria, typically around the tricuspid annulus.[6,93–97] The hallmark of atrial flutter is the flutter wave, which is usually best appreciated in the inferior leads. The classical ('saw-tooth') flutter wave is a negative deflection in the inferior leads and has a more gradual downstroke followed by a more rapid upstroke (Fig. 4.11). When flutter waves are positively identified, the diagnosis is simple, for the tachycardia can only be due

Pre-excited atrial fibrillation (single accessory pathway)

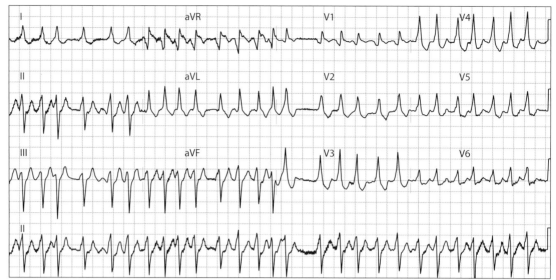

Fig. 4.9 Pre-excited atrial fibrillation (single accessory pathway). Note fairly constant pre-excitation pattern of the QRS complex.

Pre-excited atrial fibrillation (multiple accessory pathways)

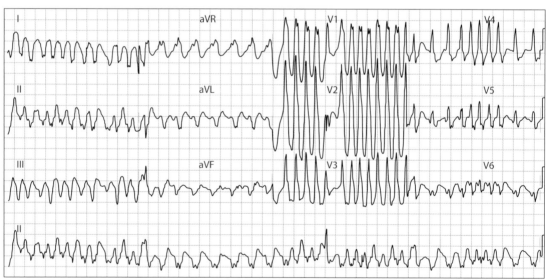

Fig. 4.10 Pre-excited atrial fibrillation (multiple accessory pathways). Note highly variable pre-excitation pattern of the QRS complex.

to atrial flutter. However, when the tachycardia is fast (e.g. atrial flutter with 2:1 AVN block), it is not always easy to decide if the negative deflection after the QRS complex is actually a flutter wave or a negative T wave. In such a situation, intravenous adenosine bolus injection to the point of inducing transient AVN block will be useful in revealing the underlying flutter waves.[98] However, both life-threatening acceleration of the ventricular response to 1:1 AVN conduction and significant bradycardia/asystole associated with hypotension have been reported in such a situation.[99–101] Because of this, due care should be exercised and resuscitation

Atrial flutter with variable atrioventricular nodal conduction

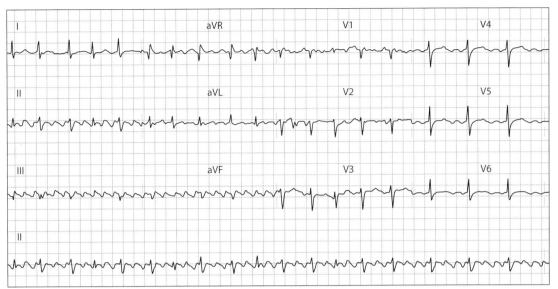

Fig. 4.11 Atrial flutter with variable atrioventricular nodal conduction.

Orthodromic atrioventricular re-entrant tachycardia

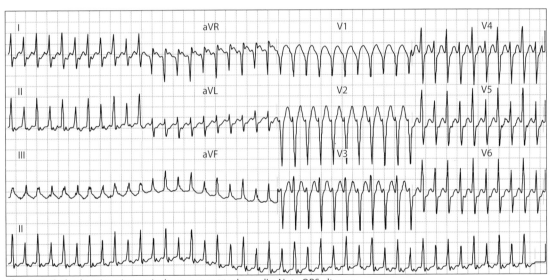

Fig. 4.12 Orthodromic atrioventricular re-entrant tachycardia. Note QRS alterans.

equipment should be readily available during the administration of adenosine for this purpose.

Atrioventricular re-entrant tachycardia

Atrioventricular re-entrant tachycardia (AVRT) is due to a macro re-entry circuit involving the atria, ventricles, (the AVN/HPS) and one or more accessory pathways. Because of re-entry, AVRT is typically of abrupt onset and termination.

AVRT can be either orthodromic (when antegrade atrioventricular conduction is via the AVN/HPS and retrograde ventriculo-atrial conduction is via an accessory pathway) or antidromic (when antegrade atrioventricular conduction is via one or more accessory pathways and retrograde ventriculoatrial conduction is via the AVN/HPS or another accessory pathway).[102] In the absence of aberrant conduction, orthodromic AVRT will have narrow QRS complexes on the ECG (Fig. 4.12). In contrast, antidromic AVRT is by definition a pre-excited reciprocating tachycardia and will have broad QRS complexes on the ECG (Fig. 4.13).

QRS alterans, or beat-to-beat fluctuation in the morphology or magnitude of the QRS complex during a narrow complex tachycardia, is associated with and highly specific for the diagnosis of orthodromic AVRT (Fig. 4.12).[103,104]

The most frequent arrhythmias seen in clinical practice

- Atrial fibrillation | narrow QRS, irregular, random re-entry
- AVNRT | narrow QRS, regular, ordered re-entry
- VT | broad QRS, monomorphic = ordered re-entry polymorphic = random re-entry bradycardia

Mahaim tachycardia: Mahaim tachycardia is a special form of pre-excited antidromic AVRT involving an atriofascicular pathway, typically situated in the right atrium around the tricuspid annulus and inserting distally into the right bundle branch or the adjacent ventricular myocardium.[9,61,62,105] The atriofascicular pathway conducts only antegradely, slowly and decrementally and hence does not give rise to pre-excitation during sinus rhythm.[106–110] Because of the insertion site of the accessory pathway, Mahaim tachycardia tends to have a relatively narrow QRS complex (≤ 150 ms) of LBBB pattern and a superior axis. The condition is associated with Ebstein's anomaly and the existence of multiple accessory pathways.[106,108,111] Mahaim tachycardia can be cured by RF ablation of the involved atriofascicular pathway.[9,12,112]

Permanent junctional re-entrant tachycardia: Permanent junctional re-entrant tachycardia (PJRT) is a special form of orthodromic AVRT involving a slowly conducting accessory pathway, which is typically situated in the inferoseptal region of the atrioventricular ring[8,113] but multiple pathways can exist.[114] The accessory

Antidromic atrioventricular nodal re-entrant tachycardia

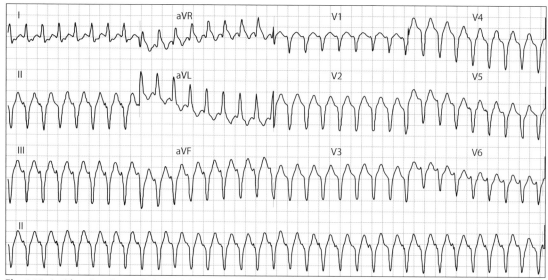

Fig. 4.13 Antidromic atrioventricular nodal re-entrant tachycardia.

pathway can either be concealed or conducts both antegradely and retrogradely.[113,115] Because of the slow conduction by the accessory pathway, PJRT typically presents as a relatively slow, long RP tachycardia. Because of the inferoseptal site of the accessory pathway, the retrograde P wave in PJRT is typically negative in the inferior leads.

PJRT typically presents as an incessant tachycardia (hence 'permanent') in childhood or adolescence but can also present later in life. Patients tend to present not with palpitations but dyspnea secondary to tachycardiomyopathy, which is reversible on treatment. PRJT is amenable to RF ablation.[8,116,117]

Atrioventricular nodal re-entrant tachycardia

Atrioventricular nodal re-entrant tachycardia (AVNRT) is a re-entrant tachycardia centered around the compact AVN and the adjacent perinodal atrial myocardium.[118] AVNRT is important as it accounts for > 70% of paroxysmal SVT encountered in clinical practice.[119]

The electrophysiological substrate of AVNRT is dual atrioventricular nodal pathways with different functional properties: a slowly conducting ('slow') pathway which is inferiorly situated and enters the compact AVN between the coronary sinus ostium and the tricuspid valve annulus, and a fast conducting ('fast') pathway which is superiorly situated in the interatrial septum.[120–122] The anatomical

substrate of dual atrioventricular nodal pathways is likely to be multiple connections between the compact AVN and adjacent atrial tissue rather than discrete intranodal pathways.[123] It is not clear whether the slow and fast pathways unite to form a common lower pathway within the compact AVN and whether the atrial myocardium forms part of the re-entrant circuit, even though there is evidence the slow pathway can be anatomically situated away from the AVN.[124]

Usually, the slow pathway has a shorter refractory period than the fast pathway. Thus after an atrial premature beat, the fast pathway blocks but the slow pathway conducts, which results in lengthening of the PR interval and initiation of typical slow-fast (antegrade conduction down the slow pathway and retrograde conduction up the fast pathway) AVNRT (Fig. 4.14). Occasionally, the slow pathway has a longer refractory period than the fast pathway, and the resulting AVNRT will be atypical in being fast-slow (antegrade conduction down the fast pathway and retrograde conduction up the slow pathway).

AVNRT is a true SVT and, in the absence of aberrant conduction or pre-excitation, will present as a regular narrow complex tachycardia (Fig. 4.15). Because the re-entrant circuit of AVNRT is comparatively small, the tachycardia rate tends to be fast (~ 170–220 bpm).[119] For typical slow-fast AVNRT, as retrograde conduction is by the fast pathway, the retrograde P wave occurs soon after the QRS complex and is often obscured. When

Atrioventricular nodal re-entrant tachycardia being initiated by a single atrial premature beat

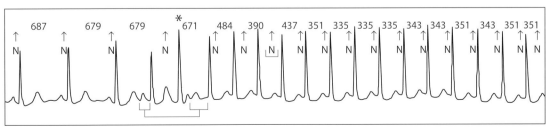

Fig. 4.14 Atrioventricular nodal re-entrant tachycardia being initiated by a single atrial premature beat. Note lengthening of the PR interval immediately after the initiation of tachycardia by a single atrial premature beat (*).

Atrioventricular nodal re-entrant tachycardia

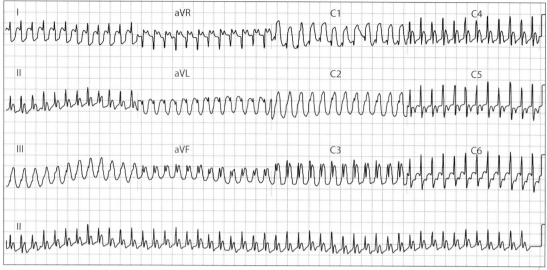

Fig. 4.15 Atrioventricular nodal re-entrant tachycardia. Note pseudo r' wave in lead V₁ and pseudo S wave in lead II.

visible, the retrograde P wave manifests as distortions to the terminal portion of the QRS complex, as pseudo r' wave in lead V_1 and pseudo S wave in lead II (Fig. 4.15).[104] For atypical fast-slow AVNRT, retrograde conduction is by the slow pathway and hence the retrograde P wave occurs relatively late in relation to the QRS complex, giving rise to a long RP tachycardia (Table 4.1).

The two main differential diagnoses of a regular narrow complex tachycardia are AVNRT and orthodromic AVRT, and QRS alterans can help to distinguish the two conditions. Unlike orthodromic AVRT, QRS alterans only occurs in AVNRT when the rate is fast (> 210 bpm).[103,119] Thus when QRS alterans occurs when the rate of a regular narrow complex tachycardia is < 210 bpm, the diagnosis is likely to be orthodromic AVRT.[103,104]

AVNRT is highly amenable to RF ablation, with the exit site of the slow pathway being the popular target. In fact, EP study and RF ablation on AVNRT have helped to define the anatomical and electrophysiological basis of the arrhythmia.[5,125–128]

Ventricular tachycardia

VT can be defined as a tachycardia whose mechanism is confined entirely to the ventricles and does not require the atria or AVN in its perpetuation. VT can be caused by re-entry (ordered or random), abnormal automaticity or triggered activity and may present as either monomorphic (i.e. one constant QRS morphology and axis) (Fig. 4.16) or polymorphic (i.e. multiple varying QRS morphologies and axes) (Fig. 4.17). Monomorphic VT is consistent with ordered re-entry, abnormal automaticity and triggered activity, but polymorphic VT is only compatible with random re-entry. By definition, a regular tachycardia can only be monomorphic and a polymorphic tachycardia must be irregular. However, because of the underlying mechanisms, a VT cannot be monomorphic and yet grossly irregular in the RR interval, or polymorphic and yet regular in the RR interval (Table 4.2). The only exception to this rule is that a VT regular in the RR interval can have slight perturbations to the QRS morphology due to intermittent capture or fusion beats. As VT originates from within the ventricular

Monomorphic ventricular tachycardia

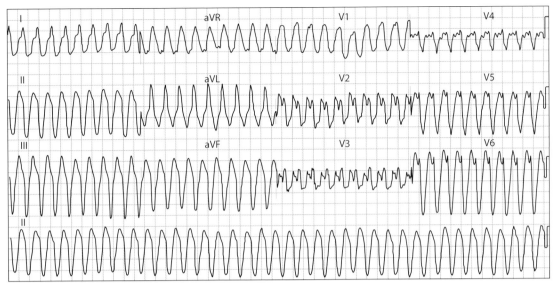

Fig. 4.16 Monomorphic ventricular tachycardia.

Polymorphic ventricular tachycardia

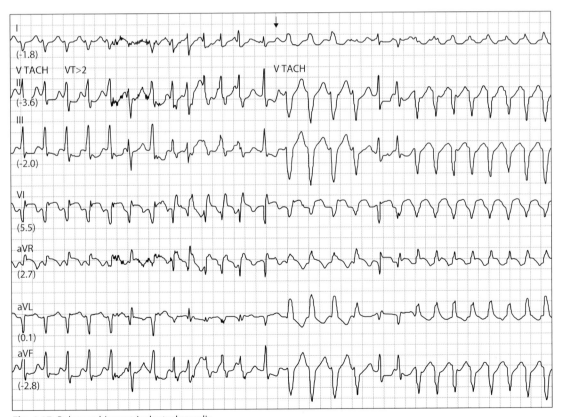

Fig. 4.17 Polymorphic ventricular tachycardia.

myocardium, unless the HPS is involved, propagation of excitation within the ventricles will be slow and the resulting QRS complex broad. Thus VT usually presents as a broad complex tachycardia on the ECG, but can also occasionally present as a narrow complex tachycardia.

Because of the prevalence of ischemic heart disease, the most common mechanism of VT is re-entry around the anatomical barrier to conduction created by the fibrous scar of a previous myocardial infarction. Thus VT most commonly presents as a regular broad complex tachycardia, of which the other two major differential diagnoses are SVT with aberrant conduction and pre-excited tachycardia. The distinction of the three conditions by the ECG is a diagnostic conundrum which perpetually confounds clinicians (Table 4.2).[129] Many different diagnostic algorithms have been proposed, but none works entirely satisfactorily.[70,130–137] The main reason for the difficulty is the myriad of manifestations possible for each of the three differential diagnoses. Of the three, SVT with aberrant conduction has the relatively more constant manifestation and can be separated from the other two on the basis of whether the QRS morphology

pattern of the tachycardia is typical of BBB,[70] but this is not absolute.[73] Features which are supposedly absolutely specific for VT such as dissociated P waves (Fig. 4.18), retrograde P waves (Fig. 4.19) or fusion/capture beats are rarely seen clinically, probably because they require a low QRS rate for them to be observed. Ultimately, the diagnosis of regular broad complex tachycardia can only be probabilistic rather than absolute.

The diagnosis of regular broad complex tachycardia of typical LBBB pattern (Fig. 4.20) deserves some special mention, as it can be due to specific forms of VT or pre-excited tachycardia with special properties and very different treatments (Table 4.3).

Polymorphic VT presents clinically as a broad complex tachycardia irregular in both QRS morphology/axis and RR interval. In fact, by definition, the QRS complex of polymorphic VT has to alter in morphology and axis once every 1–2 s.[138] Polymorphic VT is usually self-terminating, but can cause hemodynamic stability or degenerate into VF.

VT usually happens in patients with structural heart disease (e.g. previous myocardial infarction, dilated

Ventricular tachycardia with dissociated P waves

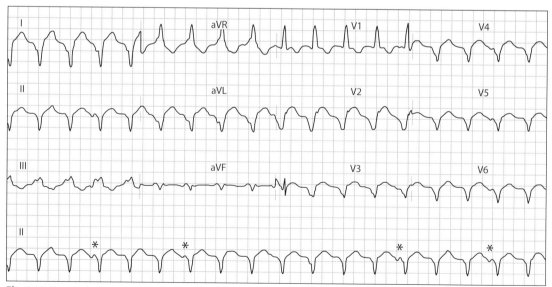

Fig. 4.18 Ventricular tachycardia with dissociated P waves. Note dissociated P waves marked by *.

Right ventricular outflow tract tachycardia with retrograde P wave

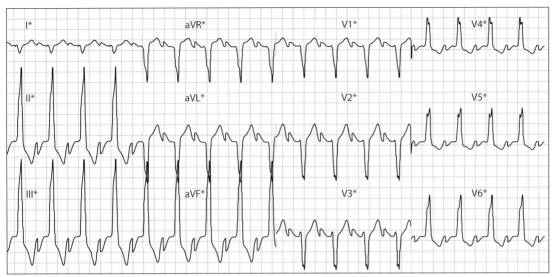

Fig. 4.19 Right ventricular outflow tract tachycardia with retrograde P wave.

Regular broad complex tachycardia of typical left bundle block pattern

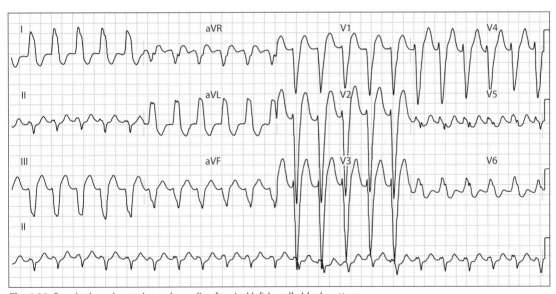

Fig. 4.20 Regular broad complex tachycardia of typical left bundle block pattern.

cardiomyopathy, hypertrophic cardiomyopathy),[135] even though a few cases happen in patients with apparently structurally normal hearts ('idiopathic' VT). VT can also be precipitated by metabolic disturbances and drug exposure.

Fascicular tachycardia

Fascicular tachycardia is a special form of VT which differs from most cases of VT in three crucial respects:

1. Fascicular tachycardia occurs in structurally normal hearts whereas most

Table 4.3 Differential diagnoses of left bundle branch block (LBBB) pattern regular broad complex tachycardia

Arrhythmia	Special properties
Ventricular tachycardia	
Right ventricular outflow tract tachycardia	In structurally normal heart
	Provoked by exertion and catecholamines
	Sensitive to adenosine and verapamil
	Amenable to radiofrequency ablation
Bundle branch re-entrant tachycardia	Associated with dilated cardiomyopathy
	Bundle branch block or intraventricular conduction defect in sinus rhythm
	Amenable to radiofrequency ablation
Pre-excited tachycardia	
Mahaim tachycardia	Typically no pre-excitation in sinus rhythm'
	Amenable to radiofrequency ablation
Supraventricular tachycardia	
Any form with LBBB	May have LBBB in sinus rhythm

cases of VT occur in structurally abnormal hearts.

2. Fascicular tachycardia has a relatively narrow QRS complex (0.11–0.14 s) and can easily be mistaken for SVT with aberrant conduction whereas most cases of VT have much broader QRS complexes (> 0.14 s);

3. Fascicular tachycardia is sensitive to verapamil whereas most cases of VT are not.[139–145]

Fascicular tachycardia originates from one of the fascicles of the left bundle (more commonly the left posterior fascicle than the left anterior fascicle) and has a relatively narrow QRS complex by virtue of utilizing the HPS, on which the tachycardia mechanism is situated, for rapid activation of the ventricular myocardium. As the left ventricle is activated before the right ventricle, the QRS complex is typically predominantly positive in lead V_1 (reminiscent of RBBB). When the source of the tachycardia is situated on the left posterior fascicle, left (superior) axis deviation is common, but when the source of the tachycardia is situated on the left anterior fascicle, right (inferior) axis deviation is common. The electrophysiological mechanism of fascicular tachycardia can be

either re-entry or triggered activity.[144,146–151] The long-term prognosis is good but if incessant, fascicular tachycardia can lead to tachycardiomyopathy reversible on treatment.[145,152] Fascicular tachycardia is amenable to RF ablation.[145,153–157]

Right ventricular outflow tract tachycardia: Right ventricular outflow tract (RVOT) tachycardia is another special form of VT which occurs in structurally normal hearts. RVOT tachycardia is caused by triggered activity (delayed afterdepolarization) emanating from an ectopic focus, most commonly within the RVOT, and hence typically has an LBBB pattern with right axis deviation on the ECG (Fig. 4.19).[158] RVOT tachycardia can be provoked by catecholamines and exertion and has an intrinsically good long-term prognosis,[159–162] but can cause tachycardiomyopathy reversible on treatment.[163–165] Unlike VT due to ischemic heart disease, for which verapamil is usually harmful,[166–168] RVOT tachycardia responds to verapamil and adenosine by either slowing or terminating.[150] RVOT tachycardia is amenable to RF ablation.[169–171]

Left ventricular outflow tract tachycardia: Left ventricular outflow tract (LVOT) tachycardia is a rare form of VT which originates from the LVOT, and appears to be driven by triggered activity.[172–177] Occasionally, LVOT tachycardia originates from the aortic root at the level of the sinuses of Valsalva and hence is not truly a 'LVOT' tachycardia.[177] LVOT tachycardia occurs in structurally normal hearts and usually presents as palpitations or presyncope.[178] LVOT tachycardia can have either an atypical LBBB or an atypical RBBB QRS morphology pattern but always an inferior axis. LVOT tachycardia can be mistaken RVOT tachycardia,[173; 179–181] but like RVOT tachycardia, is amenable to RF ablation.[172,173–175,178–180,182–184]

Bundle branch re-entrant tachycardia: Bundle branch re-entrant tachycardia (BBRT) is a specific form of macro re-entrant VT which uses the two bundle branches or the two fascicles of the left bundle branch to complete the re-entrant circuit.[185–188] The HPS has rapid conduction and short refractory periods and does not lend itself to re-entry. Even when bundle branch re-entry can be initiated, it often is not sustained.[189,190] Thus BBRT typically occurs in the presence of some form of HPS disease, be it outright BBB or intraventricular conduction defect (i.e. broadened QRS complex in sinus rhythm but not typical BBB).[191–194] BBRT most commonly occurs in patients with dilated cardiomyopathy (present in up to 95% of BBRT cases), be it caused by ischemic heart disease or not.[191,195,196] However, BBRT is much commoner among patients with non-ischemic dilated cardiomyopathy (accounting for 30–50% of VTs in such patients) than among patients with ischemic dilated cardiomyopathy (accounting for 5–6% of VTs in such patients).[197]

BBRT can present as syncope, sudden cardiac death or just palpitations.[192,195,196] The most common form of BBRT involves antegrade conduction down the right bundle branch and retrograde conduction up the left bundle branch to complete the circuit, and hence has a typical LBBB QRS morphology pattern (Table 4.3).[198] Occasionally, BBRT is due to interfascicular

macro re-entry, which involves antegrade conduction down one of the fascicles of the left bundle and retrograde conduction up the other, with the right bundle branch as a bystander. The QRS morphology pattern will be typically of RBBB in such a situation.[199,200] Interfascicular re-entry BBRT happens in structurally abnormal hearts and needs to be distinguished from fascicular tachycardia, which happens in structurally normal hearts and is sensitive to calcium antagonists. BBRT can be effectively treated by destroying one of the limbs of the re-entrant circuit, usually the right bundle branch but also occasionally the left bundle branch or one of its fascicles.[154,192,195,197,201,202]

Torsades de pointes: Torsades de pointes (TdP), or 'twisting around the point',[203] is a specific form of polymorphic VT which is initiated by triggered activity (early afterdepolarization) but perpetuated by random re-entry.[204,205] The ECG manifestation of TdP is distinct and easily recognized: the QRS complex changes in morphology and axis in a quasicyclical manner as if it is twisting around an imaginary baseline and is often preceded by a short-long-short sequence immediately prior to onset (Fig. 4.21).[206] TdP is associated with the long QT syndromes, which can be either congenital or acquired. For the congenital long QT syndromes, there might be a family history of sudden cardiac death and their molecular bases at the genetic and ion channel levels are being gradually unravelled.[207–215] The acquired long QT syndromes are associated with hypokalemia, hypomagnesemia, hypercalemia, bradycardia, nutritional deficiencies, nervous system injury and exposure to certain drugs (Table 4.4).[216] Acute treatment of TdP includes withdrawal of potentially offending medications, correction of electrolyte imbalance, intravenous magnesium infusion[217–219] or temporary overdrive pacing.[220] Long-term treatment of the long QT syndromes and TdP includes

Torsade de pointes initiated by a short-long-short sequence

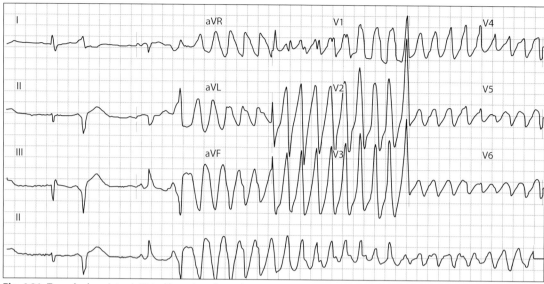

Fig. 4.21 Torsade de pointes initiated by a short-long-short sequence.

Table 4.4 Drugs causing QT prolongation

Categories	Examples
Antiarrhythmic class Ia class III	Disopyramide, procainamide, quinidine amiodarone, sotalol
Antimicrobial	Erythromycin, clarithromycin, trimethoprim-sulfamethoxazole
Antifungal	Fluclonazole, ketoconazole, itraconazole
Antimalarial or antiprotozoal	Chloroquine, halofantrine, mefloquine, pentamidine, quinine
Antihistamine	Astemizole, terfenadine, diphenydramine
Anticholinergic/gastrointestinal prokinetic	Cisapride
Psychoactive	Chloral hydrate, haloperidol, lithium, phenothiazines, pimozide, tricyclic antidepressants
Miscellaneous	Amantidine, indapamide, probucol, tacrolimus, vasopressin

beta-blockade,[221] permanent pacemaker implantation,[222–225] and the implantable cardioverter-defibrillator.[226,227]

Ventricular fibrillation

VF manifests as an irregular broad complex tachycardia on the ECG (Fig. 4.22). By definition, the electrical activity during VF has to be so disorganized that no individual QRS complexes could be recognized on the ECG, which sets VF apart from polymorphic VT (c.f. Figs 4.17 and 4.21 with Fig. 4.22).[138] VF often occur in the setting of acute myocardial infarction, cardiomyopathy (ischemic, dilated or

Ventricular fibrillation

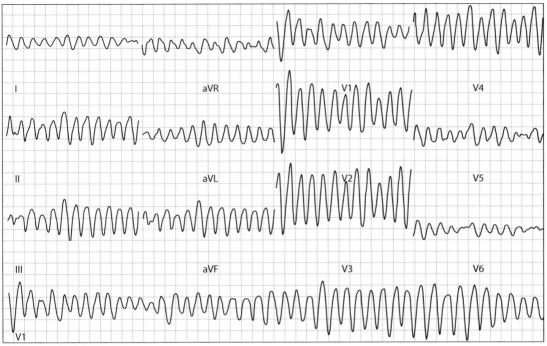

Fig. 4.22 Ventricular fibrillation.

Ventricular fibrillation which terminated spontaneously

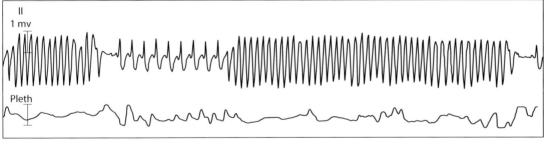

Fig. 4.23 Ventricular fibrillation which terminated spontaneously.

hypertrophic) but can also occur in apparently structurally normal hearts (the so-called 'idiopathic' VF).[228–230] VF is invariably haemodynamically unstable and the acute treatment is immediate defibrillation.[231] The long-term treatment of patients at risk of sudden cardiac death from VF rests at the moment with the implantable cardioverter-defibrillator.[27,232–235]

It is a commonly held belief that VF never self-terminates. This doctrine is not absolutely true, as demonstrated in Fig. 4.23.[236] Moreover, many sudden cardiac death survivors would have survived an episode of VF.

ACUTE TREATMENT OF TACHYCARDIAS

The treatment of a tachycardia very much depends on its diagnosis, and peculiar aspects of the treatment of specific arrhythmias have been mentioned in conjunction with their diagnoses in the section above. As mentioned at the beginning, this chapter will focus on the acute treatment of arrhythmias and a general schema for this purpose is

presented in Fig. 4.24.[142,153,217–221,237–245] This is intended only as a guideline and is by no means absolute.

The clinician must not feel compelled to act on an arrhythmia which presents acutely. Provided the arrhythmia is well

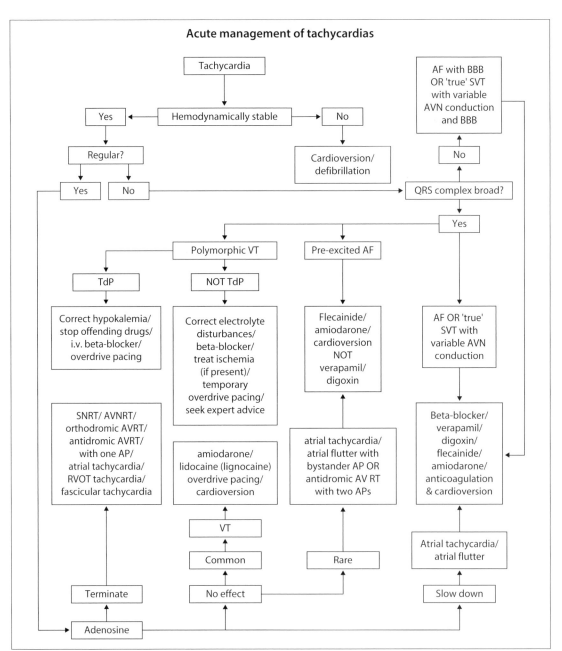

Fig. 4.24 Acute management of tachycardias. AF, atrial fibrillation; VT, ventricular tachycardia; TdP, torsade de pointes; SVT, supraventricular tachycardia; AVN, atrioventricular node; AP, accessory pathway; AVNRT, atrio-ventricular nodal re-entrant tachycardia; AVRT, atrio-ventricular re-entrant tachycardia; RVOT, right ventricular outflow tract; SNRT, sinus node re-entrant tachycardia.

tolerated, both in terms of symptoms and hemodynamic status, and has little chance of degenerating into a dangerous rhythm, then inactivity is acceptable and may be preferable. For example, most cases of paroxysmal AF which present acutely will spontaneously terminate and it is reasonable to wait for 24 h after onset of the arrhythmia before proceeding with cardioversion, provided the arrhythmia is well tolerated. On the other hand, frequent ventricular premature beats or non-sustained VT might be harbingers of more sinister arrhythmias and require immediate treatment (e.g. intravenous amiodarone, overdrive pacing).

CONCLUSIONS

Arrhythmia is a vast and rapidly evolving subject, and it is impossible to give an all encompassing review on all topics. The above account aims at providing the clinician with just enough details to make sense of the arrhythmic phenomena encountered clinically and handle their acute management confidently. Once the patient has been stabilized or the arrhythmia terminated, the patient's interest may be best served by referral to a specialist electrophysiologist.

References

1. Feld GK. Evolution of diagnostic and interventional cardiac electrophysiology: a brief historical review. Am J Cardiol 1999; 84:115R–124R.
2. Jackman WM, Friday KJ, Fitzgerald DM, et al. Localization of left free-wall and posteroseptal accessory atrioventricular pathways by direct recording of accessory pathway activation. Pacing Clin Electrophysiol 1989; 12:204–214.
3. Jackman WM, Wang XZ, Friday KJ, et al. Catheter ablation of atrioventricular junction using radiofrequency current in 17 patients. Comparison of standard and large-tip catheter electrodes. Circulation 1991; 83:1562–1576.
4. Jackman WM, Wang XZ, Friday KJ, et al. Catheter ablation of accessory atrioventricular pathways (Wolff-Parkinson-White syndrome) by radiofrequency current. N Engl J Med 1991; 324:1605–1611.
5. Jackman WM, Beckman KJ, McClelland JH, et al. Treatment of supraventricular tachycardia due to atrioventricular nodal reentry, by radiofrequency catheter ablation of slow-pathway conduction. N Engl J Med 1992; 327:313–318.
6. Feld GK, Fleck RP, Chen PS, et al. Radiofrequency catheter ablation for the treatment of human type 1 atrial flutter. Identification of a critical zone in the reentrant circuit by endocardial mapping techniques. Circulation 1992; 86:1233–1240.
7. Kay GN, Chong F, Epstein AE, et al. Radiofrequency ablation for treatment of primary atrial tachycardias. J Am Coll Cardiol 1993; 21:901–909.
8. Gaita F, Haissaguerre M, Giustetto C, et al. Catheter ablation of permanent junctional reciprocating tachycardia with radiofrequency current. J Am Coll Cardiol 1995; 25:648–654.
9. Heald SC, Davies DW, Ward DE, et al. Radiofrequency catheter ablation of Mahaim tachycardia by targeting Mahaim potentials at the tricuspid annulus. Br Heart J 1995; 73:250–257.
10. Lee RJ, Kalman JM, Fitzpatrick AP, et al. Radiofrequency catheter modification of the sinus node for 'inappropriate' sinus tachycardia. Circulation 1995; 92:2919–2928.
11. Scheinman MM, Gonzalez RP, Cooper MW, et al. Clinical and electrophysiologic features and role of catheter ablation techniques in adult patients with automatic atrioventricular junctional tachycardia. Am J Cardiol 1994; 74:565–572.
12. Grogin HR, Lee RJ, Kwasman M, et al. Radiofrequency catheter ablation of atriofascicular and nodoventricular Mahaim tracts. Circulation 1994; 90:272–281.
13. Lesh MD, Van HG, Epstein LM, et al. Radiofrequency catheter ablation of atrial arrhythmias. Results and mechanisms. Circulation 1994; 89:1074–1089.
14. Guidelines for Clinical Intracardiac Electrophysiological and Catheter Ablation Procedures. A report of the American College of Cardiology/American Heart Association Task Force on practice guidelines. (Committee on Clinical Intracardiac Electrophysiologic and Catheter Ablation Procedures). Developed in collaboration with the North American Society of Pacing and Electrophysiology. Circulation 1995; 92:673–691.
15. Fischer B, Jais P, Shah D, et al. Radiofrequency catheter ablation of common atrial flutter in 200 patients. J Cardiovasc Electrophysiol 1996; 7:1225–1233.
16. Griffith MJ, Gammage MD. Radiofrequency ablation of macro re-entrant arrhythmias: cure or adjunctive therapy? Lancet 1998; 352:1404–1405.
17. Schilling RJ. Which patient should be referred to an electrophysiologist: supraventricular tachycardia. Heart 2002; 87:299–304.
18. Peters NS, Jackman WM, Schilling RJ, et al. Images in cardiovascular medicine. Human left

ventricular endocardial activation mapping using a novel noncontact catheter. Circulation 1997; 95:1658–1660.

19. Krahn AD, Klein GJ, Yee R, et al. Randomized assessment of syncope trial: conventional diagnostic testing versus a prolonged monitoring strategy. Circulation 2001; 104:46–51.

20. Brignole M, Menozzi C, Moya A, et al. Implantable loop recorder: towards a gold standard for the diagnosis of syncope? Heart 2001; 85:610–612.

21. Krahn AD, Klein GJ, Yee R, et al. Predictive value of presyncope in patients monitored for assessment of syncope. Am Heart J 2001; 141:817–821.

22. Seidl K, Rameken M, Breunung S, Senges J, et al. Diagnostic assessment of recurrent unexplained syncope with a new subcutaneously implantable loop recorder. Reveal-Investigators. Europace 2000; 2:256–262.

23. Mirowski M, Mower MM, Staewen WS, et al. The development of the transvenous automatic defibrillator. Arch Intern Med 1972; 129:773–779.

24. Mirowski M, Mower MM, Gott VL, et al. Feasibility and effectiveness of low-energy catheter defibrillation in man. Circulation 1973; 47:79–85.

25. Mirowski M, Reid PR, Mower MM, et al. Termination of malignant ventricular arrhythmias with an implanted automatic defibrillator in human beings. N Engl J Med 1980; 303:322–324.

26. Mirowski M. Prevention of sudden arrhythmic death with implanted automatic defibrillators. Ann Intern Med 1982; 97:606–608.

27. The Antiarrhythmics versus Implantable Defibrillators (AVID) Investigators. A comparison of antiarrhythmic-drug therapy with implantable defibrillators in patients resuscitated from near-fatal ventricular arrhythmias. N Engl J Med 1997; 337:1576–1583.

28. Saksena S, Epstein AE, Lazzara R, et al. NASPE/ACC/AHA/ESC medical/scientific statement special report—clinical investigation of antiarrhythmic devices: a statement for healthcare professionals from a Joint Task Force of the North American Society of Pacing and Electrophysiology, the American College of Cardiology, the American Heart Association, and the Working Groups on Arrhythmias and Cardiac Pacing of the European Society of Cardiology. Pacing Clin Electrophysiol 1995; 18:637–654.

29. Singh S, Zoble RG, Yellen L, et al. Efficacy and safety of oral dofetilide in converting to and maintaining sinus rhythm in patients with chronic atrial fibrillation or atrial flutter: the symptomatic atrial fibrillation investigative research on dofetilide (SAFIRE-D) study. Circulation 2000; 102:2385–2390.

30. Gepstein L, Evans SJ. Electroanatomical mapping of the heart: basic concepts and implications for the treatment of cardiac arrhythmias. Pacing Clin Electrophysiol 1998; 21:1268–1278.

31. Gepstein L, Hayam G, Ben-Haim SA. A novel method for nonfluoroscopic catheter-based electroanatomical mapping of the heart. In vitro and in vivo accuracy results. Circulation 1997; 95:1611–1622.

32. Willems S, Weiss C, Ventura R, et al. Catheter ablation of atrial flutter guided by electroanatomic mapping (CARTO): a randomized comparison to the conventional approach. J Cardiovasc Electrophysiol 2000; 11:1223–1230.

33. Schilling RJ, Kadish AH, Peters NS, et al. Endocardial mapping of atrial fibrillation in the human right atrium using a non-contact catheter. Eur Heart J 2000; 21:550–564.

34. Schilling RJ, Peters NS, Davies DW. Mapping and ablation of ventricular tachycardia with the aid of a non-contact mapping system. Heart 1999; 81:570–575.

35. Schmitt C, Ndrepepa G, Weber S, et al. Biatrial multisite mapping of atrial premature complexes triggering onset of atrial fibrillation. Am J Cardiol 2002; 89:1381–1387.

36. Schmitt C, Zrenner B, Schneider M, et al. Clinical experience with a novel multielectrode basket catheter in right atrial tachycardias. Circulation 1999; 99:2414–2422.

37. Jais P, Haissaguerre M, Shah DC, et al. Successful irrigated-tip catheter ablation of atrial flutter resistant to conventional radiofrequency ablation. Circulation 1998; 98:835–838.

38. Lustgarten DL, Keane D, Ruskin J. Cryothermal ablation: mechanism of tissue injury and current experience in the treatment of tachyarrhythmias. Prog Cardiovasc Dis 1999; 41:481–498.

39. Lee LA, Simon C, Bove EL, et al. High intensity focused ultrasound effect on cardiac tissues: potential for clinical application. Echocardiography 2000; 17:563–566.

40. He DS, Zimmer JE, Hynynen K, et al. Application of ultrasound energy for intracardiac ablation of arrhythmias. Eur Heart J 1995; 16:961–966.

41. Wadhwa MK, Rahme MM, Dobak J, Li H, et al. Transcatheter cryoablation of ventricular myocardium in dogs. J Interv Card Electrophysiol 2000; 4:537–545.

42. Feld GK. Radiofrequency catheter ablation versus modification of the AV node for control of rapid ventricular response in atrial fibrillation. J Cardiovasc Electrophysiol 1995; 6:217–228.

43. Stevenson WG, Delacretaz E, Friedman PL, et al. Identification and ablation of macroreentrant ventricular tachycardia with the CARTO electroanatomical mapping system. Pacing Clin Electrophysiol 1998; 21:1448–1456.

44. Haissaguerre M, Jais P, Shah DC, et al. Spontaneous initiation of atrial fibrillation by ectopic beats originating in the pulmonary veins. N Engl J Med 1998; 339:659–666.

45. Garg A, Finneran W, Mollerus M, et al. Right atrial compartmentalization using radiofrequency

catheter ablation for management of patients with refractory atrial fibrillation. J Cardiovasc Electrophysiol 1999; 10:763–771.

46. Haissaguerre M, Shah DC, Jais P, et al. Mapping-guided ablation of pulmonary veins to cure atrial fibrillation. Am J Cardiol 2000; 86:K9–K19.

47. Della BP, Pappalardo A, Riva S, et al. Non-contact mapping to guide catheter ablation of untolerated ventricular tachycardia. Eur Heart J 2002; 23:742–752.

48. Eckardt L, Breithardt G, Haverkamp W. Idiopathic left ventricular tachycardia localised at the distal end of the posterior fascicle by non-contact activation mapping. Heart 2002; 87:374.

49. Schmitt H, Weber S, Schwab JO, et al. Diagnosis and ablation of focal right atrial tachycardia using a new high-resolution, non-contact mapping system. Am J Cardiol 2001; 87:1017–1021.

50. Haissaguerre M, Shoda M, Jais P, et al. Mapping and ablation of idiopathic ventricular fibrillation. Circulation 2002; 106:962–967.

51. Haissaguerre M, Shah DC, Jais P, et al. Role of Purkinje conducting system in triggering of idiopathic ventricular fibrillation. Lancet 2002; 359:677–678.

52. Pordon CM, Moodie DS. Adults with congenital complete heart block: 25-year follow-up. Cleve Clin J Med 1992; 59:587–590.

53. Reid JM, Coleman EN, Doig W. Complete congenital heart block. Report of 35 cases. Br Heart J 1982; 48:236–239.

54. Eronen M, Heikkila P, Teramo K. Congenital complete heart block in the fetus: hemodynamic features, antenatal treatment, and outcome in six cases. Pediatr Cardiol 2001; 22:385–392.

55. Bruckheimer E, Berul CI, Kopf GS, et al. Late recovery of surgically-induced atrioventricular block in patients with congenital heart disease. J Interv Card Electrophysiol 2002; 6:191–195.

56. Gregoratos G, Cheitlin MD, Conill A, et al. ACC/AHA Guidelines for Implantation of Cardiac Pacemakers and Antiarrhythmia Devices: Executive Summary – a report of the American College of Cardiology/American Heart Association Task Force on Practice Guidelines (Committee on Pacemaker Implantation). Circulation 1998; 97:1325–1335.

57. Wellens HJ, Durrer D. Supraventricular tachycardia with left aberrant conduction due to retrograde invasion into the left bundle branch. Circulation 1968; 38:474–479.

58. Gallagher JJ, Pritchett EL, Sealy WC, et al. The pre-excitation syndromes. Prog Cardiovasc Dis 1978; 20:285–327.

59. Becker AE, Anderson RH, Durrer D, et al. The anatomical substrates of Wolff-Parkinson-White syndrome, a clinicopathologic correlation in seven patients. Circulation 1978; 57:870–879.

60. Becker AE, Anderson RH. The Wolff-Parkinson-White syndrome and its anatomical substrates. Anat Rec 1981; 201:169–177.

61. Haissaguerre M, Cauchemez B, Marcus F, et al. Characteristics of the ventricular insertion sites of accessory pathways with anterograde decremental conduction properties. Circulation 1995; 91:1077–1085.

62. Aliot E, de Chillous C, Mabo P, et al. Mahaim tachycardias. Eur Heart J 1998; 19:E25–E31.

63. Wolff L, Parkinson J, White PD. Bundle branch block with short PR interval in healthy young people prone to paroxysmal tachycardia. Am Heart J 1930; 5:685–704.

64. Tonkin AM, Wagner GS, Gallagher JJ, et al. Initial forces of ventricular depolarization in the Wolff-Parkinson-White syndrome. Analysis based upon localization of the accessory pathway by epicardial mapping. Circulation 1975; 52:1030–1036.

65. Milstein S, Sharma AD, Guiraudon GM, et al. An algorithm for the electrocardiographic localization of accessory pathways in the Wolff-Parkinson-White syndrome. Pacing Clin Electrophysiol 1987; 10:555–563.

66. Fitzpatrick AP, Gonzales RP, Lesh MD, et al. New algorithm for the localization of accessory atrioventricular connections using a baseline electrocardiogram [published erratum appears in J Am Coll Cardiol 1994 Apr; 23(5):1272]. J Am Coll Cardiol 1994; 23:107–116.

67. Lesh MD, van Hare GF, Schamp DJ, et al. Curative percutaneous catheter ablation using radiofrequency energy for accessory pathways in all locations: results in 100 consecutive patients. J Am Coll Cardiol 1992; 19:1303–1309.

68. Garratt CJ, Antoniou A, Griffith MJ, et al. Use of intravenous adenosine in sinus rhythm as a diagnostic test for latent preexcitation. Am J Cardiol 1990; 65:868–873.

69. Tai Y-T, Campbell RWF, McComb JM. Latent functional duality in an accessory pathway. Eur Heart J 1989; 10:380–384.

70. Griffith MJ, Garratt CJ, Mounsey P, Camm AJ. Ventricular tachycardia as default diagnosis in broad complex tachycardia. Lancet 1994; 343:386–388.

71. Lau EW, Pathmanathan RK, Ng GA, Griffith MJ. Electrocardiographic criteria for diagnosis of irregular broad complex tachycardia with a high sensitivity for pre-excited atrial fibrillation. Pacing Clin Electrophysiol 2000; 23:2040–2045.

72. Littmann L, McCall MM. Ventricular tachycardia may masquerade as supraventricular tachycardia in patients with preexisting bundle-branch block. Ann Emerg Med 1995; 26:98–101.

73. Alberca T, Almendral J, Sanz P, et al. Evaluation of the specificity of morphological electrocardiographic criteria for the differential diagnosis of wide complex tachycardia in patients with intraventricular conduction defects. Circulation 1997; 96:3527–3533.

74. Morgan-Hughes NJ, Griffith MJ, McComb JM. Intravenous adenosine reveals intermittent preexcitation by direct and indirect effects on

accessory pathway conduction. Pacing Clin Electrophysiol 1993; 16:2098–2103.

75. Olshansky B. Ventricular tachyacrdia masquerading as supraventricular tachycardia: a wolf in sheep's clothing. J Electrocardiol 1986; 21:377–384.

76. Ross DL, Vohra JK, Sloman G. Similar QRS morphology in sinus rhythm and ventricular tachycardia. Pacing Clin Electrophysiol 1989; 2:486–489.

77. Lau EW, Ng GA, Griffith MJ. Variability in the manifestation of pre-excited atrial fibrillation: its quantification, theoretical origin and diagnostic potential. Ann Noninvasive Electrocardiol 2001; 6:117–122.

78. Krahn AD, Yee R, Klein GJ, et al. Inappropriate sinus tachycardia: evaluation and therapy. J Cardiovasc Electrophysiol 1995; 6:1124–1128.

79. Weisfogel GM, Batsford WP, Paulay KL, et al. Sinus node re-entrant tachycardia in man. Am Heart J 1975; 90:295–304.

80. Sanders WEJ, Sorrentino RA, Greenfield RA, et al. Catheter ablation of sinoatrial node reentrant tachycardia. J Am Coll Cardiol 1994; 23:926–934.

81. Kavthale SS, Vajifdar BU, Vora AM, et al. Reversal of tachycardia-induced cardiomyopathy following successful radiofrequency ablation of ectopic atrial tachycardia. Indian Heart J 1998; 50:548–550.

82. Lashus AG, Case CL, Gillette PC. Catheter ablation treatment of supraventricular tachycardia-induced cardiomyopathy. Arch Pediatr Adolesc Med 1997; 151:264–266.

83. Tavernier R, De PM, Trouerbach J. Incessant automatic atrial tachycardia: a reversible cause of tachycardiomyopathy. Acta Cardiologica 1999; 54:227–229.

84. Tang CW, Scheinman MM, Van HG, et al. Use of P wave configuration during atrial tachycardia to predict site of origin. J Am Coll Cardiol 1995; 26:1315–1324.

85. Moe GK. On the multiple wavelet hypothesis of atrial fibrillation. Arch Int Pharmacodyn Ther 1962; 140:183–188.

86. Konings KT, Kirchhof CJ, Smeets JR, et al. High-density mapping of electrically induced atrial fibrillation in humans. Circulation 1994; 89:1665–1680.

87. Kaplan MA, Cohen KL. Ventricular fibrillation in the Wolff-Parkinson-White syndrome. Am J Cardiol 1969; 24:259–264.

88. Dreifus LS, Haiat R, Watanabe Y. Ventricular fibrillation: a possible mechanism of sudden death in patients with Wolff-Parkinson-White syndrome. Circulation 1971; 43:520–527.

89. Jacob AS, Nielsen DH, Gianelly RE. Fatal ventricular fibrillation following verapamil in Wolff-Parkinson-White syndrome with atrial fibrillation. Ann Emerg Med 1985; 14:159–160.

90. McGovern B, Garan H, Ruskin JN. Precipitation of cardiac arrest by verapamil in patients with Wolff-Parkinson-White syndrome. Ann Intern Med 1986; 104:791–794.

91. Strasberg B, Sagie A, Rechavia E, et al. Deleterious effects of intravenous verapamil in Wolff-Parkinson-White patients and atrial fibrillation. Cardiovasc Drugs Ther 1989; 2:801–806.

92. Klein GJ, Bashore TM, Sellers TD, et al. Ventricular fibrillation in the Wolff-Parkinson-White syndrome. N Engl J Med 1979; 301:1080–1085.

93. Feld GK, Mollerus M, Birgersdotter-Green U, et al. Conduction velocity in the tricuspid valve-inferior vena cava isthmus is slower in patients with type I atrial flutter compared to those without a history of atrial flutter. J Cardiovasc Electrophysiol 1997; 8:1338–1348.

94. Nakagawa H, Jackman WM. Use of a three-dimensional, nonfluoroscopic mapping system for catheter ablation of typical atrial flutter. Pacing Clin Electrophysiol 1998; 21:1279–1286.

95. Schilling RJ, Peters NS, Goldberger J, et al. Characterization of the anatomy and conduction velocities of the human right atrial flutter circuit determined by noncontact mapping. J Am Coll Cardiol 2001; 38:385–393.

96. Schoels W, Kuebler W, Yang H, et al. A unified functional/anatomic substrate for circus movement atrial flutter: activation and refractory patterns in the canine right atrial enlargement model. J Am Coll Cardiol 1993; 21:73–84.

97. Waldo AL. Atrial flutter: entrainment characteristics. J Cardiovasc Electrophysiol 1997; 8:337–352.

98. Malcolm AD, Garratt CJ, Camm AJ. The therapeutic and diagnostic cardiac electrophysiological uses of adenosine. Cardiovasc Drugs Ther 1993; 7:139–147.

99. Rankin AC, Rae AP, Houston A. Acceleration of ventricular response to atrial flutter after intravenous adenosine. Br Heart J 1993; 69:263–265.

100. Slade AK, Garratt CJ. Proarrhythmic effect of adenosine in a patient with atrial flutter. Br Heart J 1993; 70:91–92.

101. Brodsky MA, Hwang C, Hunter D, et al. Life-threatening alterations in heart rate after the use of adenosine in atrial flutter. Am Heart J 1995; 130:564–571.

102. Bardy GH, Packer DL, German LD, et al. Preexcited reciprocating tachycardia in patients with Wolff-Parkinson-White syndrome: incidence and mechanisms. Circulation 1984; 70:377–391.

103. Green M, Heddle B, Dassen W, et al. Value of QRS alteration in determining the site of origin of narrow QRS supraventricular tachycardia. Circulation 1983; 68:368–373.

104. Kalbfleisch SJ, el-Atassi R, Calkins H, et al. Differentiation of paroxysmal narrow QRS complex tachycardias using the 12-lead electrocardiogram. J Am Coll Cardiol 1993; 21:85–89.

105. McClelland JH, Wang X, Beckman KJ, et al. Radiofrequency catheter ablation of right atriofascicular (Mahaim) accessory pathways

guided by accessory pathway activation potentials. Circulation 1994; 89:2655–2666.

106. Gallagher JJ, Smith WM, Kasell JH, et al. Role of Mahaim fibers in cardiac arrhythmias in man. Circulation 1981; 64:176–189.

107. Gillette PC, Garson A, Jr, Cooley DA, et al. Prolonged and decremental antegrade conduction properties in right anterior accessory connections: Wide QRS antidromic tachycardia of left bundle branch block pattern without Wolff-Parkinson-White configuration in sinus rhythm. Am Heart J 1982; 103:66–74.

108. Ellenbogen KA, Ramirez NM, Packer DL, et al. Accessory nodoventricular (Mahaim) fibers: a clinical review. Pacing Clin Electrophysiol 1986; 9:868–884.

109. Bardy GH, Fedor JM, German LD, et al. Surface electrocardiographic clues suggesting presence of a nodofascicular Mahaim fiber. J Am Coll Cardiol 1984; 3:1161–1168.

110. Klein GJ, Guiraudon GM, Kerr CR, et al. 'Nodoventricular' accessory pathway: evidence for a distinct accessory atrioventricular pathway with atrioventricular node-like properties. J Am Coll Cardiol 1988; 11:1035–1040.

111. Tonkin AM, Dugan FA, Svenson RH, et al. Coexistence of functional Kent and Mahaim-type tracts in the pre-excitation syndrome. Demonstration by catheter techniques and epicardial mapping. Circulation 1975; 52:193–200.

112. Klein LS, Hackett FK, Zipes DP, et al. Radiofrequency catheter ablation of Mahaim fibers at the tricuspid annulus. Circulation 1993; 87:738–747.

113. Critelli G, Gallagher JJ, Monda V, et al. Anatomic and electrophysiologic substrate of the permanent form of junctional reciprocating tachycardia. J Am Coll Cardiol 1984; 4:601–610.

114. Shih HT, Miles WM, Klein LS, et al. Multiple accessory pathways in the permanent form of junctional reciprocating tachycardia. Am J Cardiol 1994; 73:361–367.

115. Critelli G, Gallagher JJ, Monda V, et al. Catheter ablation of accessory pathway in the permanent form of junctional reciprocating tachycardia. Arch Mal.Coeur Vaiss. 1985; 78 Spec No:49-55:49–55.

116. Critelli G, Gallagher JJ, Perticone F, et al. Transvenous catheter ablation of the accessory atrioventricular pathway in the permanent form of junctional reciprocating tachycardia. Am J Cardiol 1985; 55:1639–1641.

117. Chien WW, Cohen TJ, Lee MA, et al. Electrophysiological findings and long-term follow-up of patients with the permanent form of junctional reciprocating tachycardia treated by catheter ablation. Circulation 1992; 85:1329–1336.

118. Hauer RN, Loh P. 'Para' AV nodal re-entry tachycardias. Eur Heart J 1998; 1(suppl E):E2–E9.

119. Obel OA, Camm AJ. Supraventricular tachycardia. ECG diagnosis and anatomy. Eur Heart J 1997; 18(suppl C):C2–C11.

120. Lin FC, Yeh SJ, Wu D. Determinants of simultaneous fast and slow pathway conduction in patients with dual atrioventricular nodal pathways. Am Heart J 1985; 109:963–970.

121. Lin FC, Yeh SJ, Wu D. Double atrial responses to a single ventricular impulse due to simultaneous conduction via two retrograde pathways. J Am Coll Cardiol 1985; 5:168–175.

122. Wu D, Denes P, Wyndham C, et al. Demonstration of dual atrioventricular nodal pathways utilizing a ventricular extrastimulus in patients with atrioventricular nodal re-entrant paroxysmal supraventricular tachycardia. Circulation 1975; 52:789–798.

123. McGuire MA, Janse MJ, Ross DL. 'AV nodal' reentry: Part II: AV nodal, AV junctional, or atrionodal reentry? J Cardiovasc Electrophysiol 1993; 4:573–586.

124. Olgin JE, Ursell P, Kao AK, et al. Pathological findings following slow pathway ablation for AV nodal reentrant tachycardia. J Cardiovasc Electrophysiol 1996; 7:625–631.

125. Jazayeri MR, Hempe SL, Sra JS, et al. Selective transcatheter ablation of the fast and slow pathways using radiofrequency energy in patients with atrioventricular nodal reentrant tachycardia. Circulation 1992; 85:1318–1328.

126. Haissaguerre M, Gaita F, Fischer B, et al. Elimination of atrioventricular nodal reentrant tachycardia using discrete slow potentials to guide application of radiofrequency energy. Circulation 1992; 85:2162–2175.

127. Langberg JJ, Leon A, Borganelli M, et al. A randomized, prospective comparison of anterior and posterior approaches to radiofrequency catheter ablation of atrioventricular nodal reentry tachycardia. Circulation 1993; 87:1551–1556.

128. Wang CC, Yeh SJ, Wen MS, et al. Late clinical and electrophysiologic outcome of radiofrequency ablation therapy by the inferior approach in atrioventricular node reentry tachycardia. Am Heart J 1994; 128: 219–226.

129. Lau EW, Ng GA. The reliable electrocardiographic diagnosis of regular broad complex tachycardia – a holy grail which will forever elude the clinician's grasp? Pacing Clin Electrophysiol 2002; 25(12):1756–1761.

130. Sandler A, Marriott HJL. The differential morphology of anomalous ventricular complexes of RBBB-type in lead V_1. Circulation 1965; 31:551–556.

131. Wellens HJJ. The wide QRS tachycardia. Ann Intern Med 1986; 104:879–879.

132. Dongas J, Lehmann MH, Mahmud R, et al. Value of preexisting bundle branch block in the electrocardiographic differentiation of supraventricular from ventricular origin of wide QRS tachycardia. Am J Cardiol 1985; 55:717–721.

133. Kindwall KE, Brown J, Josephson ME. Electrocardiographic criteria for ventricular tachycardia in wide complex left bundle branch

block morphology tachycardias. Am J Cardiol 1988; 61:1279–1283.

134. Brugada P, Brugada J, Mont L, et al. A new approach to the differential diagnosis of a regular tachycardia with a wide QRS complex. Circulation 1991; 83:1649–1659.

135. Griffith MJ, de Belder MA, Linker NJ, et al. Multivariate analysis to simplify the differential diagnosis of broad complex tachycardia. Br Heart J 1991; 66:166–174.

136. Drew BJ, Scheinman MM. ECG criteria to distinguish between aberrantly conducted supraventricular tachycardia and ventricular tachycardia: practical aspects for the immediate care setting. Pacing Clin Electrophysiol 1995; 18: 2194–2208.

137. Lau EW, Pathmanathan RK, Ng GA, et al. The Bayesian approach improves the electrocardiographic diagnosis of broad complex tachycardia. Pacing Clin Electrophysiol 2000; 23 [Pt I]:1519–1526.

138. Shenasa M, Borggrefe M, Haverkamp W, et al. Ventricular tachycardia. Lancet 1993; 341:1512–1519.

139. Ward DE, Nathan AW, Camm AJ. Fascicular tachycardia sensitive to calcium antagonists. Eur Heart J 1984; 5:896–905.

140. Weiss J, Stevenson WG. Narrow QRS ventricular tachycardia. Am Heart J 1986; 112:843–847.

141. Cohen HC, Gozo EGJ, Pick A. Ventricular tachycardia with narrow QRS complexes (left posterior fascicular tachycardia). Circulation 1972; 45:1035–1043.

142. Griffith MJ, Garratt CJ, Rowland E, et al. Effects of intravenous adenosine on verapamil-sensitive 'idiopathic' ventricular tachycardia. Am J Cardiol 1994; 73:759–764.

143. Andrade FR, Eslami M, Elias J, et al. Diagnostic clues from the surface ECG to identify idiopathic (fascicular) ventricular tachycardia: correlation with electrophysiologic findings. J Cardiovasc Electrophysiol 1996; 7:2–8.

144. Gonzalez RP, Scheinman MM, Lesh MD, et al. Clinical and electrophysiologic spectrum of fascicular tachycardias. Am Heart J 1994; 128:147–156.

145. Bennett DH. Experience with radiofrequency catheter ablation of fascicular tachycardia. Heart 1997; 77:104–107.

146. Tai YT, Fong PC, Lau CP, et al. Reentrant fascicular tachycardia with cycle length alternans: insights into the tachycardia mechanism and origin. Pacing Clin Electrophysiol 1990; 13:900–907.

147. Tai YT, D'Onofrio A, Bourke JP, et al. Left posterior fascicular tachycardia due to localized microreentry. Eur Heart J 1990; 11:949–953.

148. Wieland JM, Marchlinski FE. Electrocardiographic response of digoxin-toxic fascicular tachycardia to Fab fragments: implications for tachycardia mechanism. Pacing Clin Electrophysiol 1986; 9:727–738.

149. Ward DE, Nathan AW, Camm AJ. Fascicular tachycardia sensitive to calcium antagonists. Eur Heart J 1984; 5:896–905.

150. Griffith MJ, Garratt CJ, Rowland E, et al. Effects of intravenous adenosine on verapamil-sensitive 'idiopathic' ventricular tachycardia. Am J Cardiol 1994; 73:759–764.

151. Maruyama M, Tadera T, Miyamoto S, et al. Demonstration of the reentrant circuit of verapamil-sensitive idiopathic left ventricular tachycardia: direct evidence for macroreentry as the underlying mechanism. J Cardiovasc Electrophysiol 2001; 12:968–972.

152. Anselme F, Boyle N, Josephson M. Incessant fascicular tachycardia: a cause of arrhythmia induced cardiomyopathy. Pacing Clin Electrophysiol 1998; 21:760–763.

153. DeLacey WA, Nath S, Haines DE, et al. Adenosine and verapamil-sensitive ventricular tachycardia originating from the left ventricle: radiofrequency catheter ablation. Pacing Clin Electrophysiol 1992; 15:2240–2244.

154. Crijns HJ, Smeets JL, Rodriguez LM, et al. Cure of interfascicular reentrant ventricular tachycardia by ablation of the anterior fascicle of the left bundle branch. J Cardiovasc Electrophysiol 1995; 6:486–492.

155. Bogun F, el-Atassi R, Daoud E, et al. Radiofrequency ablation of idiopathic left anterior fascicular tachycardia. J Cardiovasc Electrophysiol 1995; 6:1113–1116.

156. Katritsis D, Heald S, Ahsan A, et al. Catheter ablation for successful management of left posterior fascicular tachycardia: an approach guided by recording of fascicular potentials. Heart 1996; 75:384–388.

157. Nogami A, Naito S, Tada H, et al. Verapamil-sensitive left anterior fascicular ventricular tachycardia: results of radiofrequency ablation in six patients. J Cardiovasc Electrophysiol 1998; 9:1269–1278.

158. Buxton AE, Waxman HL, Marchlinski FE, et al. Right ventricular tachycardia: clinical and electrophysiologic characteristics. Circulation 1983; 68:917–927.

159. Palileo EV, Ashley WW, Swiryn S, et al. Exercise provocable right ventricular outflow tract tachycardia. Am Heart J 1982; 104:185–193.

160. Buxton AE, Marchlinski FE, Doherty JU, et al. Repetitive, monomorphic ventricular tachycardia: clinical and electrophysiologic characteristics in patients with and patients without organic heart disease. Am J Cardiol 1984; 54:997–1002.

161. Ritchie AH, Kerr CR, Qi A, et al. Nonsustained ventricular tachycardia arising from the right ventricular outflow tract. Am J Cardiol 1989; 64:594–598.

162. Lemery R, Brugada P, Bella PD, et al. Nonischemic ventricular tachycardia. Clinical course and long-term follow-up in patients without clinically overt heart disease. Circulation 1989; 79:990–999.

163. Jaggarao NS, Nanda AS, Daubert JP. Ventricular tachycardia induced cardiomyopathy: improvement with radiofrequency ablation. Pacing Clin Electrophysiol 1996; 19:505–508.

164. Vijgen J, Hill P, Biblo LA, et al. Tachycardia-induced cardiomyopathy secondary to right ventricular outflow tract ventricular tachycardia: improvement of left ventricular systolic function after radiofrequency catheter ablation of the arrhythmia. J Cardiovasc Electrophysiol 1997; 8:445–450.

165. Grimm W, Menz V, Hoffmann J, et al. Reversal of tachycardia induced cardiomyopathy following ablation of repetitive monomorphic right ventricular outflow tract tachycardia. Pacing Clin Electrophysiol 2001; 24:166–171.

166. Dancy M, Camm AJ, Ward D. Misdiagnosis of chronic recurrent ventricular tachycardia. Lancet 1985; II:320–323.

167. Stewart RB, Bardy GH, Greene HL. Wide complex tachycardia: misdiagnosis and outcome after emergent therapy. Ann Intern Med 1986; 104:766–771.

168. Buxton AE, Marchlinski FE, Doherty JU, et al. Hazards of intravenous verapamil for sustained ventricular tachycardia. Am J Cardiol 1987; 59:1107–1110.

169. Klein LS, Shih HT, Hackett FK, et al. Radiofrequency catheter ablation of ventricular tachycardia in patients without structural heart disease. Circulation 1992; 85:1666–1674.

170. Coggins DL, Lee RJ, Sweeney J, et al. Radiofrequency catheter ablation as a cure for idiopathic tachycardia of both left and right ventricular origin. J Am Coll Cardiol 1994; 23:1333–1341.

171. Friedman PA, Asirvatham SJ, Grice S, et al. Noncontact mapping to guide ablation of right ventricular outflow tract tachycardia. J Am Coll Cardiol 2002; 39:1808–1812.

172. Shimoike E, Ueda N, Maruyama T, et al. Heart rate variability analysis of patients with idiopathic left ventricular outflow tract tachycardia: role of triggered activity. Jpn Circ J 1999; 63:629–635.

173. Shimoike E, Ohnishi Y, Ueda N, et al. Radiofrequency catheter ablation of left ventricular outflow tract tachycardia from the coronary cusp: a new approach to the tachycardia focus. J Cardiovasc Electrophysiol 1999; 10:1005–1009.

174. Frey B, Kreiner G, Fritsch S, et al. Successful treatment of idiopathic left ventricular outflow tract tachycardia by catheter ablation or minimally invasive surgical cryoablation. Pacing Clin Electrophysiol 2000; 23:870–876.

175. Kondo K, Watanabe I, Kojima T, et al. Radiofrequency catheter ablation of ventricular tachycardia from the anterobasal left ventricle. Jpn Heart J 2000; 41:215–225.

176. Hu D, Guo C, Yang J, et al. Left ventricular tachycardia originating near the left main coronary artery. J Interv Card Electrophysiol 2000; 4:423–426.

177. Kanagaratnam L, Tomassoni G, Schweikert R, et al. Ventricular tachycardias arising from the aortic sinus of valsalva: an under-recognized variant of left outflow tract ventricular tachycardia. J Am Coll Cardiol 2001; 37:1408–1414.

178. Hachiya H, Aonuma K, Yamauchi Y, et al. How to diagnose, locate, and ablate coronary cusp ventricular tachycardia. J Cardiovasc Electrophysiol 2002; 13:551–556.

179. Sadanaga T, Saeki K, Yoshimoto T, et al. Repetitive monomorphic ventricular tachycardia of left coronary cusp origin. Pacing Clin Electrophysiol 1999; 22:1553–1556.

180. Takahashi N, Saikawa T, Oribe A, et al. Radiofrequency catheter ablation from the left sinus of Valsalva in a patient with idiopathic ventricular tachycardia. Pacing Clin Electrophysiol 2000; 23:1172–1175.

181. Hachiya H, Aonuma K, Yamauchi Y, et al. Electrocardiographic characteristics of left ventricular outflow tract tachycardia. Pacing Clin Electrophysiol 2000; 23:1930–1934.

182. Asso A, Pascual ED, Lopez M, et al. Catheter ablation of repetitive monomorphic ventricular tachycardia from left ventricular outflow tract guided by unipolar mapping. J Interv Card Electrophysiol 2000; 4:435–439.

183. Merino JL, Peinado R, Ramirez L, et al. Ablation of idiopathic ventricular tachycardia by bipolar radiofrequency current application between the left aortic sinus and the left ventricle. Europace 2000; 2:350–354.

184. Ouyang F, Fotuhi P, Ho SY, et al. Repetitive monomorphic ventricular tachycardia originating from the aortic sinus cusp: electrocardiographic characterization for guiding catheter ablation. J Am Coll Cardiol 2002; 39:500–508.

185. Spurrell RA, Sowton E, Deuchar DC. Ventricular tachycardia in 4 patients evaluated by programmed electrical stimulation of heart and treated in 2 patients by surgical division of anterior radiation of left bundle-branch. Br Heart J 1973; 35:1014–1025.

186. Welch WJ, Strasberg B, Coelho A, et al. Sustained macroreentrant ventricular tachycardia. Am Heart J 1982; 104:166–169.

187. Reddy CP, Slack JD. Recurrent sustained ventricular tachycardia: report of a case with His-bundle branches reentry as the mechanism. Eur J Cardiol 1980; 11:23–31.

188. Lloyd EA, Zipes DP, Heger JJ, et al. Sustained ventricular tachycardia due to bundle branch reentry. Am Heart J 1982; 104:1095–1097.

189. Akhtar M, Damato AN, Batsford WP, et al. Demonstration of re-entry within the His-Purkinje system in man. Circulation 1974; 50:1150–1162.

190. Akhtar M, Gilbert C, Wolf FG, et al. Reentry within the His-Purkinje system. Elucidation of reentrant circuit using right bundle branch and His bundle recordings. Circulation 1978; 58:295–304.

191. Caceres J, Jazayeri M, McKinnie J, et al. Sustained bundle branch reentry as a mechanism of clinical tachycardia. Circulation 1989; 79:256–270.

192. Cohen TJ, Chien WW, Lurie KG, et al. Radiofrequency catheter ablation for treatment of bundle branch reentrant ventricular tachycardia: results and long-term follow-up. J Am Coll Cardiol 1991; 18:1767–1773.

193. Chien WW, Scheinman MM, Cohen TJ, et al. Importance of recording the right bundle branch deflection in the diagnosis of His-Purkinje reentrant tachycardia. Pacing Clin Electrophysiol 1992; 15:1015–1024.

194. Blanck Z, Jazayeri M, Dhala A, et al. Bundle branch reentry: a mechanism of ventricular tachycardia in the absence of myocardial or valvular dysfunction. J Am Coll Cardiol 1993; 22:1718–1722.

195. Tchou P, Jazayeri M, Denker S, et al. Transcatheter electrical ablation of right bundle branch. A method of treating macroreentrant ventricular tachycardia attributed to bundle branch reentry. Circulation 1988; 78:246–257.

196. Blanck Z, Dhala A, Deshpande S, et al. Bundle branch reentrant ventricular tachycardia: cumulative experience in 48 patients. J Cardiovasc Electrophysiol 1993; 4:253–262.

197. Tchou P, Mehdirad AA. Bundle branch reentry ventricular tachycardia. Pacing Clin Electrophysiol 1995; 18:1427–1437.

198. Mehdirad AA, Keim S, Rist K, et al. Asymmetry of retrograde conduction and reentry within the His-Purkinje system: a comparative analysis of left and right ventricular stimulation. J Am Coll Cardiol 1994; 24:177–184.

199. Touboul P, Kirkorian G, Atallah G, et al. Bundle branch reentry: a possible mechanism of ventricular tachycardia. Circulation 1983; 67:674–680.

200. Touboul P, Kirkorian G, Atallah G, et al. Bundle branch reentrant tachycardia treated by electrical ablation of the right bundle branch. J Am Coll Cardiol 1986; 7:1404–1409.

201. Mehdirad AA, Keim S, Rist K, et al. Long-term clinical outcome of right bundle branch radiofrequency catheter ablation for treatment of bundle branch reentrant ventricular tachycardia. Pacing Clin Electrophysiol 1995; 18:2135–2143.

202. Blanck Z, Deshpande S, Jazayeri MR, et al. Catheter ablation of the left bundle branch for the treatment of sustained bundle branch reentrant ventricular tachycardia. J Cardiovasc Electrophysiol 1995; 6:40–43.

203. Dessertenne F. La tachycardie ventriculaire a deux foyers opposes variables. Arch Mal Couer Vaiss 1966; 59:263–272.

204. El-Sherif N, Caref EB, Yin H, et al. The electrophysiological mechanism of ventricular arrhythmias in the long QT syndrome. Tridimensional mapping of activation and recovery patterns. Circ Res 1996; 79:474–492.

205. El-Sherif N, Turitto G. The long QT syndrome and torsade de pointes. Pacing Clin Electrophysiol 1999; 22:91–110.

206. El-Sherif N, Caref EB, Chinushi M, et al. Mechanism of arrhythmogenicity of the short-long cardiac sequence that precedes ventricular tachyarrhythmias in the long QT syndrome. J Am Coll Cardiol 1999; 33:1415–1423.

207. Vincent GM, Timothy K, Fox J, et al. The inherited long QT syndrome: from ion channel to bedside. Cardiol Rev. 1999; 7:44–55.

208. Splawski I, Shen J, Timothy KW, et al. Genomic structure of three long QT syndrome genes: KVLQT1, HERG, and KCNE1. Genomics 1998; 51:86–97.

209. Li H, Chen Q, Moss AJ, et al. New mutations in the KVLQT1 potassium channel that cause long-QT syndrome. Circulation 1998; 97:1264–1269.

210. Vincent GM. The molecular genetics of the long QT syndrome: genes causing fainting and sudden death. Annu Rev Med 1998; 49:263–74, 263–274.

211. Splawski I, Timothy KW, Vincent GM, et al. Molecular basis of the long-QT syndrome associated with deafness. N Engl J Med 1997; 336:1562–1567.

212. Roden DM, Lazzara R, Rosen M, et al. Multiple mechanisms in the long-QT syndrome. Current knowledge, gaps, and future directions. The SADS Foundation Task Force on LQTS. Circulation 1996; 94:1996–2012.

213. Wang Q, Curran ME, Splawski I, et al. Positional cloning of a novel potassium channel gene: KVLQT1 mutations cause cardiac arrhythmias. Nat Genet 1996; 12:17–23.

214. Curran ME, Splawski I, Timothy KW, et al. A molecular basis for cardiac arrhythmia: HERG mutations cause long QT syndrome. Cell 1995; 80:795–803.

215. Moss AJ, Zareba W, Kaufman ES, et al. Increased risk of arrhythmic events in long-QT syndrome with mutations in the pore region of the human ether-a-go-go-related gene potassium channel. Circulation 2002; 105:794–799.

216. Viskin S. Long QT syndromes and torsade de pointes. Lancet 1999; 354:1625–1633.

217. Warden T, Sacchetti A, Klodnicki WE. Magnesium sulfate termination of torsades de pointes following failure of cardioversion. Am J Emerg Med 1989; 7:126–127.

218. Bailie DS, Inoue H, Kaseda S, et al. Magnesium suppression of early afterdepolarizations and ventricular tachyarrhythmias induced by cesium in dogs. Circulation 1988; 77:1395–1402.

219. Tzivoni D, Keren A, Cohen AM, et al. Magnesium therapy for torsades de pointes. Am J Cardiol 1984; 53:528–530.

220. DiSegni E, Klein HO, David D, et al. Overdrive pacing in quinidine syncope and other long QT-interval syndromes. Arch Intern Med 1980; 140:1036–1040.

221. Schwartz PJ, Periti M, Malliani A. The long Q-T syndrome. Am Heart J 1975; 89:378–390.

222. Eldar M, Griffin JC, Abbott JA, et al. Permanent cardiac pacing in patients with the long QT syndrome. J Am Coll Cardiol 1987; 10:600–607.

223. Eldar M, Griffin JC, Van HG, et al. Combined use of beta-adrenergic blocking agents and long-term cardiac pacing for patients with the long QT syndrome. J Am Coll Cardiol 1992; 20: 830–837.

224. Moss AJ, Liu JE, Gottlieb S, et al. Efficacy of permanent pacing in the management of high-risk patients with long QT syndrome. Circulation 1991; 84:1524–1529.

225. Campanelli B, Chaudron JM. Long term follow up of long QT syndrome treated by overdrive pacing. Heart 2001; 86:E14.

226. Stefanelli CB, Bradley DJ, Leroy S, et al. Implantable cardioverter defibrillator therapy for life-threatening arrhythmias in young patients. J Interv Card Electrophysiol 2002; 6:235–244.

227. Breithardt G, Wichter T, Haverkamp W, et al. Implantable cardioverter defibrillator therapy in patients with arrhythmogenic right ventricular cardiomyopathy, long QT syndrome, or no structural heart disease. Am Heart J 1994; 127:1151–1158.

228. Viskin S, Belhassen B. Idiopathic ventricular fibrillation. Am Heart J 1990; 120:661–671.

229. Belhassen B, Shapira I, Shoshani D, et al. Idiopathic ventricular fibrillation: inducibility and beneficial effects of class I antiarrhythmic agents. Circulation 1987; 75:809–816.

230. Tung RT, Shen WK, Hammill SC, et al. Idiopathic ventricular fibrillation in out-of-hospital cardiac arrest survivors. Pacing Clin Electrophysiol 1994; 17:1405–1412.

231. de Latorre F, Nolan J, Robertson C, et al. European Resuscitation Council Guidelines 2000 for Adult Advanced Life Support. A statement from the Advanced Life Support Working Group(1) and approved by the Executive Committee of the European Resuscitation Council. Resuscitation 2001; 48:211–221.

232. Meissner MD, Lehmann MH, Steinman RT, et al. Ventricular fibrillation in patients without significant structural heart disease: a multicenter experience with implantable cardioverter-defibrillator therapy. J Am Coll Cardiol 1993; 21:1406–1412.

233. Moss AJ, Hall WJ, Cannom DS, et al. for the Multicenter Automatic Defibrillator Implantation Trial Investigators. Improved survival with an implanted defibrillator in patients with coronary disease at high risk for ventricular arrhythmia. N Engl J Med 1996; 335:1933–1940.

234. Primo J, Geelen P, Brugada J, et al. Hypertrophic cardiomyopathy: role of the implantable cardioverter-defibrillator. J Am Coll Cardiol 1998; 31:1081–1085.

235. Coats AJ. MADIT II, the Multi-center Autonomic Defibrillator Implantation Trial II stopped early for mortality reduction, has ICD therapy earned its evidence-based credentials? Int J Cardiol 2002; 82:1–5.

236. Patt MV, Podrid PJ, Friedman PL, et al. Spontaneous reversion of ventricular fibrillation. Am Heart J 1988; 115:919–923.

237. Fuster V, Ryden LE, Asinger RW, et al. ACC/AHA/ESC guidelines for the management of patients with atrial fibrillation. A report of the American College of Cardiology/American Heart Association Task Force on Practice Guidelines and the European Society of Cardiology Committee for Practice Guidelines and Policy Conferences (Committee to develop guidelines for the management of patients with atrial fibrillation) developed in collaboration with the North American Society of Pacing and Electrophysiology. Eur Heart J 2001; 22:1852–1923.

238. DiMarco JP, Sellers TD, Berne RM, et al. Adenosine: electrophysiologic effects and therapeutic use for terminating paroxysmal supraventricular tachycardia. Circulation 1983; 68:1254–1263.

239. DiMarco JP, Sellers TD, Lerman BB, et al. Diagnostic and therapeutic use of adenosine in patients with supraventricular tachyarrhythmias. J Am Coll Cardiol 1985; 6:417–425.

240. Engelstein ED, Lippman N, Stein KM, et al. Mechanism-specific effects of adenosine on atrial tachycardia. Circulation 1994; 89:2645–2654.

241. Garratt C, Linker N, Griffith M, et al. Comparison of adenosine and verapamil for termination of paroxysmal junctional tachycardia. Am J Cardiol 1989; 64:1310–1316.

242. Garratt CJ, Griffith MJ, O'Nunain S, et al. Effects of intravenous adenosine on antegrade refractoriness of accessory atrioventricular connections. Circulation 1991; 84:1962–1968.

243. Griffith MJ, Linker NJ, Ward DE, et al. Adenosine in the diagnosis of broad complex tachycardia. Lancet 1988; 1:672–675.

244. Griffith MJ, Garratt CJ, Ward DE, et al. The effects of adenosine on sinus node reentrant tachycardia. Clin Cardiol 1989; 12:409–411.

245. Rubenstein DS, Burke MC, Kall JG, et al. Adenosine-sensitive bundle branch reentry. J Cardiovasc Electrophysiol 1997; 8:80–88.

CLINICAL FEATURES

Atrial fibrillation: hemodynamics and clinical features

John Godtfredsen MD FESC
Herlev University Hospital, Herlev, Denmark

Rodney H Falk MD FRCP FACC FAHA
Boston Medical Center, Boston, MA, USA

ATRIAL FIBRILLATION is a Symptom – rarely a Disease !

Introduction

When in atrial fibrillation (AF) the atrial
walls shudder with fast undulating
movements – as already described by
William Harvey in 1628 – and a condition
exists of definite atrial contraction failure.
At the same time the ventricular rate is fast
and irregular due to the chaotic
bombardment of the AV-node by more than
700 impulses per minute from the atria
(Fig. 5.1).

It is important to realize that in AF the
hemodynamics and hence the symptoms
are extremely variable. This diversity of
clinical AF is such that in one end of the
range some patients are severely ill with
congestive heart failure (CHF) and at the
other end AF is an incidental finding in an
(usually elderly) entirely asymptomatic
patient.

The reasons for this diversity are
multiple as are the clinical presentations of
AF, encompassing several different
conditions.

Basically the hemodynamics determine
the symptoms, and in many cases AF per se
may be an accompanying symptom and
less important than the underlying
hypertensive and ischemic heart disease.

Atrial fibrillation nomenclature[1]

Types or patterns – a pragmatic taxonomy

• First episode	ECG-verified
• Paroxysmal	Acute AF, often self-limiting Recurrent episodes < 1-7 days
• Persistent	DC- or drug-convertible Recurrent episodes, usually > 7 days
• Permanent	Chronic, non-convertible

From ACC/AHA/ESC[1]

BASIC ELECTROPHYSIOLOGY

It is possible to precipitate AF in any
normal heart by mechanical means, for
instance by manipulating a catheter
(undexterously) in the right atrium.

The likely trigger of AF in this case is
acute, localized wall-stretch, and obviously
there is no underlying pathoanatomical
substrate for AF in a normal right atrium.
In such circumstances short bouts of AF are
like models of the acute onset,
self-terminating type of AF.

Predisposing factors (creating the
prefibrillatory substrates) *and* acute triggers
(generating abnormal impulses) are both
necessary to precipitate longer, and hence
clinically important paroxysmal episodes of
AF. Examples of such a pathophysiological
setting are common, like for instance
paroxysmal AF in acute myocardial
infarction (AMI) and heart surgery, or
persistent, paroxysmal AF in a (usually)
younger patient with a focal trigger
sometimes located in the ostia of the
pulmonary veins.

Atrial fibrillation

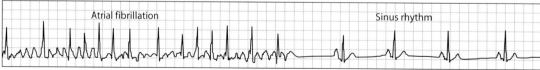

Fig. 5.1 ECG in atrial fibrillation.

In permanent, chronic AF a (prefibrillatory) substrate and a trigger still need to be present, but are not sufficient to perpetuate the arrhythmia. Chronic atrial wall stress is usually present in this situation and its electrophysiological features are certainly different from those of acute stretch.[2]

Permanency of AF requires and is associated with mechanical, histological and electrical remodeling of atrial structures, and also some underlying left ventricular or mitral valve pathology.

Thus the chain of events leading to the onset of AF may (somewhat simplified) be described as follows:[3]

Acute AF
⇑
Acute wall stretch ⇒ Trigger ⇒ Initiator ⇒ Substrate ⇒ AF-onset ⇒ Remodeling ⇒ Perpetuators ⇒ Permanent AF

The electrophysiology in AF is more complex than in most other arrhythmias where unifocal or circus movement mechanisms are present during sustained arrhythmia, and such episodes are also more clearly defined clinically and electrocardiographically.

Nonetheless AF is a good model for any tachyarrhythmia regarding the substrate-trigger interaction as well as the risk of tachycardia-induced cardiomyopathy in the case of sustained rapid heart rates.

PATHOHISTOLOGY

Until recently histological studies in AF were limited to examinations relative to the underlying heart disease, i.e. rheumatic noduli in rheumatic heart disease, amyloid depositions in elderly patients and the very rare atrial wall infarcts.

Some 30 years ago histological findings in the sinusnode of patients with chronic AF indicated severe degeneration of the normal pacemaker tissue.[4]

In the past few years atrial tissue in animals and man has been examined in cases without any underlying heart disease, so-called 'lone' AF. The results are interesting since even in AF of rather short duration the atrial walls may show changes in the myofibrillar structure as well as increased deposition of fibrotic tissue clearly indicating that AF per se leads to a kind of histological remodeling along with the electrical and mechanical changes referred to above (Fig. 5.2).

HEMODYNAMICS

Atrial contraction failure – the hemodynamic hallmark of AF – is not limited to established AF. One of the most important and frequent underlying etiologies of AF is hypertension (see Table 5.3) with ensuing and gradually developing hypertensive heart disease, a major feature of which is left atrial dilatation because of impaired left ventricular (LV) compliance. An enlarged and distended LA leads often, in its later stages, to atrial paralysis even before the advent of AF as an electrical complication verifiable on the electrocardiogram (ECG) (Table 5.1)[7].

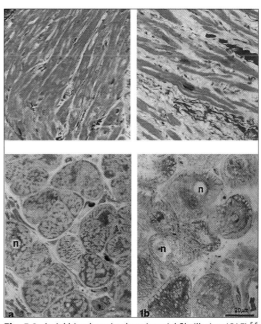

Fig. 5.2 Atrial histology in chronic atrial fibrillation (CAF).[5,6]

Table 5.1 Stepwise enlargement of left atrial size

Stages of HD	NSR –HD	NSR + HBP/HHD	PAF	Early CAF	Late CAF	CAF + RHD
LA size	normal	↑within normal limits	↑ mildly	↑ > 40 mm	↑ > 45 mm	↑↑> 5 mm
Size in mm	23	31	36	43	49	53–60

HD, heart disease; NSR, normal sinus rhythm; HBP, hypertension; HHD, hypertensive heart disease; PAF, paroxysmal AF; CAF, chronic AF; LA, left atrium; RHD, rheumatic heart disease

Permanent AF features typically both a hypertrophic LV and an enlarged left atrium with disrupted myofibrillar structure and thus furthering the chaotic electrical activity in the form of multiple wavelets perpetually meandering about in the atrial walls.

The major consequence of atrial contraction failure in established AF is of course loss of the atrial contribution to the stroke volume, in some cases amounting to as much as 50% of total stroke volume.[8]

These salient features are documented abundantly in clinical, echocardiographic and electrophysiological studies.

The ventricular rate is fast (usually > 110–120) in untreated patients with AF, and thus adding an extra hemodynamic burden to the premorbidly strained myocardium along with a shortened diastole further compromising the LV filling, already suffering from the lack of atrial systole.

In certain states, for instance the Wolff-Parkinson-White (WPW) syndrome by way of an accessory bundle, the ventricular rate may go as high as 250 imposing – even in the healthiest of hearts – a risk of degeneration into malignant arrhythmias i.e. ventricular tachycardia (VT) and ventricular fibrillation (VF).

The combined hemodynamic effect of loss of atrial systole and high ventricular heart rate is a decrease in cardiac output, as it has been amply demonstrated in invasive studies.

A sustained chronic low cardiac output may be the basis for some of the rather unpleasant symptoms in permanent AF: Decreased physical capacity and chronic fatigue (Fig. 5.3).

It has also been found that the irregularity itself interferes with the normal ventricular contractility in a negative fashion, thus contributing to a worsened hemodynamic condition already impaired by tachycardia and a low stroke volume. Normal presystolic closure of the atrioventricular valves requires a normal timing not only of atrial contraction but also of the heart rate, and when both are failing mitral valve regurgitation may occur.

Even though a dilated LA due to some underlying heart disease [e.g. hypertensive heart disease (HHD) or mitral stenosis/regurgitation] may give rise to AF, in the majority of cases it is persistent or permanent AF by it self that enlarges the atria further and possibly also the ostia of the pulmonary veins. The reason is maybe a combination of atrial wall paralysis and a sustained increase in the intra-atrial pressure.

Along with atrial contraction failure this mechanical remodeling engenders stasis in the atrial body as well as in the atrial appendage, and predisposes to thrombus formation.

Atrial wall distension has besides the above-mentioned mechanical consequences also endocrinological significance since the vasoregulatory hormone ANP is found elevated in persistent and permanent AF.

The received wisdom tells us that clinically overt CHF sooner or later in the course may precipitate AF due to increased

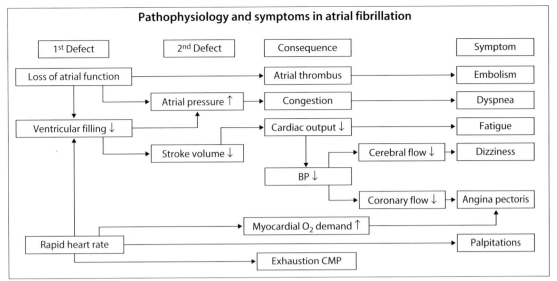

Fig. 5.3 Pathophysiology in AF. CMP, cardiomyopathy.

atrial pressure and atrial dilatation. This in turn disrupts the atrial wall structure thus creating a substrate for the electrical chain of events. This is certainly the case in many patients presenting with AF, and the trigger of AF may be some cardiac or extracardiac event adding an extra – perhaps acute – hemodynamic burden to the already diseased heart. However, even in recent-onset AF some 40% of the patients are without subjective symptoms of CHF. Therefore a revision of the mechanism of the immediate association between AF and CHF seems necessary.

Recently it has been proposed[3] that more gradual and subtle changes in the atria precede AF rather slowly over months or years without causing any (or only mild and compensated) symptoms of CHF. Such could be the case, for instance, in (poorly treated) hypertension or in old-age LV stiffness. In such cases then, the onset of AF with its attendant fast heart rate merely acts as the mechanical and hemodynamic event that precipitates overt CHF. In other words the slowly distended and disrupted atrial wall is the substrate of AF, which in its turn leads to CHF and further atrial dilatation completing a vicious circle of hemodynamic events. This perhaps more tenable theory has the appealing advantage

of making AF liable to prevention by earlier and more aggressive treatment of threatened patients for example with ACE inhibitors.

Echocardiographic and invasive studies show the feasibility of restoring improved haemodynamics by successful reversion of AF to sinus rhythm (Figs 5.4 and 5.5), and thus also indicate the possible presence of a tachycardia mediated cardiomyopathy during ongoing AF.

These features give echocardiography a prominent place in the routine evaluation, management and follow-up of AF patients, not only to detect or document some underlying heart disease, but also as a means of guiding therapy and its level of aggressiveness.

During physical exercise AF is characterized by a disproportionately fast heart rate as compared with sinus rhythm, and it is not unusual that AF patients with a controlled heart rate do rather well when at rest or performing slowly. Adding beta-blockers or calcium antagonists to digoxin with cautious respect to the LV function may very often improve the exercise capacity although not to a level found in sinus rhythm.[9]

Figures 5.4 and 5.5 show the hemodynamic improvement after

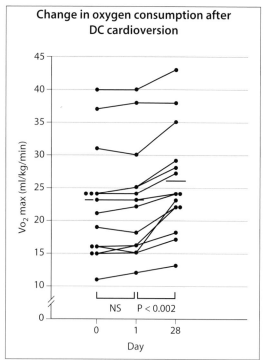

Change in oxygen consumption after DC cardioversion

Fig. 5.4 Change in maximal oxygen consumption (V_{O_2} max) after DC cardioversion of atrial fibrillation to sinus rhythm (Adapted from Lipkin[10]).

ATRIAL FIBRILLATION IN OLD AGE

There is reason to believe that the present so-called epidemic of AF in the community may partly be caused by increased longevity in the industrial countries leading to a greater number of elderly patients developing AF without any severe underlying etiological heart disease but old age by itself.

Salient features of AF in old age is shown in the box.

Atrial fibrillation in old age[16]

- Predisposing factors — Sinus node degeneration LA wall fibrosis; fatty and amyloid depositions Decreased metabolic reserve

- Hemodynamic 'chain of events'

  Myocardial stiffness increases
  ↓
  LV compliance decreases
  ↓
  LA contractile force increases
  ↓
  LA dilatation and stretch → Atrial fibrillation

conversion to sinus rhythm: return of the A-wave on Doppler M-mode echo, and an increase in exercise capacity[10] (note the very wide range of the maximal oxygen uptake when in AF). See also Table 5.2,[10–15] with data from several clinical series.

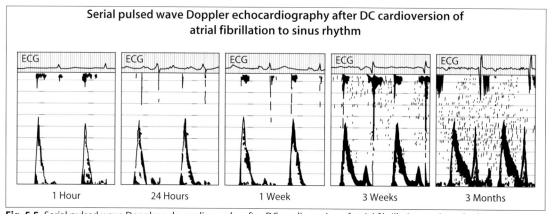

Serial pulsed wave Doppler echocardiography after DC cardioversion of atrial fibrillation to sinus rhythm

| 1 Hour | 24 Hours | 1 Week | 3 Weeks | 3 Months |

Fig. 5.5 Serial pulsed wave Doppler echocardiography after DC cardioversion of atrial fibrillation to sinus rhythm.

Table 5.2 Effect of DC conversion in AF on physical capacity and EF

Study	N	MVO$_2$ (ml/min/kg)		EF%	
		AF	SR	AF	SR
Lipkin[10]	14	23	26	–	–
Kieny[11]	17	–	–	32	53
Groningen[12]	8	20	25	36	53
Groningen[13]	63	21	24	–	–
Groningen[14]	17	21	22.3 (23.8)*	–	–
Warsaw[15]	48	–	–	59	66**

*After 2 years; ** after 1 year; MVO, maximal oxygen uptake; EF, ejection fraction.

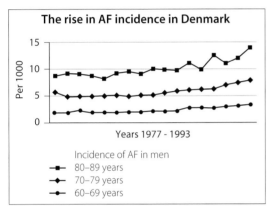

The rise in AF incidence in Denmark

Per 1000 — Years 1977 - 1993

Incidence of AF in men
- ■ 80–89 years
- ◆ 70–79 years
- ● 60–69 years

Fig. 5.6 The rise in AF incidence in Denmark (Adapted from Frost[17]).

CLINICAL FEATURES

The range of presenting complaints by the patients with AF is wide.

In the elderly with established, permanent AF many patients (up to 30% in some studies) may be mildly symptomatic or entirely without symptoms, and AF is thus an incidental finding on routine examination.

By contrast most young and middle-aged patients with the recurrent, paroxysmal form of AF usually report symptoms as being very unpleasant but rarely with dire distress.

Atrial fibrillation

Types	Clinical features
Paroxysmal (Acute)	Non-cardiac cause (Fever, alcohol, thyrotoxicosis) Cardiac cause (AMI, CHF, pericarditis, etc.)
Persistent	Independent disorder in the younger (no heart disease) Forerunner of permanent AF (± heart disease)
Permanent	Usually with underlying heart disease Old-age AF Rarely 'lone AF' Often preceded by paroxysmal AF

Figure 5.6[17] shows the rise in AF incidence in Denmark, and this same pattern of an increase in hospital incidence of AF has also been reported from Scotland[18] indicating either a true rise in the AF incidence, perhaps due to the ageing of the Western populations, or at least an increased awareness among referring physicians that AF requires more attention than previously, both regarding antiarrhythmic and preventive thromboembolic treatment.

In both permanent and persistent, paroxysmal AF symptoms of the underlying heart disease or of the precipitating cause may dominate the clinical picture, i.e. acute myocardial infarction (AMI), acute or gradually evolving heart failure, thyrotoxicosis or overt pulmonary disease such as pneumonia or exacerbations in chronic obstructive pulmonary disease (COPD).

ATRIAL FIBRILLATION AND HEART FAILURE

The relationship between AF and clinical heart failure has been examined in a number of studies in both hospitalized[19,20,21] patients and outpatients.[22–25] These data on the clinical epidemiology of AF obviously vary depending on the population studied, selection criteria and whether heart failure is documented by clinical means only or by echocardiography. But such data are helpful in any clinical situation where

judgement of the type and possible immediate course of the patient is of concern.

Thus overt CHF is present in about 40–60% of inpatients with a recent worsening just before presentation in some 30%, whereas CHF is present in only about 10–20 % of outpatients. See the boxes above and below.

PRECIPITATING FACTORS OF ATRIAL FIBRILLATION

Precipitating factors of AF are sometimes obviously present and sometimes unknown and may be cardiac or extracardiac.

Precipitating extracardiac factors in AF have been dealt with extensively in the older literature, and range from intercurrent infections, drug intoxication, stroke, thoracic surgery, and physical exertion to imbalance in the autonomic nervous system.[19,27]

Clinical congestive heart failure (CHF) at AF presentation (hospital series)

Series		CHF by history	CHF at AF-onset	Worsened CHF
Godtfredsen[19] n=534	Age 70	138 (26%)	303 (57%)	165 (31%)
Tischler et al[20] n= 87	Age 64	19 (22%)	32 (37%)	13 (15%)
Friedman et al[21] n= 98	Age 69	11 (11%)	41 (42%)	30 (31%)

Clinical CHF at AF presentation (outpatient series)

Series	n	Mean age	CHF (%)
AFI[22]	1236	69	20
EAFT[23]	669 (WF arm)	71	9
	338 (ASA arm)	77	13
AFASAK 2[24]	665	76	32*
ALFA[25]	756	69	22
AFFIRM[26]	4060	70	27

*Incl. mild CHF

Clinical extracardiac precipitating factors in atrial fibrillation,[19] n=456 (%)	
Pulmonary infection	136 (30)
Intoxications incl. alcohol	76 (17)
Stroke	70 (15)
Other infections	38 (8)
Pulmonary embolism	28 (6)
Physical exertion	24 (5)
Other causes (incl. surgery)	84 (18)

UNDERLYING HEART DISEASES OR ASSOCIATED CONDITIONS IN ATRIAL FIBRILLATION

Hypertension is certainly – as also in epidemiological studies – a very important underlying condition predisposing to and eventually even precipitating AF. The proportion of valvular heart disease, THD and diabetes are very similar across studies whereas CHF and IHD show a difference most likely because of varying definitions and populations (Table 5.3).[24,25,28]

LONE ATRIAL FIBRILLATION

This entity is probably but a subtle and longstanding minor volume/pressure overload eventually leading to decreased LV compliance and left atrial distension and finally AF (see the theory by Allessie et al[3]).

SYMPTOMS

Symptoms attributable to AF per se are sudden, shorter or longer bouts of palpitations, retrosternal or epigastrical jumps and bumps or a sensation of an uneasy fullness in the chest, often aptly described as fluctuations or fibrillations. These symptoms typically worsen when lying down or trying to exercise.

A sense of anxiety is rather common as is angina when the heart rate is very fast or when ischemic heart disease is present.

Table 5.3 Underlying heart diseases or associated conditions in atrial fibrillation in recently published clinical series[24,25,28]

Heart disease or condition	ALFA study[25] n=756	AFASAK 2*[24] n=677	CARAF study**[28] n=899
Hypertension	39.4	41.8	39.4
Valvular HD	15.2	14.5	14.8
Heart failure***	50.0	68.2	17.6****
Angina and AMI	16.6	24.7	42.0
Cardiomyopathy	15.2	-	-
Obstructive lung disease	11.2	-	-
Thyroid HD	3.1	2.5	2.9
Diabetes	10.7	13.2	9.0
None (Lone AF)	29.3	-	-

*, Chronic AF only; **, New-onset AF only; ***, NYHA 2-4; ****, By history only

Only occasionally can the patient point to a certain precipitating cause for these symptoms: after a heavy meal, during strenuous exercise or associated with some stressing psychological condition. More often than not the symptoms appear out of the blue, only sometimes with warnings in the form of scattered extrasystoles leading up to a bout of atrial fibrillation proper.

At the time of the eventual diagnosis (by ECG) many patients with paroxysmal AF can relate that they have experienced such symptoms evolving gradually and perhaps worsening over months or years, not knowing it to be heart trouble.

In the elderly with acute onset of AF such a course is much more unusual; they may present with gradually increasing shortness of breath during physical activity or sometimes overt, untreated heart failure may dominate, if not AF is just an incidental finding in an otherwise unaffected patient.

The reasons for this discrepancy in the pattern of clinical symptoms between younger and older patients are not entirely clear.

Younger patients tend to have higher (> 110) and older patients to have lower (< 110) heart rates at the AF onset, providing a possible explanation.[19] Even though the elderly typically have more often and more severe underlying heart disease, their lower heart rates and lower level of physical performance perhaps contribute to the paucity of AF symptoms per se.

Evaluation of *the quality of life (QoL)* (see Ch. 10) seems to confirm the notion of a clinically relevant difference in symptoms between the majority of (elderly > 70 years of age) patients and a smaller group of (younger) highly symptomatic patients. The preliminary results from the AFFIRM[26] study (mean age 70) indicate that only one-third perceived their QoL as poor or fair. On the other hand a recent Dutch study in younger patients (mean age 54) with one 2 h bout of AF per week found that the symptoms were significantly

related to the status of the autonomic nervous system, particularly a depressed vagal function.[27]

In the analysis of the general severity of AF, however, it is important to recognize that there are at least three ways of evaluating individuals or groups with AF, and that these are on one hand partly mutually exclusive and on the other more or less related:

1. self-reported symptoms, i.e. somatic complaints;
2. quantitatively measured QoL (perceived symptoms);
3. quantified functional cardiac disability such as New York Heart Association (NYHA) grade, degree of CHF, LV function by echocardiography, etc.

One would expect an initial reasonable agreement between these three methods of clinical judgment, but it is not so. Newer studies have found that the (semi-)quantitative relation between symptoms, QoL and for example NYHA grade is rather poor.[29]

Symptoms leading to medical attention and thus detection/verification of AF by ECG from the ALFA study are shown in Table 5.4.

The data in Table 5.4 illustrate and, to a certain degree, explain the diversity of different clinical subsets of AF:

1. at the time of presentation or detection, and
2. as perceived by the patients before medical attention or during the course of AF.

Patients with paroxysmal AF are younger and show a higher occurrence of palpitations and less heart failure. In contrast the older patients with chronic AF more often have heart failure, but there is also a significant group which have no symptoms at all. In the new-onset AF group the salient features are the complaints that led to acute medical attention and hence a diagnosis of AF, i.e. a high occurrence of both palpitations and dyspnea.

Table 5.4 Symptoms and complaints in atrial fibrillation[25]

Symptoms (%)	Chronic AF n=389	Paroxysmal AF n=167	Recent onset AF n=200
Palpitations	44.7	79.0	51.5
Dyspnea	46.8	22.8	58.0
Dizziness, syncope	8.0	17.4	9.5
Fatigue	13.1	12.6	18.0
Chest pain	8.2	13.2	11.0
Other	1.8	–	–
None	16.2	5.4	7.0
Age at presentation	69.9	65.9	68.1

IMMEDIATE COURSE AND PROGNOSIS

The prognosis regarding survival depends mainly on patient's age and the degree of heart failure so it can be said with confidence that a patient with a single, acute bout of AF precipitated by some extracardiac cause has an excellent prognosis both regarding survival and thromboembolic complications. At the other extreme is the elderly patient with overt failure, perhaps previous transitory cerebral ischemia or stroke, and certainly a bleak prognosis.

Curiously though, in (younger) patients with advanced heart failure, AF seems not to play an independent role for the prognosis[30] a finding which conflicts with the older and received wisdom, that even in severe CHF the prognosis is worsened by AF.[31]

PHYSICIANS' OBLIGATIONS AND TASKS WHEN ENCOUNTERING ATRIAL FIBRILLATION PATIENTS

- acute treatment for immediate relief of symptoms and distress
- detect and diagnose underlying etiological heart disease (Echo)
- prevent hemodynamic deterioration
- restore sinus rhythm, if possible (see box below)
- risk stratify regarding T/E risk
- antithrombotic prevention if AF continues
- improve QoL

The results of the recent AFFIRM-study[26] make it possible to refrain from trying to restore sinus rhythm in many elderly patients and opt instead for rate

---

Clinical consequences of AF

Congestive heart failure depends heavily on:

- Age of the patient
- Degree of underlying LV disease
- Degree of ventricular rate control
- Duration of AF

but depends less on:
LA function

Embolic complications depend on:

± Risk factors (LA size in some studies)

> **Reasons for restoring sinus rhythm (Modified from Waktare & Camm[32])**
>
> - Appropriate/physiological rate control
> - Regularization of heart rhythm
> - Restoration of atrial filling fraction
> - Improvements in hemodynamics
> - Maintenance of normal electrophysiology
> - Prevention of atrial dilatation
> - Prevention of left ventricular dysfunction
> - Relief of symptoms
> - Reduce thromboembolic episodes

control plus long-term anticoagulation, thus avoiding hospitalization, side-effects from antiarrhythmic drugs and the (for the patients) very often frustrating situations when one or more conversion attempts fail.

> **Reasons for *not* restoring sinus rhythm**
>
> **The AFFIRM trial found:**
>
> Increased mortality in the rhythm control arm (356 vs306), $p = 0.058$
>
> More strokes in the rhythm control arm than in the rate control arm (84 vs 79) not significant.
>
> Quality of life showed no differences
>
> Implication: Rate control is just as good as rhythm control in these patients > 65 years

TRANSITION FROM PAROXYSMAL TO PERMANENT ATRIAL FIBRILLATION[19,28,33,34]

In populations of AF (by cross-sectional analysis) the proportion of patients with paroxysmal (i.e. non-permanent) AF amounts to roughly one-third.[19] This incorporates both patients with a single, acute episode and patients with persistent AF, and it is of clinical relevance to get a measure of how many, and when they

eventually become permanent. And in these times of increasing patient participation in the choice and plan of treatment the patient may wish to know more precisely the prognosis in this regard.

Obvious and manageable risk factors for permanency may also aid the clinician in the prevention of permanency, i.e. which level of aggressive antiarrhythmic treatment is desirable and necessary in individual patients. Unfortunately the clinically significant features predictive of permanency (age and the presence of AF at baseline) are not amenable to treatment.[34]

Some clinical studies have dealt with this – see box.

Incidence of progression to chronic AF relative to PAF:		
Godtfredsen[19]	n=426	2.7%
CARAF[28,33]	n=699/896	4.6%/6.3%
Duke Univ[34]	n=231	4.5%

Thus it seems that transition from paroxysmal to permanent AF occurs in about 3–6% of the patients per year, provided the antiarrhythmic prophylactic treatment has been of current standard (which is not very effective).

THROMBOEMBOLIC COMPLICATIONS

Stasis in the left atrium induces a risk of intravascular clot formation and may eventually lead to embolization. The number of echocardiographically-detected thrombi and spontaneously occurring contrast ('smoke'), indicating stasis in the left atrium is about 15–25% in cases of permanent AF. Contributing to this rather mechanistic cause of thromboembolism in AF is the presence of a prothrombotic state involving increases in several hemostatic parameters.[35] (See Chapter 2).

This prothrombotic state may lead to refinement of the calculation of the thromboembolic risk in the individual patient (see Chapter 18).

CLINICAL FEATURES OF OTHER ARRHYTHMIAS

Atrial flutter is much less common than AF and usually less symptomatic. Very rarely it is sustained and responds easily to direct current (DC) conversion. Thromboembolic risk is calculated as in AF. Since the heart rate rarely exceeds 150, tachycardia mediated cardiomyopathy is only rarely a problem. VT is dealt with elsewhere in Chapter 19.

TACHYCARDIA-INDUCED CARDIOMYOPATHY

Incessant high heart rates for example by continuing rapid pacing is well known to be able to exhaust the myocardial metabolism and thus provoke myocardial contraction failure.[36]

Since such more or less sustained high heart rates are rare in other clinically recognized arrhythmias, AF becomes the most common arrhythmia that in some (untreated) cases may lead to the so called 'tachycardia' cardiomyopathy where the AF per se is responsible for overt heart failure at AF detection rather than CHF being a consequence of some underlying heart disease just worsened by the high heart rate.

Tachycardia mediated cardiomyopathy

- Reversible ventricular dysfunction secondary to prolonged (but not necessarily incessant) tachycardia
- Associated with cellular calcium overload
- How common is it in AF?

Suspect cases in this regard would be younger patients with a history of a possible precipitating cause (e.g. recent infection, alcohol binge, etc.) but without any underlying heart disease or hypertension. Given the methodological

No. of patients with tachycardia-induced cardiomyopathy in AF[12,19,37–39]

Series	Number of patients at AF presentation	
Charon et al[37]	17/1850	(0.9%)
Godtfredsen[19]	96/1212	(7.9%)
Grogan et al[38]	10	(prevalence ?)
Van Gelder et al[12]	8	(prevalence ?)
Redfield et al[39]	16/63	(25%) Tertiary patients Mayo Clinic

Thus the true prevalence of tachycardia-induced cardiomyopathy in AF is unknown

difficulty in the acute setting of telling whether the CHF present is a cause or an effect of AF, the truth may not be revealed until later in the course when the ventricular rate has been controlled or sinus rhythm restored (see Table 5.2).

In older subjects – as mentioned above – there is such a complex interplay between rapid heart rate and underlying prefibrillatory CHF, that the true contribution of each may never be disentangled.

Prevention and treatment of suspected tachycardia cardiomyopathy require either immediately instituted perfect control of the fast heart rate in AF (even by means of AV nodal ablation) or preferably conversion to sinus rhythm as early as possible after detection of AF. Unfortunately this hemodynamically agreeable attitude clashes with the risk of thrombus formation, which with some certainty is already in operation after AF has lasted about 12–24 h – or perhaps even earlier.[35]

Thus, postponement of conversion is detrimental from the viewpoint of establishing a lasting sinus rhythm, since it is known that a major risk factor for relapse of AF is the duration of AF before a trial of conversion, perhaps because of the electrical and mechanical remodeling referred to above.

CONCLUSIONS

- Atrial fibrillation is a symptom, rarely a disease
- Patients with AF are very heterogeneous
- Outpatients: 10–20% have CHF
- Inpatients: 40–50% have CHF
- Diastolic CHF is rather frequent in old-age AF
- Younger symptomatic patients with PAF have decreased QoL
- Mortality in AF is increased by a factor 1.5–2.0

Failure of atrial contraction is but one feature of AF:

- ventricular function
- uncontrolled ventricular rate
- thromboembolic risk
- may all be more important

References

1. Task Force Report: ACC/AHA/ESC guidelines for the management of patients with atrial fibrillation. Eur Heart J 2001; 22:1852–1923.

2. Janse MJ, Opthof T, Kléber AG. Animal models of cardiac arrhythmias. Cardiovasc Res 1998; 39:165–177.

3. Allessie MA, Boyden PA, Camm AJ, et al. Pathophysiology and prevention of atrial fibrillation. Circulation 2001; 103:769–777.

4. James TN. The sinus node. Am J Cardiol 1977; 40:965–986.

5. Mihm MJ, Yu F, Carnes CA, et al. Impaired myofibrillar energetics and oxidative injury during human atrial fibrillation. Circulation 2001; 104:174–180.

6. Ausma J, Wijffels M, Thoné F, et al. Structural changes of atrial myocardium due to sustained atrial fibrillation in the goat. Circulation 1997; 96:3157–3163.

7. Godtfredsen J. Physiology and pathophysiology of the atria: its role in atrial fibrillation. J Thrombos Thrombolys 1999; 7:13–19.

8. Upshaw CB. Hemodynamic changes after cardioversion of chronic atrial fibrillation. Arch Intern Med 1997; 157:1070–1076.

9. Hohnloser SH, Kuck KH, Lilienthal J for the PIAF investigators. Rhythm or rate control in atrial fibrillation – pharmacological intervention in atrial fibrillation (PIAF): a randomised trial. Lancet 2000; 356:1789–1794.

10. Lipkin DP, Frenneaux M, Stewart R, et al. Delayed improvement in exercise capacity after cardioversion of atrial fibrillation to sinus rhythm. Br Heart J 1988; 59:572–577.

11. Kieny JR, Sacrez A, Facello A, et al. Increase in radionuclide left ventricular ejection fraction after cardioversion of chronic atrial fibrillation in idiopathic dilated cardiomyopathy. Eu Heart J 1992; 13:1290–1295.

12. Van Gelder IC, Crijns HJ, Blanksma PK, et al. Time course of hemodynamic changes and improvement of exercise tolerance after cardioversion of chronic atrial fibrillation unassociated with cardiac valve disease. Am J Cardiol 1993; 72:560–566.

13. Gosselink ATM, Crijns HJGM, van den Berg MP, et al. Functional capacity before and after cardioversion of atrial fibrillation: a controlled study. Br Heart J 1994; 72:161–166.

14. Gosselink AT, Bijlsma EB, Landsman ML, et al. Long-term effect of cardioversion on peak oxygen consumption in chronis atrial fibrillation. A 2-year follow-up. Eur Heart J 1994; 15:1368–1372.

15. Gurba H, Kuch-Wocial A, Szulc M, et al. Does successful cardioversion favorably affect the left heart in chronic non-valvular atrial fibrillation? Long-term echocardiographic follow-up. Eur Heart J 1999; 20(suppl. August/September):211 (abstract).

16. Wei JY. Age and the cardiovascular system. N Engl J Med 1992; 327:1735–1739.

17. Frost L, Engholm G., Møller H, et al. Decrease in mortality in patients with a hospital diagnosis of atrial fibrillation in Denmark during the period 1980–1993. Eur Heart J 1999; 20:1592–1599.

18. Stewart S, MacIntyre K, MacLeod MMC, et al. Trends in hospital activity, morbidity and case fatality related to atrial fibrillation in Scotland, 1986-1996. Eur Heart J 2001; 22:693–701.

19. Godtfredsen J. Atrial fibrillation. Etiology, course and prognosis. A follow-up study of 1212 cases. Copenhagen: Munksgaard; 1975.

20. Tischler MD, Lee TH, McAndrew KA, et al. Clinical, echocardiographic and doppler correlates of clinical instability with onset of atrial fibrillation. Am J Cardiol 1990; 66:721–724.

21. Friedman HZ, Goldberg SF, Bonema JD, et al. Acute complications associated with new-onset atrial fibrillation. Am J Cardiol 1991; 67:437–439.

22. Atrial Fibrillation Investigators. Risk factors for stroke and efficacy of antithrombotic therapy in atrial fibrillation. Analysis of pooled data from five randomized controlled trials. Arch Intern Med 1994; 154:1449–1457.

23. European Atrial Fibrillation Trial (EAFT) Study Group. Secondary prevention in non-rheumatic atrial fibrillation after transient ischaemic attack or minor stroke. Lancet 1993; 342:1255–1262.

24. Gulløv AL, Koefoed BG, Petersen P, et al. Fixed minidose warfarin and aspirin alone and in combination vs adjusted-dose warfarin for stroke prevention in atrial fibrillation. Second Copenhagen Atrial Fibrillation, Aspirin, and Anticoagulation Study. Arch Intern Med 1998; 158:1513–1521.

25. Lévy S, Maarek M, Coumel P, et al. Characterization of different subsets of atrial fibrillation in general practice in France. The ALFA Study. Circulation 1999; 99: 3028–3035.
26. The Atrial Fibrillation Follow-up Investigation of Rhythm Management (AFFIRM) Investigators. A comparison of rate control and rhythm control in patients with atrial fibrillation. N Engl J Med 2002; 347:1825–1833.
27. Van den Berg MP, Hassink RJ, Tuinenburg AE, et al. Quality of life in patients with paroxysmal atrial fibrillation and its predictors: importance of the autonomic nervous system. Eur Heart J 2001; 22:247–253.
28. Humphries KH, Kerr CR, Connolly SJ, et al. New-onset atrial fibrillation. Sex differences in presentation, treatment and outcome. Circulation 2001; 103:2365–2370.
29. Dorian P, Jung W, Newman D, et al. The impairment of health-related quality of life in patients with intermittent atrial fibrillation: implications for the assessment of investigational therapy. J Am Coll Cardiol 2000; 36:1303–1309.
30. Crijns HJGM, Tjeerdsma G, de Kam PJ, et al. Prognostic value of the presence and development of atrial fibrillation in patients with advanced chronic heart failure. Eur Heart J 2000; 21:1238–1245.
31. Middlekauff HR, Stevenson WG, Stevenson LW. Prognostic significance of atrial fibrillation in advanced heart failure. A study of 390 patients. Circulation 1991; 84:40–48.
32. Waktare JEP, Camm AJ. Acute treatment of atrial fibrillation: why and when to maintain sinus rhythm. Am J Cardiol 1998; 81 (5A):3C–15C.
33. Kerr CR, Talajic M, Connolly SJ, et al. Recurrence of atrial fibrillation following its initial diagnosis: follow-up of the Canadian Registry of Atrial Fibrillation. American Heart Association 1999 (abstract 1497)
34. Al-Khatib SM, Wilkinson WE, Sanders LL, et al. Observations on the transition from intermittent to permanent atrial fibrillation. Am Heart J 2000:140; 142–145.
35. Kamath S, Blann AD, Lip GYH. Platelets and atrial fibrillation. Eur Heart J 2001; 22: 2233–2242.
36. Shinbane JS, Wood MA, Jensen DN, et al. Tachycardia-induced cardiomyopathy: a review of animal models and clinical studies. J Am Coll Cardiol 1997; 29:709–715.
37. Charon P, Himbert J, Lenegre J. Les insuffances cardiaques aiguës de la fibrillation auriculaire. Arch Mal Coeur 1968; 61: 1772–1784.
38. Grogan M, Smith HC, Gersh BJ, et al. Left ventricular dysfunction due to atrial fibrillation in patients initially believed to have idiopathic dilated cardiomyopathy. Am J Cardiol 1992;69:1570–1573.
39. Redfield MM, Kay GN, Jenkins LS, et al Tachycardia-related cardiomyopathy: a common cause of ventricular dysfunction in patients with atrial fibrillation referred for atrioventricular ablation. Mayo Clin Proc 2000; 75:790–795.

CHAPTER 6

Syncope

Aleksandras Laucevičius PhD FESC FACC

Vilnius University Hospital, Vilnius, Lithuania

Vytautas Abraitis MD

Vilnius University Hospital, Vilnius, Lithuania

> Syncope is a symptom,
> not a disease
> It is defined as a transient and
> self-limited loss of consciousness

DEFINITION

Syncope is a symptom, not a disease. It is defined as a transient and self-limited loss of consciousness. Syncope is associated with the absence of postural tone and usually leads to falling. The onset is relatively rapid and recovery is usually prompt, spontaneous and complete. The immediate cause of syncope development is a global cerebral hypoperfusion. The cerebral hypoperfusion being temporary, the restoration of consciousness is usually complete, including appropriate behavior and full orientation.

Syncope can be a sign of dangerous heart disease but in most cases it is benign. Nevertheless, injuries associated with syncopal attacks may occur in 35% of patients, and recurrent episodes can be psychologically devastating.[1]

When evaluating a patient after an episode of loss of consciousness there are several key questions to be answered: was it real or apparent transient loss of consciousness; was it syncope or a non-syncopal attack?

It is important to recognize that syncope and sudden cardiac death (SCD) are two different entities, however patients with cardiac syncope have a very high incidence of subsequent SCD (approximately 24%).[2] Patients in whom cardiopulmonary resuscitation or electric or pharmacological cardioversion have been required in restoring consciousness should be considered as having experienced sudden death but not syncope. On the other hand apart from true syncope one can encounter a syncope-resembling episode.

> Syncope can be a sign of dangerous heart disease but in most cases it is benign

PATHOPHYSIOLOGY

Transitory global cerebral hypoperfusion, manifested in syncope, can be caused by several basic underlying disturbances, including decreased cardiac output (tachyarrhythmias, bradyarrhythmias, absolute hypovolemia or relative hypovolemia because of blood pooling, intracardiac blood flow disturbances, etc.) and decreased peripheral arterial resistance. Such mechanisms of transitory hypoperfusion as obstruction to cerebral blood flow or increased intracerebral vascular resistance may play an additional role.

EPIDEMIOLOGY

Syncope is a relatively common clinical problem. As reported, the incidence of syncope over 26 years in the general population was 3% in men and 3.5% in women in Framingham study.[3] The causes of syncope differ between men and women — men more often than women have a cardiac cause for syncope.[4] Approximately one-third of individuals are likely to experience an episode of syncope during their lifetime.[2] Frequency of isolated syncopal episodes increasing with age was observed in the original cohort of patients from the Framingham study, who were followed for 26 years: the annual prevalence increased from below 10 per 1000 in those younger than 45 years up to over 30 in women and over 50 in men in the over 75-year age group.[3] In over 75% of cases in non-elderly subjects, syncope occurs as an isolated event. Data from several reports showed that 3–5% of all emergency room admissions and 1–3% of all hospital admissions were for syncope.[2,5]

RISK FACTORS FOR SYNCOPE

Risk factors for syncope in a community-based population were examined during a 20-year period in the Framingham Heart Study.[6]

CAUSES OF SYNCOPE

Several conditions may underlie a syncopal episode. Syncope may be a manifestation of

Key points

Predictors of syncope include

- a history of stroke or transient ischemic attack
- use of cardiac medications
- high blood pressure
- lower body mass index
- increased alcohol intake
- diabetes or elevated blood glucose level

neurally-mediated reflex syncopal syndromes, inadequate orthostatic reactions, cardiac arrhythmias, structural cardiopulmonary disease or malfunction of cerebrovascular system.

Determining the cause of syncope is important for both prognostic and therapeutic reasons. The listing of possible causes is provided below.

Cardiovascular:

- cardiac arrhythmias
  - sinus node dysfunction (including bradycardia-tachycardia syndrome)
  - atrioventricular (AV) conduction system disease
  - paroxysmal supraventricular tachycardia (SVT) and ventricular tachycardia (VT)
  - inherited syndromes (e.g., long QT syndrome, Brugada syndrome)
  - implanted device [pacemaker, implantable cardioverter device (ICD)] malfunction
  - drug-induced proarrhythmias;
- structural cardiac or cardiopulmonary disease
  - cardiac valvular disease
  - acute myocardial infarction/ischemia
  - obstructive cardiomyopathy
  - atrial myxoma
  - acute aortic dissection
  - pericardial disease/tamponade
  - pulmonary embolus/pulmonary hypertension;
- cerebrovascular origin
  - vascular steal syndromes.

Non-cardiovascular:

- neurally-mediated reflex (neurocardiogenic) syncopal syndromes
  - vasovagal faint (common faint)

  - carotid sinus syncope;
- situational faint
  - acute hemorrhage
  - cough, sneeze
  - gastrointestinal stimulation (swallow, defecation, visceral pain)
  - micturition (post micturition)
  - post exercise
  - others (e.g., brass instrument playing, weightlifting, postprandial); glossopharyngeal and trigeminal neuralgia

Orthostatic:

- autonomic failure
  - primary autonomic failure syndromes (e.g., pure autonomic failure, multiple system atrophy, Parkinson's disease with autonomic failure)
  - secondary autonomic failure syndromes (e.g., diabetic neuropathy, amyloid neuropathy);
- drugs and alcohol;
- volume depletion
  - hemorrhage, diarrhea, Addison's disease.

Sometimes there is more than one cause leading to the development of syncope. Especially in the elderly the development of syncope is often the result of interplay of physiological changes of aging, comorbidities and medication for the treatment of comorbid diseases.

Cardiovascular causes of syncope

Syncope resulting from cardiovascular disease (CVD) may be due to severely obstructed blood flow, such as in aortic stenosis and hypertrophic obstructive cardiomyopathy, as well as in cases of impaired left ventricular function or cardiac arrhythmias.[7]

Cardiovascular disease with blood flow obstruction

Syncope may be caused by the obstruction of blood flow, which is most frequently due to aortic stenosis or hypertrophic cardiomyopathy and less commonly due to atrial myxomas, pulmonic stenosis, primary pulmonary hypertension and pulmonary embolism.

Aortic stenosis: Although these patients rarely present with syncope, the combination of aortic stenosis and syncope can be associated with increased mortality. Syncope in these patients is associated with exertion or arrhythmia (bradyarrhythmia, paroxysmal atrial fibrillation or ventricular tachyarrhythmia).

Hypertrophic cardiomyopathy: Hypertrophic cardiomyopathy is associated with syncope, which occurs in up to 30% of patients with dynamic outflow obstruction.[8] The obstruction may intensify with exertion, postural changes, hypovolemia, drugs or tachyarrhythmia.

Cardiac arrhythmias

Key points
Most common arrhythmic causes of syncope
Sinus bradycardia
AV nodal block
Sustained VT
Pacemaker malfunction
SVT (rather rare)

Brady- or tachyarrhythmias are common causes of syncope when other causes cannot be found.[9] The most common arrhythmic causes of syncope include sinus bradycardia, AV nodal block, sustained VT, and SVT. Pacemaker malfunction with cardiac pauses is another possible cause of syncope.

Sinus bradycardia: Syncope resulting from sinus bradyarrhythmia may be caused by intrinsic sinus node disease (sick sinus syndrome, tachy-brady syndrome), drugs (beta-blockers, diltiazem, verapamil, digoxin), or autonomic imbalance (high vagal or decreased sympathetic tone). Syncope due to sinus bradycardia is

diagnosed when sinus bradycardia of < 40 beats per min (bpm) or repetitive sinoatrial blocks or sinus pauses lasting > 3 s are documented. The following findings during the electrophysiological (EP) testing are suggested as being causally related to syncope: sinus node recovery time > 2 s or corrected sinus node recovery time of >1000 ms.

Atrioventricular block: The second degree type II or third degree AV blocks can result in syncope. In general, first degree and type I (Wenckebach) second degree AV block are benign and should not be a cause of syncope. Alternating left and right bundle branch block also can be accepted as a possible cause of syncope.

Ventricular tachycardia: Sustained VT (monomorphic or polymorphic) is associated with syncope in only about 10% of patients. It is likely that recurrent syncope will be prevented if the arrhythmia is successfully treated. Syncope resulting from sustained VT is most commonly due to structural heart disease (coronary heart disease, hypertrophic cardiomyopathy, dilated cardiomyopathy and right ventricular dysplasia). An unusual form of VT, torsade de pointes, may cause syncope in patients with either the congenital or acquired long QT syndrome. Ventricular fibrillation does not cause syncope but can result in sudden cardiac death if not resuscitated.

Ventricular bigeminy: Ventricular bigeminy may result in hypotension, bradycardia, and syncope. This is seen in patients with an underlying heart disease: sinus bradycardia, advanced heart disease and significant left ventricular dysfunction.

Supraventricular tachyarrhythmias (SVT): Supraventricular tachyarrhythmias are rarely a cause of syncope. Regular SVTs are more often a cause of syncope than disorganized supraventricular rhythms (atrial fibrillation), however either can cause presyncope or syncope in patients with severe left ventricular hypertrophy, ventricular outflow obstruction, and in ventricular pre-excitation syndromes due to rapid antegrade AV conduction when the high ventricular response rate occurs.

NON-SYNCOPAL ATTACK

As already mentioned, not every episode of transitory loss of consciousness can be called syncope. Causes of such non-syncopal attacks should be taken into consideration during differential diagnostics. Most common causes of non-syncopal attacks are listed below:

- disorders with impairment or loss of consciousness
  - metabolic disorders including hypoglycemia, hypoxia, hyperventilation with hypocapnia. In such cases, syncope is probably secondary to metabolic effects on cerebrovascular tone
  - epilepsy
  - intoxications (including alcoholic)
  - vertebro-basilar transient ischemic attack;
- disorders resembling syncope without loss of consciousness
  - cataplexy
  - drop attacks
  - psychogenic 'syncope' (somatization disorders, hysteria, conversion reaction).

While differentiating syncope from non-syncopal attack it is worth taking into account the presence of conditions, associated with higher incidence of syncope, or so called risk factors for syncope, mentioned above. Among the risk factors for syncope there are variety of drugs which can provoke the development of syncope. Those being encountered more frequently are listed below:

- antihypertensive agents
  - alpha, beta-blockers
  - calcium channel blockers
  - ACE inhibitors
- nitrates, molsidomine
- antiarrhythmics (because of proarrhythmia, suppression of sinus node function, and exacerbation of conduction disturbances)
- psychotherapeutic drugs
- hypoglycemic agents
- alcohol

It is worth remembering, that identification of a condition does not always have a causal relationship with occurrence of syncope. Underlying heart disease is a cause of cardiac syncope in less than half of such patients, whereas absence of heart disease most often points to neurally-mediated syncope.

RECURRENCE OF SYNCOPE

In majority of patients (40–85%) syncope does not recur, even if untreated. Despite varying etiologies and therapies, the recurrence rate of syncope is quite similar:[10]

- 31% for patients with cardiovascular etiology;
- 36% for those with noncardiovascular cause;
- 43% for those with syncope of unknown etiology.

Thus, the absence of recurrence may simply reflect the natural history of the underlying cause and not the efficacy of treatment. Although recurrences do not predict mortality or sudden death, they may cause substantial morbidity, especially due to injury and fractures.

On the other hand, if syncope does recur, the frequency with which it will recur can be predicted. Among the patients with neurocardiogenic syncope, the time between a tilt table test and a recurrent syncopal episode predicted the frequency of syncope during a 6.5-year follow-up.[11] The frequency was 1.35 episodes per month when the first recurrence was within 1 month of a tilt table test, whereas the observed recurrence rate was 0.12 episodes per month when the first recurrence was more than 1 month after the tilt table test.

PROGNOSIS

Mortality

Although the recurrence rate of syncope does not depend on the underlying cause, the mortality rate does. The prognosis of a patient with syncope is not associated with symptoms, but is directly related to the underlying etiology. An overall reported mortality and major morbidity rate is over 7%, but among patients with an underlying cardiac cause of syncope, the reported 1-year mortality rate ranges from 18% to 33%.[2,12,13,14] As a result, patients can be categorized into different risk categories based upon the cause of syncope.

Overall, when the initial evaluation (medical history, physical exam, electrocardiogram (ECG) and blood pressure (BP) both supine and upright) reveals structural heart disease (independently of the cause of syncope), the prognosis is poor. On the other hand, excellent prognosis can be predicted for young, healthy individuals with a normal ECG, for individuals with neurally-mediated syncope, with orthostatic hypotension and with unexplained syncope.

Cardiovascular causes (organic heart disease or arrhythmia)

Patients with an underlying cardiovascular cause of syncope have higher risk of SCD than those with a non-cardiovascular cause of syncope. The mortality rate in patients with CVD largely depends on severity of the underlying disease and approaches 50% in 5 years, with a 30% incidence of death in the first year.[2,15,16] It is difficult to know whether syncope or SCD independently contribute to prognosis since such patients also have other associated chronic diseases. Long-term prognosis of the patients with and without syncope who were admitted to an intensive care unit is independent of syncope but is dependent upon the underlying disease.[3] Similarly, data from the Framingham study show that patients with cardiovascular disease and syncope had the same mortality rate as those with equivalent cardiovascular disease but without syncope.[17] Patients with coronary artery disease who do not have arrhythmia induced at EP study have a low risk of ventricular tachyarrhythmias or sudden death.

Non-cardiovascular causes (neurocardiogenic or vasovagal; situational, orthostatic, iatrogenic)

Patients with a non-cardiovascular cause of syncope usually have more favorable prognosis and lower incidence of mortality (about 6% or less in the first year).[18] This group includes some CVDs. Vasovagal syncope, for example, which is often considered a non-cardiovascular cause, is a cardiovascular reflex. In some of the patients orthostatic or iatrogenic syncope can be associated with malignant prognosis.

Unknown causes

The mortality for those patients in whom the cause is unknown (syncope of unknown etiology, comprising up to 50% of patients presented to the hospital because of syncope)[2] is approximately 5% during the first year. Although the mortality is largely due to underlying comorbidity, such patients continue to be at risk for physical injury, and may encounter employment and lifestyle restrictions.

Secondary trauma

The risk for secondary trauma is relatively high: rate of occurrence is 16–35% for injuries, 30% for minor injuries, 5–7% for fractures, and 1% for traffic accidents.[2,14]

Quality of life

The impact of syncope on the quality of patient's life can be profound. Many patients with recurrent, unexplained syncope may find the condition debilitating. Apart from the susceptibility to secondary injury, such patients often suffer from anxiety or depression, may be unable to perform their job or drive a vehicle. The reported proportion of affected patients was about 70% for anxiety or depression and for daily life activities, about 60% for driving and physical activities, 37% for employment and about 30% for sexual function and close social relationships.[19,20] Patients and their families are desperate to find out what is wrong with them and will do almost anything to get to the answer. The 'costs' of impaired quality of life are carried by both the payers' and the patients' 'budgets'.

EVALUATION

Evaluation of a patient with syncope is the same as that for presyncope, which encompasses the prodromal symptoms of lightheadedness and dizziness. The clinical features associated with the syncopal event are extremely important, the significance of every feature having been meticulously analyzed.[1,21] However, no symptoms are predictive of the 1-year mortality or recurrent syncope. Patients with syncope in whom a significant injury occurs have a higher mortality rate.

Patient history

> **Common causes of syncope elicited by patient history**
>
> Vasovagal syncope:
> Known precipitating events such as fear, severe pain, emotional distress, instrumentation and prolonged standing
>
> Situational syncope:
> If syncope occurs during or immediately after urination, defecation, coughing or swallowing
>
> Orthostatic syncope:
> Documentation of orthostatic hypotension associated with syncope or presyncope
>
> Older patients:
> Syncope after vasodilating medication

There are several signs and symptoms, which should be considered during the initial evaluation, which may yield the diagnosis or guide the direction of further investigations. These include:

- prior to attack
  - position (supine, sitting or standing)
  - activity (no, during or after exercise)
  - situation (urination, defecation, cough or swallowing)
  - predisposing factors (e.g., crowded or warm places, prolonged standing, postprandial period)
  - precipitating events (e.g., fear, intense pain, neck movements);
- onset of attack
  - occurrence of nausea, vomiting, feeling of cold, sweating, aura, pain in neck or shoulders;
- during the attack
  - skin color (pallor, cyanotic)
  - duration of loss of consciousness
  - movements (tonic, clonic, etc.)
  - tongue biting;
- end of attack
  - presence of nausea, vomiting, diaphoresis, feeling of cold, confusion, muscle aches, skin color, wounds;
- background
  - number and duration of syncopes
  - family history of arrhythmogenic disease
  - presence of cardiac disease
  - neurological history (Parkinson's disease, epilepsy, narcolepsy)
  - other relevant diseases (diabetes, etc.)
  - medication (hypotensive and antidepressant agents).

Vasovagal syncope should be suspected if precipitating events such as fear, severe pain, emotional distress, instrumentation and prolonged standing are associated with typical prodromal symptoms.

Situational syncope should be suspected if syncope occurs during or immediately after urination, defecation, coughing or swallowing.

Orthostatic syncope should be suspected when there is documentation of orthostatic hypotension (as already described) associated with syncope or presyncope.

Evaluation of older patients with syncope should include morning orthostatic blood pressure measurement and both supine and upright carotid sinus massage unless contraindicated.

Number of syncope episodes should be elucidated. Benign causes of syncope are usually associated with a single syncopal episode or with several episodes over the years. Patient with multiple episodes over a short period of time is more likely to suffer from a serious underlying disease.

Symptoms occurring in association with syncope can point toward a specific cause:

- dyspnea may suggest an acute pulmonary embolism;
- angina frequently indicates an underlying cardiac cause;
- history of focal neurological abnormalities favors a neurological origin;
- nausea, vomiting, diaphoresis, and pallor after an episode suggest high vagal tone;
- urination and defecation suggest a seizure or autonomic disorder;
- syncope accompanied by abnormal movements suggest a seizure but may also occur due to cerebral hypoxia.

Prodrome, pre-existing and concomitant conditions: vasovagal (neurocardiogenic) syncope is usually, but not always, associated with a prodrome of dizziness, nausea, pallor or diaphoresis. 'Auras' are associated with seizures and epilepsy. The sudden loss of consciousness without warning is most likely to result from an arrhythmia. Coughing, eating, drinking cold liquid, urinating and defecating can all cause syncope — these usually are situational syncopes. A vagal 'surge' immediately upon swallowing or after venous puncture can cause bradycardia and hypotension in predisposed patients. Postprandial hypotension may also reflect inadequate sympathetic compensation to meal-induced splanchnic pooling.

Coexisting illnesses can predispose a patient to syncope or can favor a specific cause. Patients with psychiatric illness may have syncope secondary to hyperventilation or panic attacks. Syncope in a patient with diabetes mellitus may result from orthostatic hypotension secondary to autonomic neuropathy. Medications can cause syncope, especially antiarrhythmic (proarrhythmic effects) and antihypertensive agents (orthostatic hypotension). Exertional syncope is always dangerous and can be associated with ventricular tachyarrhythmia or ventricular outflow tract obstruction.

Position during the syncope onset: vasovagal (neurocardiogenic) syncope commonly occurs when the patient is erect and very rarely while supine. Syncope resulting from orthostatic hypotension is frequently associated with the change from a supine to erect posture. In comparison, syncope that occurs when the patient is supine suggests an arrhythmia.

Duration of symptoms and recovery may help differentiating syncope from non-syncopal attack. A prolonged loss of consciousness may indicate epilepsy. Arrhythmias and vasovagal syncope are often associated with a brief period of syncope and the supine position reestablishes blood flow to the brain and restores the consciousness. This sequence of events can occur even if the arrhythmia is maintained. Significant neurological changes or confusion during the recovery period may be due to a stroke or seizures.

Witnessing (usually relatives) of the syncope usually describes how the loss of consciousness looked (any associated limb movements, the presence or absence of pallor or diaphoresis, etc.). Information regarding the presence or absence of a pulse is also of great diagnostic importance.

Patient's age: vasovagal syncope often occurs in young, otherwise healthy patients. However, syncope resulting from the long QT syndrome or hypertrophic cardiomyopathy can also occur in young individuals. Syncope of elderly subjects more frequently is of multifactorial origin.

Initial evaluation

Blood pressure, pulse and breathing rates should be obtained. Blood pressure measurements obtained in the supine, sitting and erect position may help to detect orthostatic hypotension. The latter is diagnosed when, within 2–5 min of quiet standing, one or more of the following is present:

- at least a 20 mmHg fall in systolic pressure;
- at least a 10 mmHg fall in diastolic pressure;
- symptoms of cerebral hypoperfusion occur.

The heart rate may be rapid or slow due to a number of possible rhythm disturbances, or irregular due to atrial fibrillation. Hyperventilation can be seen with pulmonary embolism or psychogenic causes of syncope.

Cardiac auscultation may reveal the murmur of aortic stenosis, hypertrophic obstructive cardiomyopathy, pulmonic stenosis or atrial myxoma. Pulmonary arterial hypertension may be suggested by a loud, palpable P_2. Increase in an outflow murmur with the Valsalva maneuver may help diagnose hypertrophic cardiomyopathy.

Neurological status should be evaluated. Unilateral abnormalities found upon neurological examination may reflect a cerebral vascular accident. Patients with frequent recurrent syncope also presenting a variety of other somatic complaints and raising concerns for anxiety, stress or other possible mental disturbances should undergo a psychiatric evaluation.

ECGs can be helpful diagnosing several possible underlying causes of syncope:

- sinus bradycardia;
- AV nodal disease (second or third degree heart block);
- His-Purkinje system disease (Mobitz type II AV block);
- bundle branch and/or fascicular block;
- prolonged QT interval (may favor torsade de pointes VT);
- Wolff-Parkinson-White syndrome;
- myocardial infarction;
- chronic obstructive pulmonary disease (overload of right-sided heart chambers).

Although the cause of syncope is rarely assigned following the ECG, it is a valuable test in guiding the direction of further evaluation.

Gastrointestinal bleeding should be ruled out. A positive stool blood test generally indicates gastrointestinal blood loss, which can result sequentially in anemia due to chronic blood loss, hypovolemia, orthostatic hypotension and syncope.

The following findings after obtaining patient's history and initial evaluation are accepted as diagnostic and no further testing is required unless other possible causes are considered upon the recurrence of syncope:

- if fear, emotional distress, prolonged standing, instrumentation or severe pain is associated with occurrence of typical prodromal symptoms, vasovagal syncope is diagnosed;
- if syncope develops during or shortly after urination, defecation, swallowing or coughing, situational syncope is diagnosed;
- documentation of orthostatic hypotension associated with syncope or presyncope enables diagnosing of orthostatic syncope;
- arrhythmia is accepted as a cause of syncope upon the following findings on the ECG:
  - rapid paroxysmal SVT or VT
  - sinus bradycardia below 40 bpm
  - repetitive sinoatrial blocks or sinus pauses lasting for over 3 s
  - type II second degree (Mobitz II) or third degree AV block
  - alternating right and left bundle branch block
  - cardiac pauses caused by malfunction of pacemaker.

Further testing

Useful examinations in the work-up of syncope

Carotid sinus massage

Tilt testing

Holter/loop monitoring

Electrophysiological study

Exercise stress testing

Echocardiogram

As there are no specific tests or testing for syncope, the initial evaluation of the patient provides the largest diagnostic yield of 52%. Laboratory tests elucidate the cause of another 14% of syncopes. Despite extensive testing, the cause of up to 34% of syncopal episodes remains initially unidentified, the percentage probably decreasing to an estimated 8% to 23% after the tilt table testing.

Should initial work-up fail establishing the probable cause of syncope, further diagnostic examinations should be performed. Useful examinations (when indicated) include carotid sinus massage, tilt testing, echocardiogram, Holter/loop monitoring, EP test, and exercise stress testing. One should keep in mind that some tests [including electroencephalography (EEG), computerized tomography (CT) and magnetic nuclear resonance (MNR), carotid Doppler sonography, ventricular signal-averaged electrocardiogram (SAECG), coronary angiography, and pulmonary scintigraphy] are almost never useful in establishing the cause of syncope. Expenses associated with testing for cause of syncope have been calculated. The calculated costs per diagnosis made were (in ascending order): external loop recorder ($529 per diagnosis), tilt test ($1024), Holter monitoring ($1562), internal loop recorder ($5586), EP study in patient with structural heart disease ($7044), echocardiography ($34 433), and EP study in patient without structural heart disease ($73 260).[22]

Further testing of patient after an episode of syncope is largely dependent upon the presence or absence of a heart disease. In case of certain or suspected heart disease one should proceed with cardiac evaluation (echocardiogram, Holter monitoring, exercise testing, EP study, loop monitoring), whereas in the absence of such, further testing should be directed towards the elucidation of neurally-mediated cause of syncope [carotid sinus massage, tilt testing, adenosine triphosphate (ATP) test].

Ambulatory ECG monitoring for 24–48 h or patient activated event recording is commonly obtained in the assessment of syncope. Such techniques are of limited diagnostic value because they are useful only if symptoms occur during monitoring, which rarely occurs.[2,23] An asymptomatic arrhythmia does not prove an arrhythmic cause for syncope, whereas arrhythmia may be potentially excluded as a cause of syncope in cases of occurrence of syncope symptoms and no arrhythmia on the ambulatory ECG at that time. In general, ambulatory monitoring appears to establish a diagnosis in only 2–3% of patients.[2,24,25]

Ambulatory ECG monitoring to assess syncope possibly related to arrhythmia is currently recommended in patients with unexplained syncope or presyncope in whom the cause is not obvious. The value of monitoring could not be completely ruled out in patients with symptoms such as syncope or presyncope and palpitations in whom a probable cause other than an arrhythmia has been identified but in whom symptoms recur despite treatment of the previously identified cause.

Event recorders are more helpful than 24 h ambulatory ECG monitoring. Intermittent loop recorders may store several minutes of recording if the patient activates the device immediately upon regaining consciousness.[26]

Implantable recorders can record the ECG for over 1 year, storing events when the device is activated automatically by a rapid rate or manually with magnet application. When such a device is implanted in patient with syncope of uncertain cause, transient bradycardia is found to be responsible most frequently.[22,27] Still, in up to 40% of implantations arrhythmia can not be identified as a cause of syncope.[28]

Echocardiography may disclose underlying structural heart disease such as left ventricular dysfunction, hypertrophic cardiomyopathy, significant aortic stenosis, and myxoma.

EEG is traditionally obtained in patients with syncope but is rarely useful. It can, however, be helpful in ruling out epilepsy in patients with syncope who had seizure-like episode.

Exercise testing is frequently ordered in patients with cardiac disease and also has a role in patients with a history of exertion-related syncope or exercise-induced arrhythmias.[29] Exercise testing may be useful in patients with hypertrophic cardiomyopathy. The testing proves diagnostic in case of occurrence of syncope during or shortly after exercise and also in case of development of type II second degree (Mobitz II) or third degree AV block during the exercise.

Carotid sinus massage reveals carotid sinus hypersensitivity, which is present if a cardiac pause lasting for over 3 s or a fall in systolic blood pressure of more than 50 mmHg is being evoked. Carotid sinus hypersensitivity was elicited by carotid sinus massage in the supine position in 8.7% of those with unexplained syncope; when repeated during tilt table testing, carotid hypersensitivity was observed in 60%.[30] Similar results were noted in a report of 1149 patients over 55 years of age presenting with unexplained syncope.[31] Carotid hypersensitivity provoked by carotid sinus massage was found in 19%; in one-third of these patients, a response to carotid sinus massage was elicited only during tilt table testing. The sensitivity and specificity for a positive response were 100% and 74% respectively when supine; both values were 100% during tilt testing.

Upright tilt table test has become a commonly performed test for the evaluation of syncope, particularly in young, otherwise healthy patients in whom the diagnosis of vasovagal or neurocardiogenic syncope is often entertained.[32] It is also useful in older patients with suspected neurocardiogenic syncope.[33] Although till testing is widely mentioned in the context of work-up for determining the cause of a syncope, the very procedure of tilt testing varies. We favor the protocol of a tilt testing, which can be found in the following section.

Positive tilt table test is accepted as diagnostic in patients without structural heart disease, whereas in patients with structural heart disease the cardiac causes of syncope should be ruled out prior to accepting the positive tilt table test as indicative of neurally-mediated syncope.

Identification of late potentials by means of SAECG has a sensitivity of 80% and a specificity of 90% for the prediction of inducible sustained VT in patients with heart disease and syncope.[34,35] In situations where VT is a concern in a patient with structural heart disease and syncope, a SAECG is not the most appropriate test.

Patients with syncope in whom ventricular or supraventricular arrhythmias, left ventricular dysfunction, significant coronary heart disease, or other structural heart disease have been documented are candidates for *EP testing*.[9,36] EP testing also has an important role in the establishment of a diagnosis of syncope of unknown etiology, particularly (up to 70%) among patients with structural heart disease. Syncope associated with a ventricular tachyarrhythmia induced during an EP study indicates increased risk of death.

A prolonged sinus node recovery time or sinoatrial conduction time detected during EP studies may suggest sinus node dysfunction; however, a relationship with syncope must be established clinically to verify any possible causative association. Similarly, establishing a causal role in syncope for AV nodal dysfunction is difficult unless there is documented ECG evidence of high degree AV block.

The EP induction of an SVT associated with hypotension is presumptive evidence for the tachycardia as the cause for syncope.

Administration of ATP provokes a short and potent cardioinhibitory response of vagal origin. Since ATP has a depressant effect on the AV node, it may be of particular use in patients with syncope due to paroxysmal AV nodal block. The ATP and tilt tests may provide valuable information in different patient groups.[37,38]

Overall, the following tests should be considered as suggested by findings of initial patient's evaluation:

- If a metabolic cause of syncope or blood loss is suspected, basic laboratory tests are recommended.
- If structural heart disease is suspected, echocardiography and prolonged ECG monitoring should be performed. If these are non-diagnostic, EP study should be considered.
- Patients with syncope associated with ischemic chest pain should undergo stress testing, echocardiography and ECG monitoring
- Palpitations in association with syncope require ECG monitoring and echocardiography.
- Occurrence of syncope during or after physical exertion require echocardiographic evaluation and stress testing.
- If there is no suspicion of heart or neurological disease and syncope is recurrent, tilt testing is recommended. In older individuals this should be complemented by carotid sinus massage.
- If development of syncope is associated with neck turning, carotid sinus massage is recommended.

Tilt testing

Indications for tilt table testing

Recommendations concerning indications for diagnostic tilt testing are:

- single occurrence of unexplained syncope in high risk settings (e.g. possibly resulting in physical injury or with occupational implications);

- recurrence of syncope after organic heart diseases have been ruled out;
- after cardiac causes of syncope have been excluded despite of the presence of organic heart disease;
- when the patient will benefit from demonstration of susceptibility to neurally-mediated syncope.

The tilt testing may also be considered provided that:

- an understanding of the hemodynamic pattern in syncope would alter the anticipated treatment;
- there is a necessity of differentiating syncope with seizure-like movements from fit of epilepsy;
- the patient is experiencing recurrent unexplained falls, presyncope or dizziness.

The tilt testing is not valuable for assessment of treatment effectiveness and is not reasonable when elucidation of a susceptibility to neurally-mediated syncope would not alter treatment. Also, the tilt testing would not be recommended after a single episode that did not lead to an injury and where the possibility of injury upon the recurrence of syncope is remote.

Tilt testing technique

The technique of tilt testing is illustrated with Fig. 6.1 and should be as follows:

- The test should be performed after at least 2 h of fasting.
- Pretilt for 5 min in the supine position is sufficient if vein is not cannulated (foreseeing drug provocation with nitroglycerin if required). If vein is to be cannulated, this should be followed by a 20 min supine rest.
- The angle of tilt should be between 60 and 70 degrees
- Passive testing phase should last for 20–45 min.
- If the passive phase has been negative, i.v. isoproterenol or sublingual

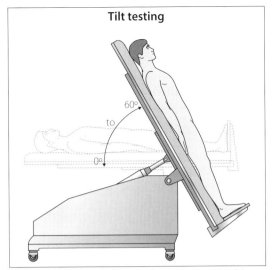

Tilt testing

Fig. 6.1 Tilt testing. Patient rest for 5 min on a tilt table should be followed by the inclination of the tilt table to 60–70 degrees for 20–45 min.

nitroglycerin for syncope provocation should be administered. Drug phase duration of 15–20 min in the upright position is recommended employing one of the two drug challenge regimens:

1. isoproterenol: incremental infusion rate starting with 1.0 µg/min and increased up to 3 µg/min in order to increase average heart rate by about 20–25% as compared to baseline value. The patient should remain tilted for the whole duration of the drug challenge.
2. Nitroglycerin – a fixed dose of 400 µg in spray should be administrated sublingually while patient remaining tilted.

The test is considered positive and terminated upon induction of syncope. If the planned duration of tilt including drug provocation is completed without development of syncope, the test is considered negative. Significance of presyncope occurring during the tilt testing is ambiguous.

Response to tilt table test

Physiology of head-up tilt includes displacement of blood from the intrathoracic vascular compartment to more dependent vascular structures. This results in drop of central venous pressure, cardiac stroke volume, and systemic arterial pressure. Normally, head-up tilt activates cardiovascular and cardiopulmonary reflexes resulting in vasoconstriction and both increased chronotropy and inotropy, which in turn restore systemic arterial pressure.

Classification of abnormal responses to tilt table testing:

- cardioinhibitory (mainly bradycardia, sinus, junctional, or AV nodal block, asystole);
- vasodepressor (marked hypotension without marked bradycardia);
- mixed: cardio-inhibitory + vasodepressor (hypotension with bradycardia).

HOSPITALIZATION

One of immediate questions to be answered at the emergency room after the episode of syncope is whether to hospitalize a patient. The hospitalization is recommended for either further testing or treatment in cases where initial evaluation raises the following concerns:

- suspected or known cardiac cause of a syncope (including arrhythmia suggested by patient history or ECG, family history of sudden death, signs of cardiac ischemia);
- stroke or other focal neurological disorder;
- presence of severe injury;
- need for pacemaker implantation

Key points
Hospitalization is recommended in cases suspected of
Cardiac cause of syncope (arrhythmia, family history of SCD, signs of ischemia)
Stroke
Presence of severe injury
Need for pacemaker implantation

MANAGEMENT

Metabolic or iatrogenic syncope

Metabolic abnormalities, anemia and hypovolemia can be effectively managed by correction of these abnormalities. In addition, iatrogenic syncope resulting from drug therapy is a treatable and preventable condition, especially in the elderly or in those with coexisting chronic diseases, and diminished or blunted cardiovascular reflexes. In this setting, such interventions as elimination of the drug or substitution with an alternative agent, changing the dose, or altering the timing of drug administration are usually effective.

Orthostatic hypotension

Orthostatic hypotension is due to volume depletion or autonomic neuropathy. Avoiding volume depletion and administration of beta-blockers and antidepressants are the first line measures. Tensing the legs by crossing them while actively standing on both legs is of major benefit as well. In one report of patients with autonomic neuropathy, this procedure raised the cardiac output by 16% and the systemic blood pressure by 13%.[39]

Other physical measures that may be helpful include:

- arising slowly in stages from supine to seated to standing;
- performing dorsiflexion of the feet or handgrip exercise before standing;
- wearing Jobst stockings, up to and including the thighs, to minimize venous pooling.

Should these measures prove insufficient in preventing further syncopes, medicamental treatment of orthostatic hypotension should be considered. These include:

- Fludrocortisone and high salt diet. The most common treatment is induction of volume expansion with a combination of fludrocortisone (an oral mineralocorticoid given in a dose of 0.1 mg/day to 1.0 mg/day) and a high salt diet. Patients must be carefully monitored for the development of edema or worsening of seated or supine hypertension. Long-term therapy with this drug, even when administered in low doses, is poorly tolerated in patients over the age of 65 years.[40] Furthermore, incremental doses may be needed over time because of escape from the sodium retaining effects of the mineralocorticoid.
- Midodrine (an alpha-1-adrenergic agonist) is used 2.5 mg to 10 mg t.i.d. and can be tried if fludrocortisone does not work or is not well tolerated.
- Phenylephrine may be administrated in dose of 60 mg every 6 to 12 h.
- Non-steroidal antiinflammatory drugs.
- Caffeine.
- Serotonin uptake inhibitors (fluoxetine).

Neurocardiogenic (neurally-mediated) syncope

Treatment of neurally-mediated syncope includes both drugs and non-medicamental measures. Volume expansion by liberalizing salt intake is encouraged, and occasionally fludrocortisone is prescribed (similar to the regimen used in treatment of orthostatic hypotension). The majority of patients are started on a cardioselective beta-blocker, such as metoprolol or atenolol. In younger patients with a high baseline vagal tone, as demonstrated by profound resting sinus bradycardia, beta-blocker with intrinsic sympathomimetic effect (pindolol, acebutolol) may be effective. An alternative agent disopyramide is often effective and well tolerated. The use of serotonin uptake inhibitors is reserved for symptomatic patients who do not respond to this regimen. Combinations of therapies may be necessary in conjunction with an AV sequential pacemaker in patients refractory to these therapies.

Drugs, which are most commonly used in patients with episodes of neurally-mediated syncope, are listed below, followed by some non-pharmacological measures.

Pharmacological measures

- Beta-blockers appear to act upon the ill-defined afferent limb of the reflex arc involved in the Bezold-Jarisch reflex. They also inhibit the discharge frequency of the C fibers originating from the cardiac mechanoreceptors and chemoreceptors. They are currently the most common and effective therapy for neurocardiogenic syncope, including those who have asystole with a tilt test.[41,42] In one study of 193 patients with syncope and a positive tilt test, oral beta-blockers were effective in 118 of 125 patients (94%) in whom repeat tilt testing was performed.[42] Long-term oral beta-blocker therapy was effective in preventing recurrent syncope in 90% of such patients at a mean follow-up of 28 months. The bradycardia that can result from beta-blockade does not increase the frequency of syncope. Beta-blockers with intrinsic sympathomimetic activity (pindolol, acebutolol) that maintain resting heart rate and blood pressure, may be of particular benefit in patients developing bradycardia or in patients who fail therapy with other beta-blockers.
- Disopyramide — anticholinergic, alpha-adrenergic, and negative inotropic — may be useful due to its negative inotropic (inhibition of myocardial mechanoreceptors) and anticholinergic properties.[43]
- Scopolamine may be useful because of its vagolytic properties that modify autonomic outflow.
- Theophylline, aminophylline and ephedrine may be effective, although their mechanism of action is not established. One of the possible explanations of their effectiveness is the maintenance of vessel tone in the presence of increased vagal activity.
- Vasoconstrictive substances (Midodrine, Etilephrine). Midodrine (5 mg t.i.d.), an alpha-1-adrenergic agonist, has had a beneficial effect on symptoms during head-up tilt and on symptom frequency during a short follow-up period.[44] This agent prevented syncopal episodes in 95% of previously untreated patients. Another study found that the drug was effective in 64% of patients who failed to respond to a beta-blocker.[45] Etilephrine (Effortil, 5–10 mg t.i.d.), an alpha-1, beta-1 and a weak beta-2 agonist, can be used in neurocardiogenic syncope as well. Vasoconstrictor drugs are potentially more effective in orthostatic hypotension caused by autonomic dysfunction than in the neurally-mediated syncopes.
- Serotonin uptake inhibitors (sertraline, fluoxetine or paroxetine) act at the level of the central nervous system, but it is unclear if they act on the afferent or efferent limb of the reflex arc.[46,47]

Non-pharmacological measures

- The North American Vasovagal Pacemaker Study (VPS) revealed the significant reduction in the incidence of recurrent syncope with dual-chamber pacing (22% versus 70% for no pacemaker, $p < 0.00002$) and a significant increase in the time to first syncope (112 versus 54 days) in 54 patients with syncope studied.[48] It seems important to document whether the predominant cause of symptoms is cardioinhibitory (bradycardia) or vasodepressor (hypotension) in origin because therapy will differ. It appears that dual-chamber permanent pacing is appropriate and should eliminate most, if not all, symptoms in patients with a pure cardioinhibitory response. In contrast, patients with pure vasodepression should be treated with drugs and compressive stockings. In the patient with a mixed response with a significant vasodepressor component, dual-chamber permanent pacing can blunt the vasodepressor-related symptoms.[49] Permanent implantation of pacemaker could be considered when hypersensitive cardioinhibitory response is demonstrated, syncope is recurrent, and clear provocative events are not elucidated or when the EP study demonstrates major abnormalities of sinus node function or AV conduction in patients with unexplained syncope.

- Orthostatic training program may help those young patients with neurocardiogenic syncope who respond to medical therapy poorly. Orthostatic training may be an effective approach in this group.[50] One of the evaluated training methods includes five in-hospital upright tilt table studies (the duration of the study was initially 10 min and was increased by 10 min each day up to 50 min), continued by the standing against a wall for up to 40 min twice a day at home. After a mean follow-up of 18 months, almost all patients of the training group became tilt-negative (96% versus 26% of the control group); none of the trained patients had spontaneous recurrent syncope, while 57% of controls experienced a recurrent episode.
- Driving restrictions should be considered because the potential for car accident and injury is a concern.
- Other measures include volume expansion by liberalizing and encouraging salt intake. Newer therapeutic agents are also being evaluated. One study, for example, has suggested the use of methylphenidate in refractory patients.[51] This agent shares some properties with the amphetamines: it is a peripheral vasoconstrictor and stimulates the central nervous system.

Carotid sinus hypersensitivity

Carotid sinus hypersensitivity is often considered to be a variant of neurocardiogenic syncope and many of the same therapies have been used. Pacemakers are of benefit for patients with only cardioinhibitory responses but are not effective for patients with a vasodepressor response. Implantation of pacemaker is indicated if light pressure on the carotid sinus induces ventricular asystole lasting for over 3 s in the absence of any medication that depresses the sinus node or AV conduction in the setting of recurrent carotid sinus pressure induced syncope.

The serotonin uptake inhibitors have been helpful for patients with syncope due to carotid sinus hypersensitivity in several small series.[52]

Situational vasovagal syncope

In situational vasovagal syncope, the most frequently effective action is avoidance of triggers responsible for syncope. Many such patients experience warning symptoms of variable duration. In this setting, they should be advised to assume a supine position with legs raised at the onset of such symptoms. In some patients, treatment with fludrocortisone, aminophylline, theophylline, support stockings, or ephedrine may also be helpful.

Cardiovascular disease with obstruction

Cardiac diseases that obstruct the flow of blood generally require surgical correction or attenuation of the obstruction. As an example, aortic valve replacement for aortic stenosis will alleviate symptoms, prevent syncope and prolong survival. Dynamic outflow obstruction resulting from hypertrophic cardiomyopathy is treated pharmacologically with beta-blockers or calcium channel blockers. The use of right ventricular pacing, alcoholic septum ablation, surgical myomectomy and mitral valve replacement also may be effective in this setting.

Patients with advanced heart failure due to non-ischemic cardiomyopathy who also have syncope, regardless of the cause, have a high 1-year risk of sudden death (45% versus 12% in those without syncope in one series).[7] The possible efficacy of an ICD in this group was evaluated in a small study of 14 patients with a non-ischemic cardiomyopathy, unexplained syncope and a negative EP test.[53] After ICD implantation, 50% had an appropriate shock for a sustained ventricular arrhythmia during a mean follow-up of 24 months. In a comparison group of 19 patients with non-ischemic cardiomyopathy, who had an ICD implanted because of a cardiac arrest, the incidence of appropriate shocks was 42% during a 45-month follow-up. The mortality of those receiving an ICD for syncope and a cardiac arrest was the same (28% and 32%). Another study of 147 patients with non-ischemic cardiomyopathy, unexplained syncope, and no prior history of a sustained ventricular tachyarrhythmia or cardiac arrest found that the actuarial survival at 2 years was higher among the 25 patients treated with an ICD than in the 122 patients managed with conventional medical therapy (85% versus 67%); 40% of those receiving an ICD experienced an appropriate shock.[54]

Arrhythmias

Ventricular arrhythmias

Patients with syncope due to a documented VT that is inducible during an EP evaluation or those with unexplained syncope and inducible ventricular arrhythmias are usually candidates for antiarrhythmic drug therapy guided by this technique. Additional therapeutic options in patients with documented or inducible ventricular arrhythmias include an ICD, radiofrequency ablation, and EP guided surgery. The outcome with an ICD is the same in patients with syncope and no documented VT/VF and those with documented VT/VF. As an example, one study compared the outcome with an ICD in 178 patients with unexplained syncope and no documented VT, but arrhythmia that was induced, and 568 patients with documented VT/VF. Recurrent syncope was associated with a ventricular tachyarrhythmia in most patients in both groups (85% and 92% for the VT/VF group).[55] At 2 years, the actuarial probability of appropriate ICD therapy (55% and 58%) and the actuarial survival was equivalent (91% and 93%).

However, regardless of therapy, some studies have found that the mortality remains high in these patients. In one study of 67 patients with coronary heart disease and syncope, 29 of whom had monomorphic VT induced during EP studies and then received an ICD, the total mortality in patients with inducible VT was significantly higher compared to those who did not have VT; the 1- and 2-year survival rates were 77% and 45% versus 94% and 84% for those without VT.[56]

Currently the implantation of an ICD for syncope-associated arrhythmia is indicated in cases of documented syncopal VT or VF and in cases of undocumented syncope in the setting of previous myocardial infarction and inducible sustained monomorphic VT (both are class I indications).

Patients with the congenital long QT syndrome often respond to beta-blockers, although in some patients stellate ganglion ablation or an ICD are necessary.

Supraventricular arrhythmias

Although supraventricular arrhythmias can be treated with antiarrhythmic drugs, radio frequency ablation has become a preferred therapy for the majority of such arrhythmias, especially those that involve the AV node or an accessory pathway. Surgery or antitachycardia pacemakers are infrequently used.

Bradycardia due to conduction abnormalities

Permanent pacemaker implantation is indicated when sinus node dysfunction or a high grade AV block is the documented cause for syncope. In some cases, however, a permanent pacemaker is used empirically when the EP study strongly suggests a conduction abnormality as the cause for syncope. In addition to general guidelines for pacemaker implantation, patients with syncope should be treated with a pacemaker if:

- bifascicular or trifascicular disease is present on the baseline electrocardiogram; and
- a prolonged His-ventricular (HV) interval or infranodal block occurs during atrial pacing, or there is evidence of significant AV nodal disease uncovered during EP testing.

References

1. Olshansky B. Evaluation of the patient with syncope. Up To Date v10.1 (CD-ROM). Up To Date, Wellesley 2001.
2. Kapoor WN. Evaluation and outcome of patients with syncope. Medicine 1990; 69:160–175.
3. Savage DD, Corwin L, McGee DL, et al. Epidemiologic features of isolated syncope: The Framingham study. Stroke 1985; 16:626–628.
4. Freed LA, Eagle KA, Mahjoub ZA, et al. Gender differences in presentation, management, and cardiac event-free survival in patients with syncope. Am J Cardiol 1997; 80:1183–1187.
5. Manolis AS, Linzer M, Salem D. Syncope: current diagnostic evaluation and management. Ann Intern Med 1990; 112:850–863.
6. Chen L, Chen MH, Larson MG, et al. Risk factors for syncope in a community-based sample (the Framingham Heart Study). Am J Cardiol 2000; 85:1189–1193.
7. Middlekauff HR, Stevenson WG, Stevenson LW, et al. Syncope in advanced heart failure: High risk of sudden death regardless of the origin of syncope. J Am Coll Cardiol 1993; 21:110–116.
8. Nienaber CA, Hiller S, Spielmann RP, et al. Syncope in hypertrophic cardiomyopathy: Multivariate analysis of prognostic determinants. J Am Coll Cardiol 1990; 15:948–955.
9. Olshansky B, Mazuz M, Martins JB. Significance of inducible tachycardia in patients with syncope of unknown origin: A long-term follow-up. J Am Coll Cardiol 1985; 5:216–233.
10. Kapoor WN, Peterson JR, Wieand HS, et al. The diagnostic and prognostic implications of recurrences in patients with syncope. Am J Med 1987; 83:700–708.
11. Malik P, Koshman ML, Sheldon R. Timing of first recurrence of syncope predicts syncopal frequency after a positive tilt table test result. J Am Coll Cardiol 1997; 29:1284–1289.
12. Silverstein M, Singer D, Mulley A. Patients with syncope admitted to medical intensive care units. JAMA 1982; 248:1185–1189.
13. Martin G, Adams S, Martin H. Prospective evaluation of syncope. Ann Emerg Med 1984; 13:499–504.
14. Day S, Cook EF, Funkenstein H, et al. Evaluation and outcome of emergency room patients with transient loss of consciousness Am J Med. 1982;73:15–23.
15. Kapoor WN, Karpf M, Levey GS. Issues in evaluating patients with syncope. Ann Intern Med 1984; 100:755–757.
16. Kapoor WN, Karpf M, Wieand S, et al. A prospective evaluation and follow-up of patients with syncope. N Engl J Med 1983; 309:197–208.
17. Link MS, Kim K-MS, Homoud MK, et al. Long-term outcome of patients with syncope associated with coronary artery disease and a nondiagnostic electrophysiologic evaluation. Am J Cardiol 1999; 83:1334–1337.
18. Wayne HH. Syncope: Physiological considerations and an analysis of the clinical characteristics in 510 patients. Am J Med 1961; 30:418–438.
19. Linzer M. Impairment of physical and psychosocial function in recurrent syncope. J Clin Epidemiol 1991;44:1037–1043.
20. Linzer M, Gold DT, Pontinen M, et al. Recurrent Syncope as a Chronic Disease. J Gen Intern Med 1994;9:181–186.
21. Olshansky B. Syncope: overview and approach to management. In: Grubb BP, Olshansky B, eds. Syncope: Mechanisms and Management. New York: Futura; 1998:15–71.
22. Krahn AD, Klein GJ, Yee R, et al. The high cost of syncope: cost implications of a new insertable loop recorder in the investigation of recurrent syncope. Am Heart J 1999; 137:870–877.
23. Gibson TC, Heitzman MR. Diagnostic efficacy of 24 hour electrocardiographic testing for syncope. Am J Cardiol 1984; 53:1013–1017.
24. Clark PI, Glasser SP, Spoto E, et al. Arrhythmias detected by ambulatory monitoring. Lack of correlation with symptoms of dizziness and syncope. Chest 1980; 77:722–725.
25. Kapoor WN, Cha R, Peterson JR, et al. Prolonged electrocardiographic monitoring in patients with syncope. Am J Med 1987; 82:20–28.
26. Linzer M, Pritchett ELC, Pontinen M, et al. Incremental diagnostic yield of loop electrocardiographic recorders in unexplained syncope. Am J Cardiol 1990; 66:214–219.

27. Krahn AD, Klein GJ, Yee R, et al for the Reveal Investigators. Use of an extended monitoring strategy in patients with problematic syncope. Circulation 1999; 99:406–410.

28. Krahn AD, Klein GJ, Norris C, et al. The etiology of syncope in patients with negative tilt table and electrophysiological testing. Circulation. 1995; 92:1819–1824.

29. Edward C, Hyucke MD, Harold G, et al. Post-exertional cardiac asystole in a young man without organic heart disease. Ann Intern Med 1987; 106:844–845.

30. Morillo CA, Camacho ME, Wood MA, et al. Diagnostic utility of mechanical, pharmacological and orthostatic stimulation of the carotid sinus in patients with unexplained syncope. J Am Coll Cardiol 1999; 34:1587–1594.

31. Parry SW, Richardson DA, O'Shea D, et al. Diagnosis of carotid sinus hypersensitivity in older adults: carotid sinus massage in the upright position is essential. Heart 2000; 83:22–23.

32. Strasberg B, Rechavia E, Sagie A, et al. The head-up tilt table test in patients with syncope of unknown origin. Am Heart J 1989; 118:923–927.

33. Oribe E, Caro S, Perera R, et al. Syncope: the diagnostic value of head-up tilt testing. Pacing Clin Electrophysiol 1997; 20:874–879.

34. Kuchar DL, Thorburn CW, Sammel NL. Signal-averaged electrocardiogram for evaluation of recurrent syncope. Am J Cardiol 1986; 58:949–953.

35. Steinberg JS, Prystowsky E, Freedman RA, et al. Use of signal averaged electrocardiogram for predicting inducible ventricular tachycardia in patients with unexplained syncope: relation to clinical variables in a multivariate analysis. J Am Coll Cardiol 1994; 23:99–106.

36. Bachinsky WB, Linzer M, Weld L, et al. Usefulness of clinical characteristics in predicting the outcome of electrophysiologic studies in unexplained syncope. Am J Cardiol 1992; 69:1044–1049.

37. Flammang D, Church T, Waynberger M, et al. Can adenosine 5'-triphosphate be used to select treatment in severe vasovagal syndrome? Circulation 1997; 96:1201–1208.

38. Brignole M, Gaggioli G, Menozzi C, et al. Adenosine-induced atrioventricular block in patients with unexplained syncope. The diagnostic value of ATP testing. Circulation 1997; 96:3921–3927.

39. Ten Harkel AD, van Lieshout JJ, Wieling W. Effects of leg muscle pumping and tensing on orthostatic arterial pressure: A study in normal subjects and patients with autonomic failure. Clin Sci 1994; 87:553–558.

40. Hussain RM, McIntosh SJ, Lawson J, et al. Fludrocortisone in the treatment of hypotensive disorders in the elderly. Heart 1996; 76:507–509.

41. Lacroix D, Kouakam C, Klug D, et al. Asystolic cardiac arrest during head-up tilt test: Incidence and therapeutic implications. Pacing Clin Electrophysiol 1997; 20:2746–2754.

42. Cox MM, Perlman BA, Mayor MR, et al. Acute and long-term beta adrenergic blockade in patients with neurocardiogenic syncope. J Am Coll Cardiol 1995; 26:1293–1298.

43. Grubb BP, Temsey-Armos P, Hahn H, et al. Utility of upright tilt-table testing in the evaluation and management of syncope of unknown origin. Am J Med 1991; 90:6–10.

44. Ward CR, Gray JC, Gilroy JJ, et al. Midodrine: A role in the management of neurocardiogenic syncope. Heart 1998; 79:45–49.

45. Klingenheben T, Credner S, Hohnloser SH. Prospective evaluation of a two-step therapeutic strategy in neurocardiogenic syncope: Midodrine as a second line treatment in patients refractory to β-blockers. Pacing Clin Electrophysiol 1999; 22:276–281.

46. Grubb BP, Samoil D, Kosinski D, et al. Use of sertraline hydrochloride in the treatment of refractory neurocardiogenic syncope in children and adolescents. J Am Coll Cardiol 1994; 24:490–494.

47. Di Girolamo E, Di Iorio C, Sabatini P, et al. Effects of paroxetine hydrochloride, a selective serotonin reuptake inhibitor in refractory vasovagal syncope: A randomized, double-blind, placebo-controlled study. J Am Coll Cardiol 1999; 33:1227–1230.

48. Connolly SJ, Sheldon R, Roberts RS, et al on behalf of the Vasovagal Pacemaker Study Investigators. The North American Vasovagal Pacemaker Study (VPS): A randomized trial of permanent cardiac pacing for the prevention of vasovagal syncope. J Am Coll Cardiol 1999; 33:16–20.

49. Sutton R, Brignole M, Menozzi C, et al. Dual-chamber pacing in the treatment of neurally-mediated tilt-positive cardioinhibitory syncope : pacemaker versus no therapy: a multicenter randomized study. Circulation 2000; 102:294–299.

50. Di Girolamo E, Di Iorio C, Leonzio L, et al. Usefulness of a tilt training program for the prevention of refractory neurocardiogenic syncope in adolescents : a controlled study. Circulation 1999; 100:1798–1801.

51. Grubb BP, Kosinski D, Mouhaffel A, et al. The use of methylphenidate in the treatment of refractory neurocardiogenic syncope. Pacing Clin Electrophysiol 1996; 19:836–840.

52. Dan S, Grubb BP, Mouhaffel AH, et al. Use of serotonin re-uptake inhibitors as primary therapy for carotid sinus hypersensitivity. Pacing Clin Electrophysiol 1997; 20:1633–1635.

53. Knight BP, Goyal R, Pelosi F, et al. Outcome of patients with nonischemic dilated cardiomyopathy and unexplained syncope treated with an implantable defibrillator. J Am Coll Cardiol 1999; 33:1964–1970.

54. Fonarow GC, Feliciano Z, Boyle NG, et al. Improved survival in patients with nonischemic advanced heart failure and syncope treated with an implantable cardioverter-defibrillator. Am J Cardiol 2000; 85:981–985.

55. Pires LA, May LM, Ravi S, et al. Comparison of event rates and survival in patients with unexplained syncope without documented ventricular tachyarrhythmias versus patients with documented sustained ventricular tachyarrhythmias both treated with implantable cardioverter-difibrillators. Am J Cardiol 2000; 85:725–728.

56. Mittal S, Iwai S, Stein KM, et al. Long-term outcome of patients with unexplained syncope treated with an electrophysiologic-guided approach in the implantable cardioverter-defibrillator era. J Am Coll Cardiol 1999; 34:1082–1089.

Stroke in atrial fibrillation: epidemiology, risk factors and prognosis

John Godtfredsen MD FESC

Herlev University Hospital, Herlev, Denmark

Atrial Fibrillation accounts for about 20% of all strokes and stroke in atrial fibrillation is the most feared and calamitous complication

Introduction

In the course of atrial fibrillation stroke plays a major role as the most feared and calamitous complication.

The importance of stroke occurrence and estimation of stroke risk derives from the fact that compared with sinus rhythm, atrial fibrillation (AF) carries an increased mortality of about 1.5–1.9-fold, independent of heart disease and age, and part of this increased mortality is likely due to stroke in its various presentations.[1,2]

It must, however, be borne in mind that the concept of risk factors has different meanings in theoretical statistics, clinical epidemiology, clinical practice, and not the least in the patients' perception, respectively.

The risk factor concept has its background in epidemiological and clinical studies in which precursors and statistical predictors of subsequent events are identified. The aim of dealing with the risk factor concept in clinical cardiology is the hope that altering a particular risk factor will really change the risk. In fact, most of the recognized risk factors for stroke in AF are not alterable at all, i.e. the age of the patient, a past history of hypertension, previous cerebrovascular events etc.

This means that the purpose of risk estimation in a given patient rather than giving a promise of event elimination, is to enable the physician and the patient – after a qualified conference on the subject – to choose and guide an empirical, preventive treatment at a certain level of aggressiveness relative to the patient's estimated quantitative risk.

The basic neurological stroke taxonomy is shown in the following two boxes.

Types of stroke

By clinical course
  Transient ischemic attack (TIA)
  Stroke in progression
  Completed stroke
  Silent cerebral infarct(s)

By prognosis
  Minor, major, fatal

Table 7.1 Stroke rates in populations (%/year)

Copenhagen, DK 55–84 years	Males 0.8	Females 0.6
Göteborg, SE 50–69 years	Males 0.4	
Framingham, US 50–89 years	Males and females	0.5

Stroke mechanisms and etiology

Ischemic stroke	85%
Cardioembolic 20% AF, valve disease, ventricular thrombi	
Atherosclerotic 45% Vasoembolic: aortic, carotid intracranial thrombosis, hypoperfusion	
Cryptogenic, other 35%	
Hemorrhagic stroke	15%
Intracerebral, subarachnoid	

EPIDEMIOLOGY

The stroke rate in the background population is known from several studies, and amounts to about 0.4–0.8%/year, the general yardstick against which the stroke rate in AF must be measured and compared (Table 7.1).

Figures 7.1 and 7.2 show the stroke incidence in selected epidemiological series.

This incidence is heavily age dependent as can be seen in both sinus rhythm and AF in the Framingham Study[3] (population-based), and in a recent Danish hospital-based study[4] of patients discharged with a diagnosis of AF where the fivefold increased risk in patients over 70 years of age compares well with the results indicated in Table 7.2 from The Framingham Study.[5]

RISK FACTORS

Levels of risks: there is no definite unanimity as to what constitutes a low, intermediate or high risk in clinical,

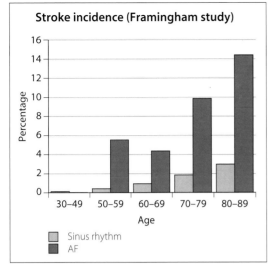

Fig. 7.1 Stroke incidence (Framingham Study) (From Wolf et al[3]).

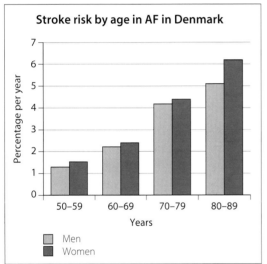

Fig. 7.2 Stroke risk by age in AF (% per year) in Denmark (From Frost et al[4])

Table 7.2 Risk factors for stroke (Framingham 1991: 34 years follow-up in 5070 subjects) (From Wolf et al[5])

Etiology	Factor increase
Atrial fibrillation	> 5
Congestive heart failure	> 4
Hypertension	> 3
Ischemic heart disease	> 2
Age (etiological fraction)	
50–59 years	1.5%
80–89 years	23.5%

cardiovascular medicine, but Table 7.3[6] indicates a reasonable quantitative approach which has gained a more or less time-honored acceptance over the years. Examples of established risks in subgroups of AF are also shown in this table.

In clinical epidemiology generally and in AF specifically, it is possible to set up a rather clear and well-defined *hierarchy* of risk factors (Fig. 7.3) which is necessary to estimate the particular level of risk in a patient as low, intermediate or high, regarding any future event.

The relation, however, between this cascade of risk factors obtained from statistical analysis, and the causative stroke mechanisms in individual cases is not immediately apparent. Compared to, for example, an i.v. injection of insulin causing indisputable severe hypoglycemia, it is far more obscure why hypertension, diabetes and the age of the patient are quantitative and significant risk factors for stroke in AF. Clearly age per se does not in any way

Table 7.3 Time honored (semi-)quantitative risk factor estimation (From Stein et al[6]). Risk for thromboembolic complications has been graded:

Low	< 2%/year	'Lone'AF; patients < 65 years w/o RF; many PAF patients
Medium	2–6%/year	Patients > 65 years or patients with ≥ one RF
High*	> 6%/year	Patients with previous stroke or TIA; AF with mitral stenosis

* in Atrial Fibrillation Investigators (AFI) analysis all upper 95% confidence intervals > 6%
RF, risk factors; PAF, paroxysmal AF; TIA, transient ischemic attack

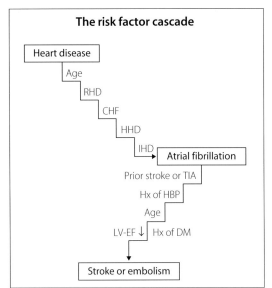

Fig. 7.3 The risk factor cascade. RHD, rheumatic heart disease; CHF, congestive heart failure; HHD, hypertensive heart disease; IHD, ischemic heart disease; TIA, transient ischemic attack; HBP, high blood pressure; DM, diabetes; LV-EF, left ventricular ejection fraction.

Table 7.4 Risk factors for chronic atrial fibrillation – 2-year relative risk in men (Framingham 1983)

Etiology	Relative risk (RR)
Rheumatic heart disease	9.9
Congestive heart failure	8.5
Hypertensive heart disease	4.7
Ischemic heart disease	2.2
Any heart disease	3.2

For women and paroxysmal AF the same ranking applies

Table 7.5 Risk factors for stroke (multivariate analysis) in 1236 control patients in the AFI Study[7]

Risk factor	Relative risk
Prior stroke or TIA	2. 5
History of Hypertension	1.6
Age (per decade)	1.4
History of diabetes	1.7
History of CHF	1.4 (ns)

CHF, congestive heart failure; TIA, transient ischemic attack

enter into a mechanism whereby clots are formed and transported from the heart/aorta to the brain vessels. The same goes for hypertension and diabetes, yet the presence of these conditions is predisposing a given patient to an increased stroke risk.

Thus the whole process of individual stroke risk estimation and the weighing against the bleeding risk of anticoagulation has the character of an exercise in clinical statistics, and the effort to reduce the stroke risk leads to the implementation of a prophylactic treatment, and certainly not an absolute cure (as many elderly patients would probably like it to be).

As can be seen in Table 7.4 compared with Table 7.2 there is a certain overlap between risk factors, since hypertension, congestive heart failure and ischemic heart disease all are risk factors both for chronic AF and stroke, thus illustrating the notion of a cascade of risk factors (Fig. 7.3). An interesting and clinically important feature about increasing age as a risk factor is that whereas all other risk factors become weakened with age, this in itself

independently increases stroke risk in the very elderly, i.e. 80–89 years (Table 7.2).[5]

Randomized clinical studies of AF particularly aiming at risk stratification for the purpose of comparing placebo with anticoagulant treatment also indicate the very same pattern and magnitude of risk factors for stroke (see Table 7.5 from the Atrial Fibrillation Investigators meta-analysis 1994[7]) and further add the important feature of a previous cerebrovascular accident as a powerful, independent risk factor. The problem of increasing age as a risk factor is particularly important, since various prominent risk stratification schemes for stroke have been published with the result that the proportion of low-risk patients ranges from about 11–23% to 29% in the Atrial Investigation Investigators, American College of Chest Physicians (ACCP) and Stroke Prevention in Atrial Fibrillation (SPAF) schemes respectively (Table 7.6).[8]

Table 7.6 Risk stratification schemes[8]

AFI Study 1994	SPAF Study 1996	ACCP 1998
Previous stroke or TIA	Previous stroke or TIA	Previous stroke or TIA
LV dysfunction (echo)	LV fractional shortening < 25% or recent CHF	Heart failure or CAD
Previous hypertension	Current SBP > 160 mmHg	Previous hypertension
Increasing age	Women > 75 years of age	Age > 75 years
Diabetes	-	Diabetes

ACCP; American College of Chest Physicians; CAD, coronary artery disease; CHF, congestive heart failure; SBP, systolic blood pressure; SPAF, Stroke Prevention in Atrial Fibrillation; TIA, transient ischemic attack

This variation is dependent upon whether patients in the age group 65–75 years and men over 75 years without other clinical risk factors are included or not.

The ability of these three risk schemes to successfully predict the absolute stroke rate was tested prospectively by the SPAF group in acetyl salicylic acid (ASA)-treated patients. Low-risk patients were accurately identified, whereas high-risk patients were less precisely identified with an incidence rate ranging from 3.5 to 7.2%, depending upon which age group was used. In this study the proportion of low-risk patients also ranged widely from 14 to 45%.[9]

Risk of stroke in 'lone AF'

When AF is encountered in patients without any history or signs of underlying heart disease (clinically or echocardiographically) it is often termed 'lone AF' (LAF). Whatever the justification of this denomination LAF may be considered a definite low-risk group, yet the prognostic implications regarding both stroke and mortality are contradictory.

Four recent studies from 1999 found the following: The Italian study[10] found that paroxysmal LAF had an excellent prognosis whereas LAF patients with chronic AF had an increased risk of both embolic complications and mortality; the Mayo

Clinic study[11] found that LAF in patients over age 60 is a risk marker for cardiovascular events of a comparable magnitude to that of AF patients with an underlying heart disease, i.e. of about 5%/year. The Paris Study[12] found, with a 23-year follow-up in men, that cardiovascular mortality was increased with a relative risk of 4.2 whereas no stroke-related deaths occurred. In a French cohort[13] of almost 200,000 patients and 14.5 years of follow-up the group with LAF did not show a significantly increased cardiovascular mortality.

Risk factors and stroke mechanism

As mentioned above none of these epidemiologically derived risk factors bear any clear relationship to the supposed mechanism(s) of thrombus formation and transport (embolization) as viewed by a more mechanistic approach (Fig. 7.4).

The type of stroke and its mechanism seems to have some bearing on the best and most appropriate way of prevention. In a retrospective analysis from the SPAF study, presumed cardioembolic stroke was significantly better prevented by antithrombotic therapy with warfarin (83% reduction) than with ASA, and the

Stroke mechanisms in atrial fibrillation	
1.	R/F → Thrombus formation in LA, LV or central arteries (Virchow's triad)
2.	R/F → Cerebral (systemic) embolism (migration of thrombus or vasoembolic)
3.	R/F → Intracranial thrombosis
4.	The R/F cascade (or the hierarchy of R/Fs)

Fig. 7.4 Simplified mechanisms of stroke in AF. LA: left atrium; LV: Left ventricle; R/F: Risk factor.

proportion of putative vasoembolic stroke was lower in ASA patients than in those on warfarin.[14]

Unfortunately it is not possible to know in advance which type of stroke will occur in any given patient. Only by statistical risk factor analysis can we choose between ASA and warfarin for low-risk and high-risk patients respectively. Combining ASA with adjusted dose warfarin would seem to be the logical choice for full, primary prevention, but no data are available from prospective trials on this treatment modality.

Risk factors determined multifactorially in big trials

The thromboembolic risk in AF as related to the presence of defined risk factors and the various age groups is particularly important because of its immediate utility in the daily clinical work.

All published guidelines are in agreement when deeming it mandatory that every patient with AF must be individually evaluated regarding the embolic risk and managed accordingly with the apropriate preventive antithrombotic treatment[15]

Tables 7.7[7] and 7.8 indicate the current, absolute annual risk rate to be compared with the anticipated bleeding risk gleaned from available sources, or better, from the records of one's own anticoagulation clinic. Regarding the difficult group of patients with permanent, chronic AF and one or

Table 7.7 Annual risk of thromboembolic (T/E) complications (endpoints) in AF: 1236 control patients from Atrial Fibrillation Investigators study[7])

Age	Risk factor	Endpoint (%/ year)
< 65	0	1.0
	≥ 1	4.9
65–75	0	4.3
	≥ 1	5.7
> 75	0	3.5
	≥ 1	8.1

more established risk factor (Table 7.8), where the risk range is rather wide (3.0–8.0%) it may be necessary to include echocardiographic variables as well as the patient's preference after a full discussion about the pros and cons of warfarin treatment, including its logistics, before a final decision is arrived at.

Bleeding risk

The bleeding risk is highly dependent upon the experience and quality of care in any particular setting as is available locally (patient's self-management of anticoagulant treatment is increasingly used in some areas), Table 7.9[16] shows results from a US study regarding pertinent risk factors for bleeding.

Other risk factors

In a few observational studies the finding of spontaneous echo contrast ('smoke') or thrombus by echocardiography in the left atrium has had prognostic implications [17] (Fig. 7.5), and this has been translated into clinical use by the guidelines afforded by for instance the ACUTE study.[18]

Thrombus formation, in the classical notion of Virchow's triad, requires that abnormalities are present in all three of the contributing factors: Vessel wall, blood flow and blood constituents (Table 7.10). Endothelial pathology has been

Table 7.8 Thromboembolic risk in various types of AF

	Annual risk (%)	Comments
Acute AF spontaneous conversion	0.8	Conversion within 48 h
Acute AF and flutter DC/drug conversion	0.2–1.5	On warfarin
Persistent, PAF	1.3–5.6	Depending on risk factor
	1.6–2.9	AFFIRM Study, on warfarin
Permanent, chronic AF		
without risk factors	1.0	
with risk factors	3.0–8.0	AFI and EAFT
with previous TIA/stroke	12.0	

AFFIRM, Atrial Fibrillation Follow-up Investigation of Rhythm Management; AFI, Atrial Fibrillation Investigators; DC, direct current; EAFT, European Atrial Fibrillation Trial; PAF, paroxysmal AF; TIA, transient ischemic attack

Table 7.9 Risk score for major bleedings in anticoagulant treatment (From Beyth et al[16])

Risk factors (1 point per box: Max. 0–4 points):
- Age > 65
- Previous stroke
- Previous gastrointestinal bleeding
- Recent acute myocardial infarction; Diabetes; Haematocrit < 30%; Creatinin > 130 mmol/L

	Risk for major bleeding	% Bleedings/year
Low risk:	0 points	3
Medium risk	1–2 points	7
High risk	3–4 points	30

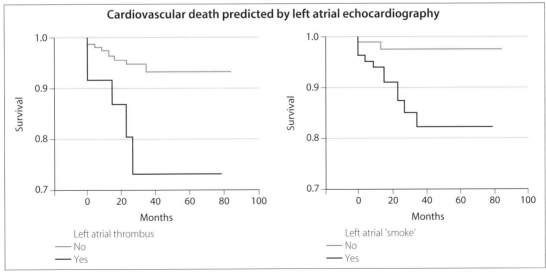

Fig. 7.5 Cardiovascular death as predicted from echocardiographic findings of thrombus and 'smoke' in AF.

Table 7.10 Virchow's triad in AF[31]	
Thrombogenicity in AF	
Virchow's triad is fullfilled...	
Vessel walls	LA immobility; LA endothelial lesions
Blood flow	low CO; local stasis (LA)
Blood components	↑ D-dimer; fibrinogen; vWF

CO: Cardiac output; LA: Left atrium; vWF: von Willebrand factor.

demonstrated recently in both histological and ultrastructural studies. [19,20]

The third factor of Virchow's triad i.e. the hypercoagulable state has been extensively examined and researched in clinical AF[21] but as yet the results have not been able to fit into any algorithm aiming at risk stratifying patients before choosing an anticoagulant treatment.

PROGNOSIS OF STROKE IN ATRIAL FIBRILLATION

The neurologists are the unfortunate colleagues who have to deal with the cardiologists' sins of omission regarding the selection of patients for anticoagulant treatment, however, even if AF patients are anticoagulated properly, strokes do occur[22] and it has been known for many years, and recently confirmed in the International Stroke Trial,[23] that strokes due to embolism are particularly severe.

These rather sad facts are shown in Table 7.11 with data from five representative studies[23–27] on the prognosis of stroke in AF as compared with stroke in sinus rhythm. The acute mortality from stroke in AF ranges from 17 to 37% as compared to the mortality in sinus rhythm of 6–20%, but it should be noted that AF patients with stroke are 6–7 years older than the patients in sinus rhythm.

As indicated in Figure 7.6, detailing the Stockholm experience, the early mortality is high, but also regarding functional status poststroke the clinical outcome is worse in AF patients as can be seen in Table 7.12 from the Copenhagen Stroke Study:[24] The Barthel Index is significantly lower in AF than in sinus rhythm.

Essentially the same figures were found in the recent and much larger European Community Stroke Project[27] where in AF the 3-month mortality was 33% and the

Table 7.11 Acute stroke: proportion of patients with AF and mortality (The neurologist's view)						
Series	N	% AF	Atrial fibrillation		Sinus rhythm	
			Age	% mortality	Age	% mortality
CPH	1197	18	80	33	73	17
Stockholm	276	32	76	37	70	6
Oxfordshire	675	17	77	23	71	8
ECSP	4462	18	77	33	71	20
IST	18451	17	78	17	71	8

CPH, Copenhagen Study; ECSP, European Concerted Stroke Prevention; IST, International Stroke Trial

Table 7.12 Copenhagen stroke study[24]			
N: 1,185 patients (AF present in 18%)			
Acute mortality	SR 171 (17%)	AF 72 (33%)	p < .0001
Barthel Index	78	67	p < .0007
Rec. Stroke	5%	6%	n.s.

odds ratio for both disability and handicap was 1.5. In the International Stroke Trial the acute 14-day mortality was 17% in AF. [23]

The long-term follow-up is seen in Figures 7.6[25] and 7.7[26] (from Stockholm and Oxford) indicating that in these elderly patients only about 25–40% are alive after 5 years. Age at baseline in these two studies was 76 and 77 years respectively, so one-quarter of the patients attained an age of over 80 years even at a time when

Table 7.13 Stroke: late mortality in various AF series

Series	Age	Average (%/year)
Godtfredsen (DK)[28] 1956–1967	67	25
Gustafsson (SE)[25] 1976–1979	76	15
Oxfordshire (UK)[26] 1981–1988	77	12
EAFT (EU)[29] 1987–1992	73	9–13
AFI (US, DK, CAN)[7] 1985–1991	69	< 5

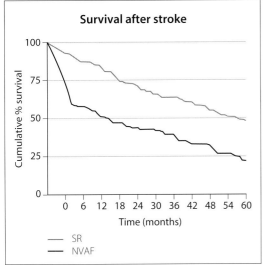

Fig. 7.6 Survival after stroke. SR, sinus rhythm; NVAF, non-vascular AF. (From Gustafsson et al[25]). © 1991 Blackwell Science.

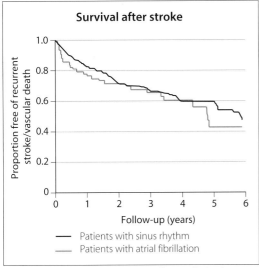

Fig. 7.7 Survival (30 days–6 years) after stroke in the Oxfordshire Project. (From Sandercock et al[26]).

antithrombotic prevention was not in widespread use. Whereas both studies found early mortality significantly higher in AF, the Oxfordshire data, representing patients from general practice as opposed to the Stockholm hospital series, indicate that versus sinus rhythm AF is a rather weak predictor of all cause death in the long term.

Table 7.13[25–29] seems to convey the message that there has been some improvement over the years regarding the long-term annual stroke mortality, declining from about 25% in the 1960s to about 5–12% during the 1990s. Of note is the annual total mortality rate of 4.8% in the recently published Atrial Fibrillation Follow-up Investigation (AFFIRM) study, [30] suggesting that also the stroke mortality has declined in the new millenium.

The stroke severity as regards functional recovery is shown in Table 7.14,[7,29] where about one-third of all strokes in AF are major and leave the patient in a state of invalidity, a fact which is one of the strongest arguments for increasing the clinical use of proper anticoagulant treatment.

The rate of stroke recurrence in AF has been debated over the years. Earlier it was believed that it was higher than in sinus

Table 7.14 Rates of major stroke* in various clinical series of AF (%)

AFASAK[7]	33
SPAF 2 (ASA + WF)[7]	50
SPAF 1 (placebo)[7]	33
SPINAF[7]	16
BAATAF[7]	38
EAFT[29]	38
All Studies (mean)	35

* Major stroke = invalidating stroke
AFASAK, Atrial Fibrillation Aspirin and Anticoagulation, København Study (note: København is Copenhagen in Danish); SPAF, Stroke Prevention in Atrial Fibrillation; SPINAF, Stroke Prevention in Non-valvular Atrial Fibrillation; BAATAF, Boston Area Anticoagulation Trial in Atrial Fibrillation; EAFT, European Atrial Fibrillation Trial Study Group

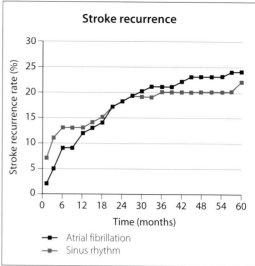

Fig. 7.8 Stroke recurrence in the Stockholm study (From Gustafsson et al[25]). © 1991 Blackwell Science.

rhythm, but the results from Stockholm[25] and Copenhagen[24], as well as the recent International Stroke Trial[23] seem to refute this notion (see Table 7.12 and Fig. 7.8).

CONCLUSIONS

- **Stroke risk in AF is increased fivefold compared with sinus rhythm**

- **Major stroke**   35%

- **Acute mortality**   17–30%

- **Annual mortality**   5–15%

- **Various AF-types have very different stroke risk**

- **Stroke risk shows a substantial age gradient**

- **Risk factors for stroke are well identified**

- **Some stroke risk factors are amenable to prevention**

References

1. Benjamin EJ, Wolf PA, D'Agostino RB, et al. Impact of atrial fibrillation on the risk of death: the Framingham Heart Study. Circulation 1998; 98:946–952.
2. Lip GYH. Atrial fibrillation and mortality. Eur Heart J 1999; 20:1525–1527.
3. Wolf PA, Abbott RD, Kannel WB. Atrial fibrillation: a major contribution to stroke in the elderly. The Framingham Study. Arch Intern Med 1987; 147:1561–1564.
4. Frost L, Engholm G, Johnsen S, et al. Incident stroke after discharge from the hospital with a diagnosis of atrial fibrillation. Am J Med 2000; 108:36–40.
5. Wolf PA, Abbott RD, Kannel WB. Atrial fibrillation as an independent risk factor for stroke: The Framingham Study. Stroke 1991; 22:983–988.
6. Stein B, Fuster V, Halperin JV, et al. Antithrombotic therapy in cardiac disease. An emerging approach based on pathogenesis and risk. Circulation 1989; 80:1501–1513.
7. Atrial Fibrillation Investigators. Risk factors for stroke and efficacy of antithrombotic therapy in atrial fibrillation. Analysis of pooled data from five randomized controlled trials. Arch Intern Med 1994; 154:1449–1457.
8. Go AS, Hylek EM, Phillips KA, et al. Implications of the stroke risk criteria on the anticoagulation decision in nonvalvular atrial fibrillation. The anticoagulation and risk factors in atrial fibrillation (ATRIA) study. Circulation 2000; 102:11–13.
9. Pearce LA, Hart RG, Halperin JL. Assessment of three schemes for stratifying stroke risk in patients with nonvalvular atrial fibrillation. Am J Med 2000; 109:45–51.
10. Scardi S, Mazzone C, Pandullo C, et al. Lone atrial fibrillation: prognostic differences between paroxysmal and chronic forms after 10 years of follow-up. Am Heart J 1999; 137:592–595.
11. Kopecky SL, Gersh BJ, McGoon MD, et al. Lone atrial fibrillation in elderly persons. A marker for cardiovascular risk. Arch Intern Med 1999; 159:1118–1122.
12. Jouven X, Desnos M, Guerot C, et al. Idiopathic atrial fibrillation as a risk factor for mortality. The Paris Prospective Study. Eur Heart J 1999; 20:896–899.

13. Guize L, Thomas F, Lavergne T, et al. Prevalence, associated factors and mortality of atrial fibrillation in a large french cohort. Eur Heart J 1999; 20(suppl. August/September):467. (Abstract)

14. Hart RG, Pearce LA, Miller VT, et al. Cardioembolic vs. Noncardioembolic strokes in atrial fibrillation: frequency and effect of antithrombotic agents in the stroke prevention in atrial fibrillation studies. Cerebrovasc Dis 2000; 10:39–43.

15. Task Force Report– American College of Cardiology/American Heart Association/European Society of Cardiology guidelines for the management of patients with atrial fibrillation. Eur Heart J 2001; 22:1852–1923.

16. Beyth RJ, Quinn LM, Landefeld CS. Prospective evaluation of an index for predicting the risk of major bleeding in outpatients treated with warfarin. Am J Med 1998; 105:91–99.

17. Dawn B, Singh P, Stoddard MF, et al. Cardiovascular death in patients with atrial fibrillation is better predicted by left atrial thrombus and spontaneous echo contrast as compared to clinical parameters. American College of Cardiology 1998; abstract 872–5.

18. Klein AL, Grimm RA, Murray RD, et al. Use of transesophageal echocardiography to guide cardioversion in patients with atrial fibrillation. N Engl J Med 2001; 344:1411–1420.

19. Shirani J, Alaeddini J. Structural remodeling of the left atrial appendage in patients with chronic non-valvular atrial fibrillation. Implications for thrombus formation, systemic embolism, and assessment by transesophgeal echocardiography. Cardiovasc Pathol 2000; 9:95–101.

20. Goldsmith I, Kumar P, Carter P, et al. Atrial endocardial changes in mitral valve disease: a scanning electron microscopy study. Am Heart J 2000; 140:777–784.

21. Kamath S, Blann AD, Lip GYH. Platelets and atrial fibrillation. Eur Heart J 2001; 22:2233–2242.

22. Thibault B, Talajic M, Dubuc M, et al. Thromboembolic events occur in patients with atrial fibrillation despite maintenance of sinus rhythm or use of anticoagulation: The Canadian Trial of Atrial Fibrillation experience. American Heart Association, November 2000; (Abstract):31528.

23. Saxena R, Lewis S, Berge E, et al. Risk of early death and recurrent stroke and effect of heparin in 3169 patients with acute ischemic stroke and atrial fibrillation in the International Stroke Trial. Stroke 2001; 32:2333–2337.

24. Jørgensen HS, Nakayama H, Reith J, et al. Acute stroke with atrial fibrillation. The Copenhagen Stroke Study. Stroke 1996; 10:1765–1769.

25. Gustafsson C, Britton M. Pathogenetic mechanism of stroke in non-valvular atrial fibrillation: follow-up of stroke patients with and without atrial fibrillation. J Intern Med 1991; 230:11–16.

26. Sandercock P, Bamford J, Dennis M, et al. Atrial fibrillation and stroke: prevalence in different types of stroke and influence on early and long term prognosis (Oxfordshire community stroke project). Br Med J 1992; 305:1460–1465.

27. Lamassa M, Di Carlo AA, Pracucci G, et al. Characteristics, outcome, and care of stroke associated with atrial fibrillation in Europe: data from a multicenter multinational hospital-based registry (The European Community Stroke Project). Stroke 2001; 32:392–398.

28. Godtfredsen J. Atrial fibrillation. Etiology, course and prognosis. A follow-up study of 1212 cases. Copenhagen: Munksgaard; 1975.

29. European Atrial Fibrillation Trial (EAFT) Study Group. Secondary prevention in non-rheumatic atrial fibrillation after transient ischaemic attack or minor stroke. Lancet 1993; 342:1255–1262.

30. The Atrial Fibrillation Follow-up Investigation of Rhythm Management (AFFIRM) Investigators. A comparison of rate control and rhythm control in patients with atrial fibrillation. N Engl J Med 2002; 347:1825–1833.

31. Lip GY. Does atrial fibrillation confer a hypercoagulable state? Lancet 1995; 346(8986):1313–1314.

Wide QRS complex tachycardias: principles of diagnosis and management

Germanas Marinskis PhD

Vilnius University Hospital, Vilnius, Lithuania

Wide QRS complex tachycardias represent a significant number of cardiac emergencies Ventricular tachycardias make up about 80% of these cases

Introduction

Wide QRS complex tachycardias represent a significant part of cardiac emergencies. This clinical entity (QRS complex width >120 ms in adults and >80 ms in children, depending on age[1]) can be related to several electrophysiological mechanisms:

- ventricular tachycardias (about 80% of cases);
- supraventricular tachycardias with aberrant conduction (15%);
- tachycardias with anterograde conduction via accessory pathways (5%).

Since ventricular tachycardias (VT) contribute to majority of wide QRS complex tachycardias and are often related to structural heart disease (scars after myocardial infarction, cardiomyopathies), patients presenting with wide QRS complex tachycardia require prompt diagnosis and therapy, and are likely to deteriorate hemodynamically in case of delayed or improper therapy. Knowing the exact etiology and mechanism of wide QRS complex tachycardia allows selection of the most appropriate method of treatment [implantable cardioverter-defibrillators (ICDs), catheter ablation, or drug therapy]. Differentiating VTs from other wide QRS complex tachycardias is also of paramount importance because of different prognosis and treatment strategies. Contemporary experience with invasive electrophysiological studies and catheter ablation enables us to choose the most informative signs that could help to distinguish and classify various forms of wide QRS complex tachycardia.

MECHANISMS OF NORMAL AND WIDE QRS COMPLEXES

Narrow QRS complexes require simultaneous activation of the left and right ventricles starting from the basal septum (Fig. 8.1). Conduction velocity via the Purkinje system is several times faster compared to that in the ventricular myocardium. Therefore, conduction block in one of the bundle branches leads to additional time required for activation to spread via the ventricular muscle and enter specialized conduction fibers below the level of block. Activation originating in the ventricular myocardium as during VT or conduction via the accessory pathway (AP) would prolong the total duration of QRS complex because of eccentric (sequential rather than simultaneous) pattern of ventricular activation. For these reasons, VTs originating in the septal part, especially in the Purkinje system (for example, left fascicular tachycardias) result in less asynchronic ventricular activation pattern and narrower QRS complexes that are difficult or impossible to distinguish from aberrant ones using a 12-lead electrocardiogram (ECG) in about 10% cases of VT.[2]

INVASIVE ELECTRO-PHYSIOLOGICAL DIAGNOSTIC TECHNIQUES

Invasive electrophysiological study (EPS) is a 'gold standard', and often the only method establishing the correct mechanism of wide QRS complex tachycardia. For example, short or negative HV interval rules out supraventricular tachycardia (SVT) with bundle branch block, but can present both during VT and tachycardia with anterograde conduction via AP. It is necessary to emphasize that there are numerous criteria for diagnosing particular tachycardia mechanisms, but few absolutely specific ones (Table 8.1), and rather than using single criterion for establishing the diagnosis of VT or other arrhythmia, it is necessary to use combination of several features favoring or ruling out the specific mechanism. One of possible causes is combination of two tachycardia mechanisms (atrial tachycardia and VT, VT with bystander AP).

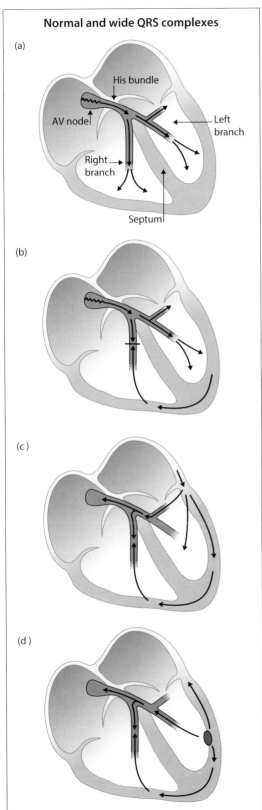

Normal and wide QRS complexes

(a)

(b)

(c)

(d)

Fig. 8.1 Mechanisms of normal ventricular activation and widening of QRS complexes. (*a*) Narrow QRS complex is a result of synchronous activation of both ventricles. (*b*) Block in one of bundle branches results in QRS widening because of trans-septal conduction time and an unusual activation pattern of the corresponding ventricle. (*c*) Ventricular activation via the accessory pathway (preexcitation) leads to eccentric ventricular activation and wide QRS complexes. (*d*) Ventricular origin of activation (ventricular tachycardia) also leads to eccentric ventricular activation and wide QRS complexes.

Atrioventricular (AV) dissociation is 100% specific for VT (Fig. 8.2), and there are reported single cases of WQRSCT with participation of nodoventricular conduction pathway and occasional ventriculoatrial (VA) block. Fusion and capture beats, as signs of AV dissociation, are rarely seen (mostly at lower VT rates, Fig. 8.2). AV dissociation is seen in about 50% of VT cases.[3] In others, character of VA conduction (1:1, 2:1 or more complex pattern) is merely the product of tachycardia rate and VA conduction capabilities. For these reasons, idiopathic VTs that usually have slower ventricular rate, in young patients can exhibit 1:1 VA conduction (Fig. 8.3). SVTs with bundle branch aberration always show normal or prolonged HV interval (Fig. 8.4). Some diagnostic difficulties may arise when dealing with accessory pathway-mediated antidromic tachycardias (1:1 AV conduction and unusual timings on the His bundle electrogram). These rare cases require various pacing maneuvers, and their diagnostics, being beyond the scope of this chapter, are described in detail elsewhere.[4–6] Sometimes only successful catheter ablation with subsequent changes of electrophysiological parameters (AV or VA conduction) allow us to make sure that a particular diagnosis is correct ('learning when burning').

Key points

Diagnosis of wide QRS complex tachycardia

Invasive electrophysiological study is the 'gold standard' and it is necessary to emphasize that there are numerous criteria for diagnosing particular tachycardia mechanisms, but few are absolutely specific

Table 8.1 Electrophysiological features that are specific for or exclude various wide QRS complex tachycardia mechanisms

	Ventricular tachycardias	SVTs with aberrant conduction	Tachycardias with anterograde conduction over AP
AV dissociation (VA block)	Quite common and very specific	Excludes this mechanism	Possible yet extremely rare (tends to exclude this mechanism)
Fusion and capture beats	Rare (more often seen at lower tachycardia rates) and specific	Excludes this mechanism but may be simulated by ventricular premature beats or intermittent nature of bundle branch block	Excludes this mechanism but may be simulated by ventricular premature beats
HV dissociation	Rare and extremely specific	Excludes this mechanism	Possible (multiple APs) but extremely rare
Short or negative HV interval	Possible	Excludes this mechanism	Possible
Termination of tachycardia by atrial extrastimulus not advancing ventricular activation	Excludes this mechanism	Possible	Possible

AP, accessory pathway; AV, atrioventricular; SVT, supraventricular tachycardia; VA, ventriculoatrial

ELECTROCARDIO-GRAPHIC DIAGNOSTICS

The first step in the analysis of a 12-lead ECG of wide QRS complex tachycardia is to determine whether it is rhythmic (regular) or arrhythmic (irregular) using the mechanisms shown in Table 8.2.

Regular wide QRS complex tachycardia

Key points

Important clinical advice in an emergency situation

Clinical experience has shown that the worst mistake is to consider VT as SVT with aberration and to administer drugs such as verapamil that could lead to hemodynamic deterioration in cases of VT

Electrocardiographic diagnosis of wide QRS complex tachycardia was extensively described in the literature. Starting from paper of Wellens and co-workers published in 1978,[7] many electrocardiographic criteria of VT and aberration were proposed and re-evaluated. The importance of 12-lead ECG for diagnosis of wide QRS complex tachycardia follows from the fact that it is the only diagnostic tool available in emergency settings and upon patient arrival to cardiology center for further evaluation. Diagnostic criteria of VT proposed by Wellens et al[7] (and often referred to as 'classical') were as follows:

- AV dissociation;
- superior (leftward) frontal plane QRS axis ($-90°$ to $\pm180°$);
- QRS duration > 140 ms;
- specific QRS configurations and R/S wave duration in leads V_1 and V_6.

Diagnostic criteria of ventricular tachycardia

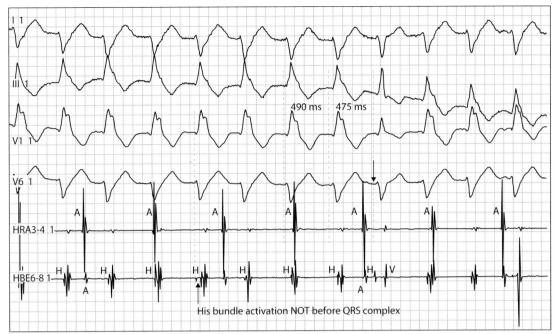

Fig. 8.2 Diagnostic criteria of VT during invasive electrophysiological study. ECG leads I, III, V$_1$ and V$_6$ are presented together with the high right atrial electrogram (HRA) and His bundle electrogram (HBE). Note that this idiopathic left ventricular tachycardia has pretty slow heart rate of about 120 bpm. The following diagnostic signs of VT are seen: AV dissociation is present (A waves 'marching' between QRS complexes); His bundle activation is within QRS complex, i.e. its activation is retrograde; one of atrial activations (in RR of 475 ms) is conducted to the ventricles, and ventricular activation is partly of supraventricular origin ('fusion beat', upper arrow).

Table 8.2 Mechanisms of regular and irregular wide QRS complex tachycardia

Regular wide QRS complex tachycardia	Irregular wide QRS complex tachycardia
Ventricular tachycardia	Atrial fibrillation/flutter with aberrant conduction
Supraventricular tachycardia with aberrant conduction	Atrial fibrillation/flutter with anterograde conduction
Tachycardias with anterograde conduction via accessory pathways (antidromic)	Polymorphic ventricular tachycardia

These QRS configurations in leads V$_1$ and V$_6$ specific for VT are presented in Figure 8.5. Later Wellens reported that retrospective analysis of 100 cases of wide QRS complex tachycardia with application of these criteria has led to correct diagnosis in 90%.[8]

Subsequent analysis of a larger number of wide QRS complex tachycardias has led to other publications evaluating classical criteria and offering some new ones. It was shown that some of these criteria could present in SVT with pre-existing bundle branch block.[9] Clinical experience has shown that the worst mistake is to consider VT as SVT with aberration and to administer drugs such as verapamil that could lead to hemodynamic deterioration in cases of VT.[10] An algorithm proposed by Brugada and co-workers[11] offered a safer

1:1 ventriculoatrial conduction during ventricular tachycardia

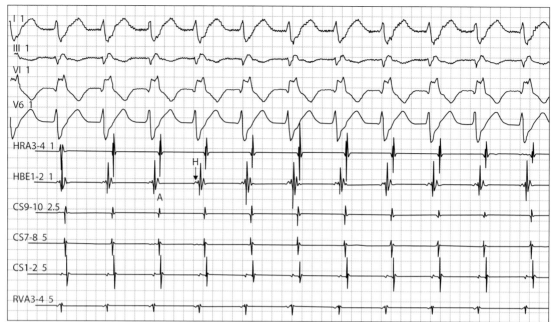

Fig. 8.3 Absence of AV dissociation in a 38-year-old patient with idiopathic left ventricular tachycardia. Heart rate is about 125 bpm (RR intervals of 460–480 ms). ECG leads I, III, V_1 and V_6 are presented together with the high right atrial electrogram (HRA), His bundle electrogram (HBE), proximal to distal coronary sinus (CS9–10, CS7–8, and CS1–2), and right ventricular apex (RVA) electrograms. VA conduction 1:1 is present during tachycardia, with normal retrograde atrial activation sequence [the earliest atrial activation (A) on HBE]. Note however, that His bundle deflection on the HBE is within the QRS complex, i.e. its activation is retrograde.

Bundle branch block aberration

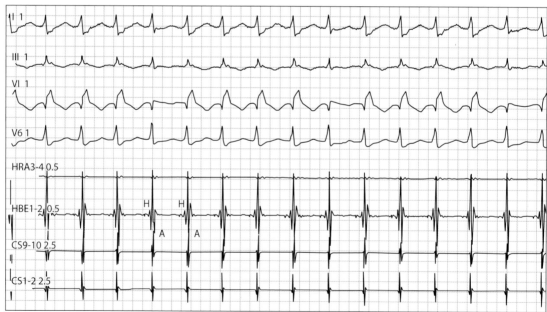

Fig. 8.4 Atrioventricular nodal tachycardia with intermittent right bundle branch block (RBBB) aberration. ECG leads I, III, V_1 and V_6 are presented together with the high right atrial electrogram (HRA), His bundle electrogram (HBE), proximal to distal coronary sinus (CS9–10 and CS1–2) electrograms. Tachycardia is characterized by 1:1 AV conduction (atrial activation is within ventricular activation on the HBE). Both narrow (95 ms) and wide (RBBB with QRS width of 125 ms) QRS complexes show normal HV interval of 45 ms.

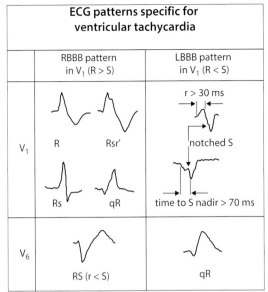

ECG patterns specific for ventricular tachycardia

	RBBB pattern in V₁ (R > S)	LBBB pattern in V₁ (R < S)
V₁	R Rsr' Rs qR	r > 30 ms notched S time to S nadir > 70 ms
V₆	RS (r < S)	qR

Fig. 8.5 ECG patterns specific for ventricular tachycardia in leads V₁ and V₆.

way to diagnose SVT with aberration with exclusion of VT. This algorithm led to the diagnosis of VT if the answer to any of the following questions was positive:

- are RS complexes absent in all precordial leads?
- R to S interval >100 ms in any precordial lead?
- is atrioventricular dissociation present?
- morphology criteria for VT present both in precordial leads V₁₋₂ and V₆?

Some of these criteria still have not 100% specificity for VT (for example, RS-shaped complexes in precordial leads may be absent in pre-excited tachycardia). Some idiopathic right ventricular outflow tract and left fascicular VTs are impossible to distinguish from aberration using 12-lead ECG.[2]

Other authors suggested that the algorithm based on a decisional tree could lead to incorrect diagnosis or stop in the middle if one is unable to answer a particular question with certainty. For example, sometimes it is impossible to answer any or most of the questions (Fig. 8.6). To solve this problem, they analyzed diagnostic weight (likelihood ratio) of various criteria and multiplied

ECG of ventricular tachycardia - difficult to interpret

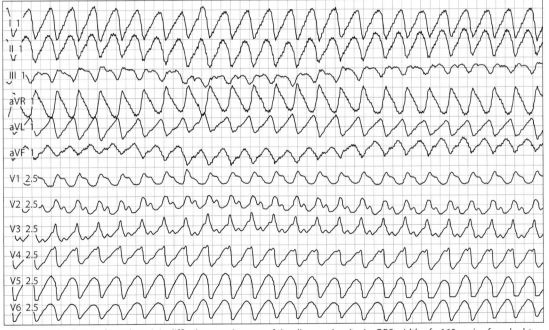

Fig. 8.6 12-lead ECG of VT where it is difficult to apply most of the diagnostic criteria. QRS width of >160 ms is of no doubt, but QRS axis, presence or absence of RS complexes, AV dissociation and others are hardly usable.

Bayesian approach for differentiation between ventricular tachycardia and aberrant supraventricular tachycardia

ECG features	Likelihood ratio (LR)	ECG features	Likelihood ratio (LR)
QRS width		**QRS width**	
≤ 0.14 second	0.31	≤ 0.14 second	
> 0.14 and ≤ 0.16 second	0.46	> 0.14 and ≤ 0.16 second	0.46
> 0.16 second	22.86	> 0.16 second	
QRS axis		**QRS axis**	
Right superior (-90º to ± 180º)	7.86	Right superior (-90º to ± 180º)	
Left (-60º to - 90º) (RBBB type)	8.21	Left (-60º to - 90º) (RBBB type)	
Right (+120º to ± 180º) (LBBB type)	3.93	Right (+120º to ± 180º) (LBBB type)	
None of the above	0.47	None of the above	0.47
V_1 morphology in RBBB pattern		**V_1 morphology in RBBB pattern**	
Taller left peak	50	**V_1 or V_2 morphology in LBBB pattern**	
Biphasic Rs or qR	4.03	r ≥ 0.04 second, or	
Triphasic rsR' or rR'	0.21	notched S downstroke, or	
None of the above	1.41	delayed S nadir > 0.06 second	
V_1 or V_2 morphology in LBBB pattern		None of the above	0.13
r ≥ 0.04 second, or		**Interval to intrinsicoid deflection in V_6**	
notched S downstroke, or	50	≥ 0.08 second	
delayed S nadir > 0.06 second		< 0.08 second	0.46
None of the above	0.13	**V_6 morphology**	
Interval to intrinsicoid deflection in V_6		Monophasic QS	
≥ 0.08 second	19.30	Biphasic rS (R/S < 1) (RBBB type)	
< 0.08 second	0.46	Triphasic qRs (R/S > 1) (RBBB type)	
V_6 morphology		None of the above	0.57
Monophasic QS	50		
Biphasic rS (R/S < 1) (RBBB type)	50		
Triphasic qRs (R/S > 1) (RBBB type)	0.13		
None of the above	0.57		

After choosing applicable criteria, their LR values are multiplied and the result is multiplied by 4 (because VT is 4 times more common than SVT in wide QRS tachycardias).

If the final result is less than 1, SVT is more probable.

If the final result equals 1 or more, VT is more probable.

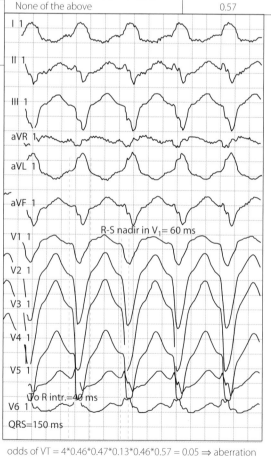

R-S nadir in V_1= 60 ms

To R intr.=40 ms

QRS=150 ms

odds of VT = 4*0.46*0.47*0.13*0.46*0.57 = 0.05 ⟹ aberration

Fig. 8.7 Bayesian approach for differentiation between VT and aberrant SVT and its uses for analysis of 12-lead ECG. (*Left panel*) List of proposed criteria and their respective likelihood ratios favoring VT, and principles of calculating the final likelihood ratio. (Modified from Lau et al.[12]) (*Right panel*) An example of applying this approach for LBBB-shaped tachycardia (SVT with LBBB aberration as confirmed during invasive electrophysiological study).

those ratios, then the result was multiplied by four (VT is approximately four times as frequent as aberrant SVT), and the final result was evaluated (VT is diagnosed if the result equals one or more).[12] A criterion such as AV dissociation is omitted using this approach, because its likelihood ratio for VT is infinite, and further work-up is not necessary. If none of the criteria is applicable, the result equals four, and VT is diagnosed. Application of this approach is illustrated in Figure 8.7.

It is extremely difficult to memorize and apply most of the previously-mentioned systems in an emergency situation. To solve this problem and make less harm to a patient with wide QRS complex tachycardia (that in 80% or more is VT), another simple rule was offered: *if QRS shape of regular wide QRS complex tachycardia is not absolutely typical for left bundle branch block (LBBB) or right bundle branch block (RBBB), VT is diagnosed.*[13] ECG patterns typical for bundle branch blocks and this simple rule are presented in Figure 8.8.

Irregular wide QRS complex tachycardia

Key points

Irregular wide QRS complex tachycardia

Main entities:
Atrial fibrillation with QRS aberration
Atrial fibrillation with ventricular pre-excitation
(do not ever use verapamil or digoxin in this arrhythmia)
Polymorphic VT is rare

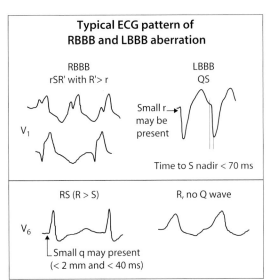

Fig. 8.8 Typical ECG pattern of RBBB and LBBB aberration. If QRS shape of regular wide QRS complex tachycardia does not match one of these variants, diagnosis of VT should be made.[13]

Analysis of QRS shape described above is also applicable for irregular wide QRS complex tachycardia. However, in this group of tachycardias two main entities are atrial fibrillation with QRS aberration and atrial fibrillation with ventricular pre-excitation. Polymorphic VT is rare and quite easily diagnosed by specific electrocardiographic patterns (Fig. 8.9). For this reason, and because the treatment of two previously mentioned entities (atrial fibrillation with aberrant and pre-excited QRS complexes) is so different (AV nodal-blocking drugs as verapamil and digoxin can be used in atrial fibrillation with aberrant QRS complexes to slow conduction via the AV node, but are absolutely contraindicated in pre-excited atrial fibrillation), the main task of a

Polymorphic ventricular tachycardia

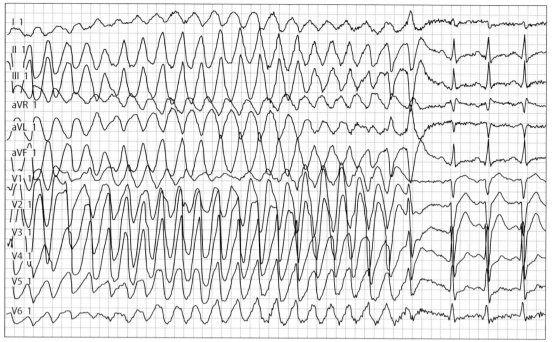

Fig. 8.9 Polymorphic VT in a patient with a normal QT interval. This clinical entity is characterized by changing QRS morphology and twisting QRS axis.

clinician is to differentiate between these two forms of atrial arrhythmia. Many ECG criteria were proposed for this purpose, but the safest way is to think about the most dangerous (pre-excited QRS) arrhythmia. Therefore, *if the ECG pattern of irregular wide QRS complex tachycardia is not absolutely typical for aberration, pre-excited atrial arrhythmia is diagnosed* and appropriate treatment is given (Fig. 8.10). This approach is shown to be both safe and specific to establish correct diagnosis.[14] It is also important to emphasize that tachycardia is considered irregular if RR intervals are not just not equal, but 'irregularly irregular'. RR interval changes as RR alternans can be seen in some VTs and aberrant SVTs (Fig. 8.11).

OTHER NON-INVASIVE TECHNIQUES

Analysis of the clinical history and bedside signs can provide important information about the tachycardia mechanism (Table 8.3) and can lead to correct diagnosis when 12-lead ECG during the paroxysm is unavailable or inconclusive. Indeed, 80% of wide QRS complex tachycardia is of ventricular origin, and probably the percentage of VT in emergency settings is even greater.[15]

A very useful and possibly underused non-invasive technique for differentiating between different wide QRS complex tachycardia mechanisms is transesophageal recording and pacing. It can easily detect AV dissociation (Fig. 8.12) or VA block that is specific for VT but hardly discernible on surface ECG tracings (Fig. 8.13). Detection of atrial fibrillation (or the possibility to consistently capture atria by pacing) in cases of rhythmic wide QRS complex tachycardia also makes diagnosis other than VT unlikely. This technique is also useful in detecting changes in VA interval and tachycardia rate with changing QRS shape which can sometimes help to establish an exact diagnosis of wide QRS complex tachycardia (Fig. 8.14).

Pre-excited atrial fibrillation

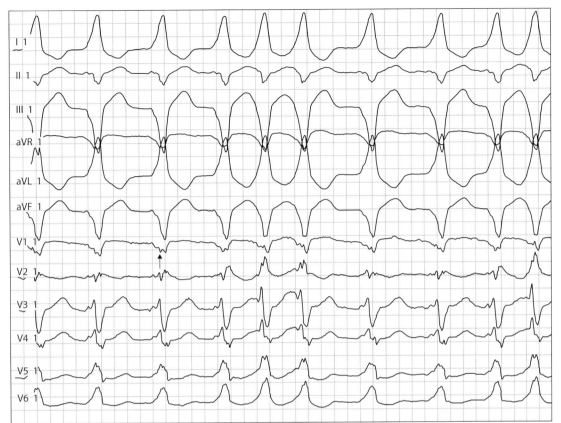

Fig. 8.10 Atrial fibrillation with anterograde conduction via an accessory pathway. Analysis of QRS shape in lead V$_1$ shows a notched S wave which is not typical for left bundle branch block (see Fig. 8.8). Therefore, diagnosis of preexcited atrial fibrillation is made.

Table 8.3 Clinical history and bedside signs that indicate various mechanisms of wide QRS complex tachycardias

Sign	Meaning
History of WPW syndrome	Pre-excited tachycardia is most probable diagnosis, but coexisting VT may also be present
History of cardiomyopathy or congestive heart failure	High probability of VT
Wide QRS complex tachycardia appears after myocardial infarction	High probability of VT
Jugular venous pulse rate does not match arterial pulse rate	AV dissociation – high probability of VT
Irregular filling of rhythmic arterial pulse not dependent on breathing	AV dissociation – high probability of VT

VT, ventricular tachycardia; WPW, Wolf-Parkinson-White

Ventricular tachycardia with RR alternans

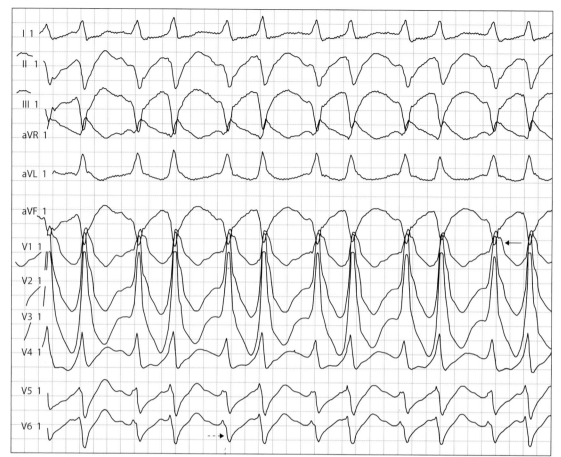

Fig. 8.11 Left ventricular VT with RR alternans. Morphological criteria specific for VT are seen in lead V_1 (RR' with R > R', solid arrow) and V_6 (R < S in RBBB shape, dashed arrow). If this tachycardia was considered irregular, pre-excited atrial fibrillation would be diagnosed. Emergency treatment of VT and pre-excited AF would not differ.

Adenosine intravenous bolus injection in conjunction with 12-lead ECG or especially with transesophageal recording is valuable tool to differentiate mechanisms of wide QRS complex tachycardia. Its effect primarily on AV and sinoatrial nodes, and to far lesser extent, on atrial and ventricular arrythmias, is summarized in Table 8.4. In emergency settings, however, its value is not as great as was thought earlier, simply due to the fact that most patients who arrive in the emergency room suffer from VT. Because adenosine usually does not terminate VT, its administration delays effective therapy and may destabilize borderline hemodynamics in VTs and pre-excited tachycardias. These days its usage is therefore discouraged if the tachycardia is not proven to be SVT.[16]

APPROACH TO WIDE QRS COMPLEX TACHYCARDIA

Contemporary guidelines and tachycardia management algorithms[16] emphasize the importance of the hemodynamic status of the patient and possible proarrhythmic effects of antiarrhythmic drugs. If the patient is hemodynamically unstable,

AV dissociation during ventricular tachycardia

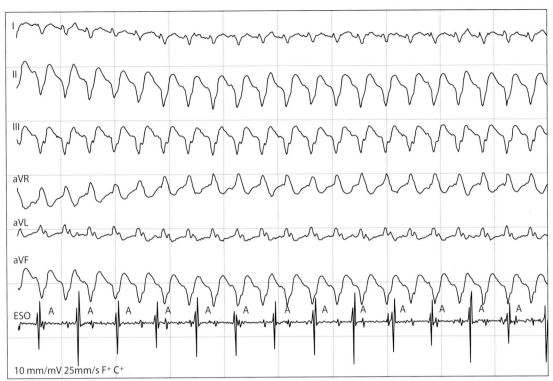

Fig. 8.12 Transesophageal signal recording in VT related to scarring after myocardial infarction. Surface ECG leads I–aVF are presented together with esophageal lead (ESO). Esophageal lead shows AV dissociation (atrial activity is not related to QRS complexes and has a lower rate). P waves are hardly seen on surface ECG leads and can be easily confused with artifacts.

Table 8.4 Diagnostic clues given by effects of adenosine in various wide QRS complex tachycardias

Tachycardia is terminated	Tachycardias with participation of AV node (AV nodal, orthodromic tachycardias with participation of APs), sinus node reciprocal tachycardia, some automatic atrial tachycardias, some right ventricular outflow tract tachycardias
AV node is blocked and tachycardia is ongoing in atria ('unmasking of atrial activity')	Atrial flutter and intra-atrial tachycardias
No effect	VT, pre-excited tachycardias, insufficient dose or inappropriate administration of adenosine

AP, accessory pathway; AV, atrioventricular; VT, ventricular tachycardia

synchronized direct current cardioversion should be performed immediately despite the width of QRS complex and heart rate. Use of more than one antiarrhythmic agent per patient is not recommended because of a high probability of proarrhythmia, especially in failing hearts. However, sometimes the combination of two drugs may be used (for example, if tachycardia recurs after cardioversion and is resistant to one antiarrhythmic drug). Correction of electrolyte balance and other deteriorating factors like ischemia should always be performed in these cases.

2:1 VA block during ventricular tachycardia

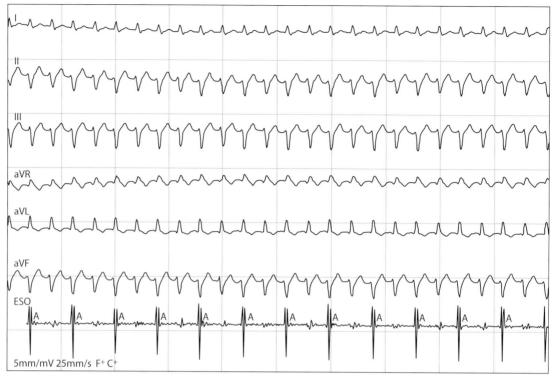

Fig. 8.13 Transesophageal signal recording in idiopathic left ventricular tachycardia. Surface ECG leads I–aVF are presented together with the esophageal lead (ESO). The esophageal lead shows 2:1 VA block (each second atrial complex is within QRS complex).The resulting QRS alternans ECG pattern (negative part of QRS accentuated by negative retrograde P waves in inferior leads II, III and aVF) is not specific for VT.

Re-evaluation of the role of one drug [lidocaine (lignocaine)] and growing experience with others (such as amiodarone) has changed recommendations for emergency therapy of wide QRS complex tachycardia.[16] These recommendations are summarized in Table 8.5. Newer guidelines also emphasize the role of establishing as an exact diagnosis as possible, including the use of esophageal recording.

An algorithmic approach to evaluate clinical signs of a patient with tachycardia including wide QRS complex tachycardia is presented in Figure 8.15, and approach to the patient with wide QRS complex tachycardia is presented in Figure 8.16.

An invasive electrophysiological study is often indicated in wide QRS complex tachycardia patients, both to establish correct diagnosis and to study the possibility of ablation and other treatment options.[17] Long-term usage of antiarrhythmic drugs is not indicated if the exact mechanism of tachycardia is unknown and is only safe in low-risk patients (with preserved ventricular function). Treatment options for wide QRS complex tachycardia and other tachycardias (ablation, ICD) are discussed in other chapters.

Emergency treatment of wide QRS complex tachycardia

When the patient is hemodynamically unstable, synchronized direct current cardioversion should be the treatment of choice and performed immediately regardless of the width of QRS complex and heart rate

Accessory pathway-mediated tachycardia

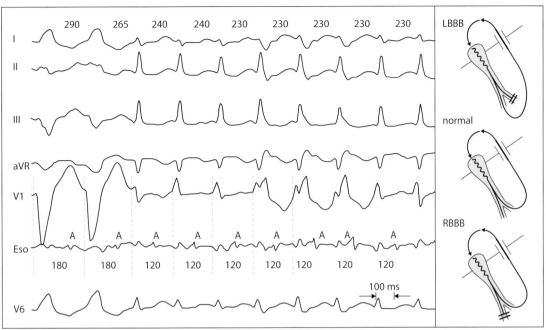

Fig. 8.14 Transesophageal recording in a patient with left-sided accessory pathway-mediated tachycardia showing intermittent LBBB (two first QRS complexes) and RBBB (three middle QRS complexes). ECG leads I, II, III, aVR, V_1 and V_6 are presented together with esophageal lead (Eso). RR intervals (figures above the lead I tracing) and VA intervals (figures below Eso tracing) are shown in ms. LBBB aberration prolongs VA interval (measured from the onset of QRS complex on the surface ECG leads to A potential on the Eso tracing) by 60 ms and slows the tachycardia. RBBB aberration has no effect on VA and RR intervals. Corresponding diagrams are shown on the right. The fact that LBBB influences the VA and RR intervals (ipsilateral bundle branch block) allows a diagnosis to be established.

Table 8.5 Recommendations for emergency therapeutic interventions in wide QRS complex tachycardias	
Hemodynamically unstable wide QRS complex tachycardia irrespective of mechanism	Direct current cardioversion if serious signs are related to tachycardia
Wide QRS complex tachycardia of unknown type	Procainamide (if cardiac function preserved), amiodarone
SVT with aberration	Vagal maneuvers, adenosine, then all other antiarrhythmics can be considered according to hemodynamic state and possibility of proarrhythmia in depressed left ventricular function
Monomorphic VT	Procainamide, sotalol, amiodarone, lidocaine (lignocaine). Class IC antiarrhythmias are contraindicated in case of ischemia or depressed left ventricular function
Polymorphic VT	Correction of electrolyte imbalance and/or ischemia – normal baseline QT interval: beta-blockers, lidocaine (lignocaine), amiodarone, procainamide, sotalol – prolonged baseline QT interval: magnesium, overdrive pacing, isoproterenol, phenytoin, lidocaine (lignocaine)

AV, atrioventricular; AP, accessory pathway; VT, ventricular tachycardia.

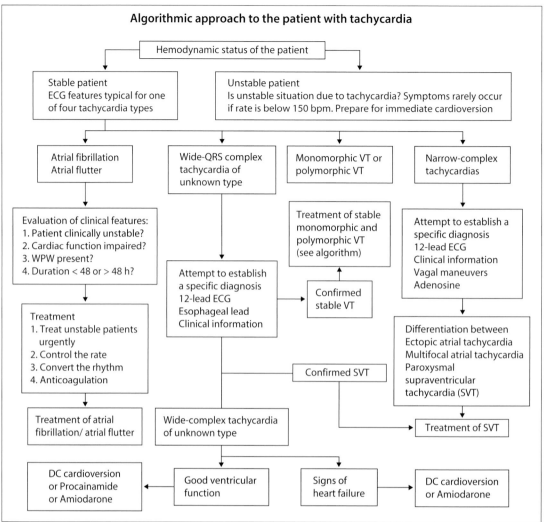

Fig. 8.15 Algorithmic approach to the patient with tachycardia. WPW, Wolff-Parkinson-White syndrome. (Tachycardia overview algorithm modified from the European Resuscitation Council[16]).

References

1. European Resusctation Council. Part 10: Pediatric advanced life support. Resuscitation 2000; 46:343–399.

2. Drew BJ, Scheinman MM. ECG criteria to distinguish between aberrantly conducted supraventricular tachycardia and ventricular tachycardia. PACE 1995; 18:2194–2208.

3. Wellens HJJ, Brugada P. Diagnosis of ventricular tachycardia from the 12-lead electrocardiogram. Cardiol Clin 1987; 5:511–525.

4. Prystowsky EN, Packer DL. Pre-excited tachycardias. In: Zipes DP, Jalife J, eds. Cardiac electrophysiology from cell to bedside. Philadelphia: WB Saunders; 1990: 472–479.

5. Akhtar M, Jazayeri M, Avitall B, et al. Electrophysiological spectrum of wide QRS complex tachycardia. In: Zipes DP, Jalife J, eds. Cardiac electrophysiology from cell to bedside. Philadelphia: WB Saunders Company; 1990:635–646.

6. Prystowsky E. Diagnosis and management of the preexcitation syndromes. Curr Probl Cardiol 1988; 13:231–310.

7. Wellens HJ, Bar FW, Lie KL. The value of the electrocardiogram in the differential diagnosis of a tachycardia with a widened QRS complex. Am J Med 1978; 64:27–33.

8. Wellens HJJ. The wide QRS tachycardia. (editorial). Ann Intern Med 1986; 104:879.

9. Alberca T, Almendral J, Sanz P, et al. Evaluation of the specificity of morphological electrocardiographic

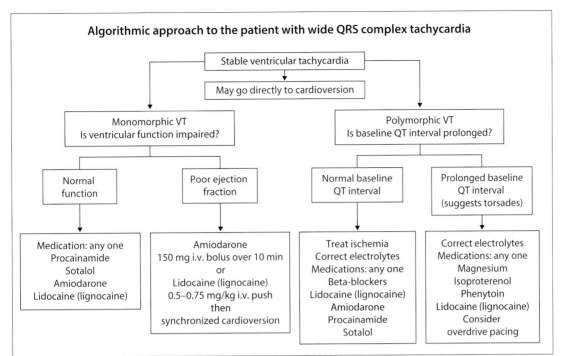

Algorithmic approach to the patient with wide QRS complex tachycardia

Fig. 8.16 Algorithmic approach to the patient with wide QRS complex tachycardias (stable ventricular tachycardia (monomorphic or polymorphic) algorithm modified from the European Resuscitation Council[16]).

criteria for the differential diagnosis of wide QRS complex tachycardia in patients with intraventricular conduction defects. Circulation 1997; 96:3527–3533.

10. Buxton AE, Marchlinski FE, Doherty JU. Hazards of intravenous verapamil for sustained ventricular tachycardia. Am J Cardiol 1987; 59:1107.

11. Brugada P, Brugada J, Mont L, et al. A new approach to the differential diagnosis of a regular tachycardia with a wide QRS complex. Circulation 1991; 83:1649–1659.

12. Lau EW, Pathamanathan RK, Ng GA, et al. The Bayesian approach improves the electrocardiographic diagnosis of broad complex tachycardia. PACE 2000; 23:1519–1526.

13. Griffith MJ, Garratt CJ, Mounsey P, et al. Ventricular tachycardia as default diagnosis in broad complex tachycardia. Lancet 1994; 343:386–388.

14. Lau EW, Pathamanathan RK, Ng GA, et al. Electrocardiographic criteria for diagnosis of irregular broad complex tachycardia with a high sensitivity for preexcited atrial fibrillation. PACE 2000; 23:2040–2045.

15. Barold SS. Bedside diagnosis of wide QRS tachycardia (editorial). PACE 1995; 18:2109–2115.

16. European Resuscitation Council. Part 6: Advanced cardiovascular life support. Section 7: Algorithm approach to ACLS emergencies. 7D: The tachycardia algorithms. Resuscitation 2000; 46:185–193.

17. Zipes D, Di Marco JP, Gillette PC, et al. ACC/AHA task force report: guidelines for clinical intracardiac electrophysiological and catheter ablation procedures. J Am Coll Cardiol 1995:555–573.

Postsurgical atrial fibrillation

Arjun V Gururaj MD
Boston Medical Center, Boston, MA, USA

Rodney H Falk MD FRCP FACC FAHA
Boston Medical Center, Boston, MA, USA

> **Prevalence of atrial fibrillation in cardiothoracic surgery is high: 20–50% with a steep age gradient**

Introduction

The development of supraventricular arrhythmias (predominantly atrial fibrillation) after surgery is not uncommon. For major non-thoracic surgery the prevalence is about 3%, whereas following cardiothoracic procedures the prevalence of atrial fibrillation is as high as 17–50%. Although many attempts have been made to identify and to modify risk factors associated with postsurgical atrial fibrillation, the prevalence of this condition has remained essentially unchanged since the introduction of coronary artery bypass grafting. Indeed although minimally-invasive coronary artery grafting was initially thought to significantly reduce postoperative atrial fibrillation, this is probably related to patient selection.[1]

Under most circumstances, the hemodynamic consequences of postsurgical atrial fibrillation are minimal. However, the risk of a stroke [cerebrovascular accident (CVA)] after surgery may be increased, and the duration of hospitalization is often increased by an average of 2 to 3 days while the arrhythmia is being corrected prior to patient discharge. Thus, postsurgical atrial arrhythmias may pose a significant burden upon healthcare costs and, occasionally, on patient well-being.

EPIDEMIOLOGY

Although atrial arrhythmias may occur after any surgical procedure, the association with cardiothoracic surgery is most robust. The prevalence of atrial fibrillation in major non-thoracic surgery is about 3% while in non-cardiac surgery requiring thoracotomy it approaches 10–20%.[2] Shortly after the advent of modern coronary artery bypass grafting (CABG) surgery, pioneered by Favalaro in the late 1960s, many investigators reported that atrial fibrillation post-CABG was not uncommon. Although Favaloro reported a prevalence of 12% in his first 100 patients[3]

post-CABG atrial fibrillation now approaches (and sometimes exceeds) 30%, possibly because of the inclusion of older and sicker patients. The peak onset of atrial fibrillation occurs around the second day after the operation, with almost one-half of patients who are destined to have the arrhythmia developing it by then. By day 3 there is a halving of the peak incidence and after that there is a rapid decrease in onset.

Among the known risk factors for post-CABG atrial fibrillation, the most powerful include older age and the lack of perioperative use of beta-adrenergic antagonists. The increased risk of atrial fibrillation in elderly patients probably relates to the increased atrial fibrosis that is associated with increasing age. The protective effect of beta-blockade suggests a triggering role of catecholamines and is discussed below.

MECHANISMS OF ARRHYTHMOGENESIS

Although several characteristics of postoperative atrial fibrillation differ from other forms of the arrhythmia (Table 9.1), the electrophysiological features of the established episode is likely to be similar to the mechanisms postulated by Moe and investigators four decades ago. Most episodes of this arrhythmia can be considered a micro-re-entrant rhythm that is dependent on the presence of multiple propagating electrical wavefronts. These constantly collide and produce new wavefronts (daughter wavelets). The process usually occurs in an abnormal atrium (ischemic, fibrosed, dilated, etc.) and is characterized by an abnormal dispersion of atrial refractoriness. Patients advanced in age have a higher risk of atrial fibrillation regardless of any surgical manipulation, due simply to the greater likelihood of possessing abnormal atria. Thus, the many postulated risks factors for atrial fibrillation may provide appropriate triggers (in the form of atrial premature

Table 9.1 Is post-CABG AF a different entity from non-surgical AF?

POSTSURGICAL AF	NON-SURGICAL AF
Limited time frame (2 days to ?6 weeks) postoperatively	Generally time independent
Prophylactic beta-blockade effective	Beta-blockade minimally effective
Normal atrial size	Variable atrial size
Associated with older age	Associated with older age
Commoner with preoperative P wave prolongation	P wave prolongation common when in sinus rhythm
May occur early post-Maze operation	Maze operation used as therapy

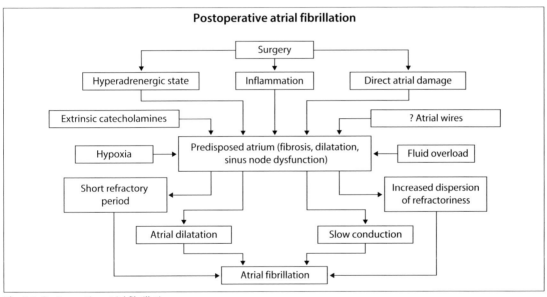

Fig. 9.1 Postoperative atrial fibrillation.

beats, further increasing the heterogeneity of atrial refractoriness, etc.) that can induce postoperative atrial fibrillation. This is illustrated in Figure 9.1.

A likely common link between all patients undergoing surgery and the development of atrial fibrillation is the level of sympathetic tone and the presence of circulating catecholamines. The significant reduction in post-CABG atrial fibrillation by perioperative beta-blockade contrasts with the modest antifibrillatory role of beta-blockers in non-surgical atrial fibrillation, and suggests that the

mechanisms differ. Several other risk factors for post-CABG atrial fibrillation have been postulated, and these are detailed in Table 9.2. Of interest, is the finding that a prolonged preoperative P wave duration is correlated with post-CABG atrial fibrillation. Buxton and Josephson measured preoperative P wave duration on a standard 12-lead ECG and initially reported this finding.[4] Subsequent studies using signal averaging of the P wave confirmed these observations [5] and suggest that, as in other types of atrial fibrillation, a *substrate* (slow or

Table 9.2 Proposed risk-factors for post-CABG AF

- Patient-related
  Age
  P wave duration
  Coronary anatomy
  Pulmonary status
  Pre-op beta-blocker
  Valve disease
- Procedure-related
  Type of surgery
  Cardioplegia type
  Cross-clamp time
  Atrial ischemia
- Postoperative factors
  Beta-blocker
  withdrawal
  Pericarditis/effusion

inhomogeneous inter- or intra-atrial conduction) may be a necessary component of atrial fibrillation development in addition to the *triggers* surrounding surgery. Table 9.2 illustrates some of the potential factors involved in the development of post-CABG atrial fibrillation

TREATMENT OPTIONS

Figure 9.2 illustrates an approach to the management of post-CABG atrial fibrillation. This arrhythmia is generally a self-limiting condition, frequently occurring in patients who have been fully revascularized and who are therefore unlikely to experience tachycardia-mediated ischemia. Thus, before discussing the various therapeutic options available to the clinician for the prevention and treatment of postoperative atrial fibrillation, one might question whether therapy is warranted, and if it is, whether there is a subgroup of patients in whom the arrhythmia is more likely to produce problems.

The hemodynamic response to post-CABG atrial fibrillation varies, with some patients remaining asymptomatic and a small minority developing severe cardiac compromise. Although no published data exist, it is likely that those patients most at risk of symptoms are those with left ventricular hypertrophy due to hypertension or aortic valve disease, as well as those with incomplete myocardial revascularization. A rapid ventricular response to atrial fibrillation is probably the

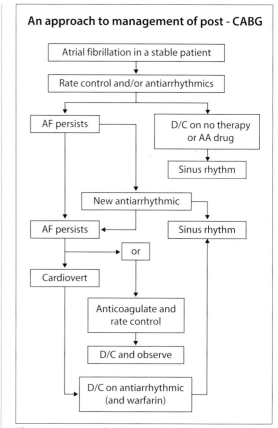

An approach to management of post - CABG

Fig. 9.2 An approach to management of post-coronary artery bypass grafting (CABG). D/C, discharge.

most significant contributor to symptoms and thus rate control is an important part of initial management if atrial fibrillation develops.

Another potential morbidity of postsurgical atrial fibrillation is the risk of embolic stroke.[6] The prevalence of stroke in the post-CABG population with atrial fibrillation has been estimated at 3.5–7%. Although this is about twofold greater than those who do not experience atrial fibrillation, the question has been raised whether atrial fibrillation is a risk factor for stroke, or merely a marker in an older population who also have vascular disease with a likelihood of aortic plaques and cerebrovascular disease. In a large group of patients from the Cleveland Clinic, the role of vascular disease as a stroke risk factor was confirmed and it conferred a twofold relative risk of stroke. An unstable preoperative state was associated with a

2.2-fold risk and postoperative atrial fibrillation increased stroke prevalence from 3.5% to 6.6%, a relative risk of 1.8. However, the risk of stroke increases with age and older patients may have other risk factors to develop a stroke. Thus, although for many patients, postoperative atrial fibrillation is no more than a nuisance, elevated postoperative stroke risk remains a major argument for therapies aimed at preventing post-CABG atrial fibrillation and for early aggressive management if atrial fibrillation occurs.

Prophylaxis

Several pharmacological therapies have been evaluated for prophylaxis against post-CABG atrial arrhythmias. These can be divided into trials of prophylactic antiarrhythmic drugs and trials of beta blockers, digoxin, or calcium-channel antagonists. Andrews et al[7] performed a pooled analysis of 26 studies using beta blockade, digoxin, or verapamil preoperatively in an attempt to reduce the incidence of postoperative atrial fibrillation. Those investigators demonstrated that only beta blockers (commenced preoperatively and continued postoperatively) were efficacious in preventing postoperative atrial fibrillation. In the 18 studies with patients receiving beta blockers (n=1549), the relative risk of developing postoperative atrial fibrillation was 0.28 ($p < 0.0001$) – an approximately 70% reduction in risk.

Sotalol and amiodarone are the main antiarrhythmic agents that have been evaluated for prophylaxis of atrial fibrillation. Sotalol, started 24–48 h prior to surgery at doses of 80 to 120 mg twice daily, effectively reduced the incidence of post-CABG atrial fibrillation.[8] However sotalol is a potent beta blocking agent and it is not clear whether the class III properties of the drug add anything to this property. Studies evaluating amiodarone have generally demonstrated that preoperative amiodarone prophylaxis is effective in reducing postoperative atrial fibrillation.[9] Prophylaxis with oral amiodarone was, however, started 7–14 days preoperatively in some of these studies. This is impractical for patients who are undergoing urgent surgery, as in many centers in the USA the time between angiography and surgery is often only a day or two. An alternate regimen of intravenous amiodarone, administered immediately preoperatively has had demonstrated efficacy in small studies.[10] When considering amiodarone prophylaxis, the small but potentially very serious complication of postoperative respiratory distress syndrome which has been linked to amiodarone should not be ignored.[11]

Whether or not these regimens reduce hospital stay by reducing the incidence of atrial fibrillation is debatable, with some studies showing a reduction, but most demonstrating no effect on length of stay (Fig. 9.3).[12,13]

At present, it is unclear whether an attempt to reduce postoperative atrial fibrillation by the use of preoperative antiarrhythmic agents is warranted. While it is prudent to attempt to treat all patients with beta blockers perioperatively, it may be reasonable to limit perioperative antiarrhythmic therapy to patients in whom there is a concern that postoperative atrial fibrillation is most likely to occur[14] or in whom it may cause hemodynamic compromise. The latter patients might include those with significant impairment of ventricular function and those with left ventricular hypertrophy (who may be dependent upon the atrial contribution to ventricular filling).

An alternative, non-pharmacological approach to the prevention of atrial fibrillation is the use of bi-atrial pacing, via temporary epicardial pacing wires implanted during CABG. Bi-atrial pacing may (among other mechanisms) prevent atrial fibrillation by overdrive suppression of atrial premature depolarizations or by reduction in heterogeneity of atrial refractoriness. Several studies have demonstrated the efficacy of this

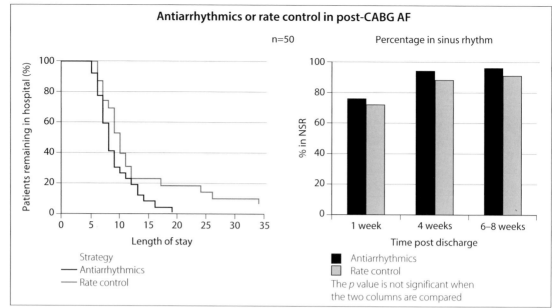

Fig. 9.3 Antiarrhythmics or rate control in post-coronary artery bypass grafting (CABG) AF. Reproduced with permission from Lee et al.[13]

approach,[15] but complications may occur, and precise positioning and stability of the pacing electrodes appears to be of great importance.[16] Although bi-atrial pacing holds promise for therapy of postoperative atrial fibrillation, the additional cost and potential risks involved warrant larger, multicenter studies before it can be generally recommended.

Oral beta-blockade prophylaxis in cardiac surgery

Dose:	To an HR-target about 60 ± 5 bpm
Duration:	Several days preoperatively to postoperatively long term
Contra-indications:	Chronic obstructive lung disease, A-V block, severe congestive heart failure

HR, heart rate; A-V, atrioventricular

Oral amiodarone prophylaxis in cardiac surgery

Dose:	6 g over 6 days beginning on preoperative day 1, or 7 g over 10 days beginning on preoperative day 5. Thereafter 200 mg per day
Duration:	Until discharge, or longer if indicated
Contraindications:	Risk of proarrhythmia

Treatment of an acute episode

Acute management of postoperative atrial fibrillation is similar to treatment of non-surgical atrial fibrillation. The cornerstones of therapy consists of:

1. control of ventricular rate
2. consideration of anticoagulation therapy
3. determination whether to attempt cardioversion

Slowing of the ventricular rate is best achieved with beta-blockers and calcium channel antagonists. Digoxin, used as monotherapy, has a limited role in this circumstance as this agent's predominant mode of action is to augment parasympathetic tone, which is generally suppressed in most postoperative patients. Nevertheless, digoxin may be synergistic with beta-blockers and calcium-channel antagonists and also may be of value in patients with impaired ventricular function.

Most episodes of postoperative atrial fibrillation are self-terminating. However, they may last for several days and they may be quite sensitive to antiarrhythmic drugs because of the short duration of the arrhythmia. Therefore, many physicians attempt to terminate atrial fibrillation pharmacologically. The choice of agent is dependent on the clinician's preference and experience, and high rates of conversion have been demonstrated with quinidine, intravenous flecainide and intravenous amiodarone, among other drugs. Because of the concern about proarrhythmia if the drug is continued long term, it is best to avoid flecainide particularly as most postcardiac surgery patients have coronary artery disease. Quinidine is also potentially problematic and amiodarone has probably become the drug of choice. If the patient has been converted to sinus rhythm with an antiarrhythmic agent and is in sinus rhythm at the time of hospital discharge, it is unclear whether or not such a drug needs to be continued. Generally, recurrences of atrial fibrillation are relatively uncommon but they can occur and it may be prudent to continue an agent for 4 weeks after discharge.

The risk–benefit ratio of anticoagulant therapy following an episode of postoperative atrial fibrillation is also unknown. Data from patients who have had prosthetic valves implanted indicate that warfarin can be initiated early without significant risk of bleeding and it is reasonable to consider warfarin therapy in a patient with recurrent episodes of postoperative atrial fibrillation. However, as the risk of stroke in the few weeks following surgery is probably low, it is generally our policy to use anticoagulation in such patients, but if a contraindication exists we have a low threshold for stopping or for not initiating the drug. The treatment of an episode of atrial fibrillation that is not, or cannot be, terminated by antiarrhythmic drugs is also subject to debate. The role of cardioversion prior to hospital discharge is unclear and is dependent on the individual clinician. Many of these patients, if untreated, will be found to have reverted to sinus rhythm at follow-up (Fig. 9.3) and if they are anticoagulated and have adequate rate control at the time of discharge, cardioversion seems unnecessary. Should atrial fibrillation persist at the first postoperative visit, electrical cardioversion may be considered at that time.

CONCLUSIONS

Atrial fibrillation affects as many as 40% of patients following cardiac surgery, and may lead to greater duration of hospital stay. Despite its high prevalence among patients who have undergone cardiac surgery, its clinical significance remains unclear, although increasing evidence suggests that it is a risk factor for postoperative stroke. Postoperative atrial fibrillation differs from other forms of atrial fibrillation by virtue of its self-limiting nature, the marked preventive effect produced by beta-blockers and the uncertainties that surround the risks and benefits of treatment. It remains a challenging arrhythmia that is attracting an increasing focus of attention, from cost analyses through drug prevention and treatment strategies to sophisticated approaches to prevention by pacing that may offer deeper insights into the mechanism of this common condition.

Key points

Potential risk factors for postsurgical atrial fibrillation

- Age
- Absence of perioperative beta-blockers
- Presence of obstructive lung disease
- Presence of significant valvular disease
- Extent of coronary artery disease
- Prolonged P wave duration on the surface electrocardiogram

References

1. Tamis-Holland JE, Homel P, Durani M, et al. Atrial fibrillation after minimally invasive direct coronary artery bypass surgery. J Am Coll Cardiol 2000; 36:1884–1888.
2. Neustein SM, Kahn P, Krellenstein DJ, et al. Incidence of arrhythmias after thoracic surgery: Thoracotomy versus video-assisted thoracoscopy. J Cardiothorac Vasc Anesth 1998; 12:659–661.
3. Favaloro R. Direct myocardial revascularization: a 10 year journey. Myths and realities. Am J Cardiol 1979; 43:109–129.

4. Buxton AE, Josephson ME. The role of P wave duration as a predictor of postoperative atrial arrhythmias. Chest 1981; 80:68–73.

5. Stafford PJ, Kolvekar S, Cooper J, et al. Signal averaged P wave compared with standard electrocardiography or echocardiography for prediction of atrial fibrillation after coronary bypass grafting. Heart 1997; 77:417–422.

6. Stamou SC, Hill PC, Dangas G, et al. Stroke after coronary artery bypass – Incidence, predictors, and clinical outcome. Stroke 2001; 32:1508–1512.

7. Andrews T, Reimold S, Berlin J, et al. Prevention of supraventicular arrhythmias after coronary artery bypass surgery. A meta-analysis of randomized controlled trials. Circulation 1991; 84(suppl III):III 236–III 244.

8. Gomes JA, Ip J, Santoni-Rugiu F, et al. Oral d,l sotalol reduces the incidence of postoperative atrial fibrillation in coronary artery bypass surgery patients: A randomized, double-blind, placebo-controlled study. J Am Coll Cardiol 1999; 34:334–339.

9. Giri S, White CM, Dunn AB, et al. Oral amiodarone for prevention of atrial fibrillation after open heart surgery, the Atrial Fibrillation Suppression Trial (AFIST): a randomised placebo-controlled trial. Lancet 2001; 357:830–836.

10. Solomon AJ, Greenberg MD, Kilborn MJ, et al. Amiodarone versus a beta-blocker to prevent atrial fibrillation after cardiovascular surgery. Am Heart J 2001; 142:811–815.

11. Ashrafian H, Davey P. Is amiodarone an underrecognized cause of acute respiratory failure in the ICU? Chest 2001; 120:275–282.

12. Reddy P. Does prophylaxis against atrial fibrillation after cardiac surgery reduce length of stay or hospital costs? Pharmacotherapy 2001; 21:338–344.

13. Lee J, Klein G, Krahn A, et al. Rate-control versus conversion strategy in postoperative atrial fibrillation: a prospective randomized pilot study. Am Heart J 2000; 140:871–877.

14. Weber UK, Osswald S, Huber M, et al. Selective versus non-selective antiarrhythmic approach for prevention of atrial fibrillation after coronary surgery – is there a need for pre-operative risk stratification – a prospective placebo-controlled study using low-dose sotalol. Eur Heart J 1998; 19:794–800.

15. Gerstenfeld EP, Khoo M, Martin RC, et al. Effectiveness of bi-atrial pacing for reducing atrial fibrillation after coronary artery bypass graft surgery. J Intervent Cardiac Electrophysiol 2001; 5:275–283.

16. Daubert JC, Mabo P. Atrial pacing for the prevention of postoperative atrial fibrillation: How and where to pace? J Am Coll Cardiol 2000; 35:1423–1427.

Quality of life in atrial fibrillation

Mads D M Engelmann MD PhD
Herlev University Hospital, Herlev, Denmark

John Godtfredsen MD FESC
Herlev University Hospital, Herlev, Denmark

Quality of life is impaired
in atrial fibrillation

Introduction

It is now widely acknowledged that quality of life (QoL) should be measured as an integral component of clinical trails, particularly where treatments are given with an intention to palliate or reduce symptoms.[1] Several factors have contributed to the growing interest in QoL. QoL issues are becoming central to the management of chronic conditions that accompany the growth of an aging population. Patients expect to participate as partners in therapeutic decisions and QoL measures facilitate informed choice in making these decisions. Furthermore, regulatory authorities are requesting QoL data as part of new drug approval. And, finally the growing fields of outcome research and health-technology assessment evaluate the efficacy, cost effectiveness and net benefit of new therapeutic strategies to determine whether the associated increases in expenditures for healthcare are justified.[2]

Reasons for the growing interest in quality of life assessment

- central in the management of chronic conditions
- patient expectations
- requested by regulatory authorities
- requested by healthcare planners

Since QoL assessment may be unfamiliar to some readers the first part of the present chapter is an introduction of basic definitions and instruments used in QoL research. The objective of the remaining part of the chapter is to accentuate some of the more recent as well as ongoing studies on QoL in AF in an attempt to review what is currently known and perhaps more important what still has to be learned in regard to QoL in AF.

DEFINITION OF QUALITY OF LIFE

The evaluation of QoL is inherently subjective and no consensus on the definition exists. Most approaches used in medical contexts do not attempt to include more general notions such as life satisfaction or living standards[3] and tend rather to concentrate on four broad domains: physical condition, psychological well-being, social activities and everyday activities.

Key points

There is an emerging consensus that quality of life is a multidimensional construct based on four components:

1. physical condition
2. psychological well-being
3. social activities
4. everyday activities.

(From Lüderitz[4])

Constructing scales of measurement

The majority of QoL questionnaires measure each QoL domain separately by asking a series of questions known as 'items'. The answers to each item are then converted to numerical scores that are

Delineation of terms

- *Item*: a single question, such as 'How severe is your shortness of breath'.
- *Scale*: contains the available categories or other mechanisms for expressing the response to the question. The foregoing question might be answered with a set of three categories such as mild, moderate or extreme.
- *Domain*: identifies a particular focus of attention such as cardiovascular symptoms or cognitive functioning, it may comprise the response to a single item or responses to several related items.
- *Instrument*: a collection of items used for obtaining the desired data.

(From Gill & Feinstein[6])

combined to 'scale scores' which may also be combined to yield summary scores known as 'domain scores'.[5] The objective for this method is that each domain score reflects the most important components of the overall QoL.

SELECTING AN INSTRUMENT

The lack of a clear definition of QoL is reflected in the many instruments that have been proposed to measure it.[6] Indeed a state of the art review identified some 150 different QoL measures.[7] Several factors affect the selection of appropriate instruments to assess QoL. There are two basic approaches to measure QoL: generic instruments and disease specific instruments.

Generic instruments are used in the general population to assess a wide range of domains applicable to a variety of health states, conditions and diseases. They are usually not specific to any particular disease state or susceptible population of patients and are therefore most useful in conducting general survey research on health and making comparisons between disease states.[5] The generic instruments facilitate comparisons among different disease groups, however the broad approach may reduce responsiveness to effects of healthcare.

Disease-specific instruments focus on the domains most relevant to the disease or condition under study and on the characteristics of patients in whom the condition is most prevalent. Disease-specific instruments are most appropriate for clinical trials in which specific therapeutic interventions are being evaluated. Disease-specific instruments have several theoretical advantages. They reduce patient burden and increase acceptability by including only relevant dimensions. Disadvantages are the lack of comparability of results with those from other disease groups and the possibility of missing effects in dimensions that are not included.[8]

Psychometric properties

Apart from being generic or disease-specific the instrument should possess several important properties, which include coverage, reliability, validity, responsiveness, sensitivity and practicality.

Basic requirements of quality of life assessments

- *multidimensional construct*: the instrument reflects several dimensions of QoL
- *coverage*: the measurement of QoL should address each objective and subjective component (symptom, condition, or social role) that is important to members of the patient population and susceptible to being affected, positively or negatively, by interventions
- *reliability*: does the measure produce the same results when repeated in the same population under the same conditions
- *validity*: does the instrument measure what it is intended to measure, such as QoL
- *responsiveness*: is a measure of the association between the change in the observed score and the true value of the construct[5]
- *sensitivity*: refers to the ability of a measurement to reflect true changes or differences in QoL[5]
- *practicality*: for a measure to be useful in clinical practice it must not only be valid, appropriate, reliable, responsive and sensitive, but it must be simple, quick to complete, easy to score and provide useful clinical data.[9]

PREVIOUS STUDIES OF QUALITY OF LIFE IN PATIENTS WITH ATRIAL FIBRILLATION

Although the number of studies on QoL in atrial fibrillation (AF) are rapidly increasing, the impact of AF on QoL is far from established. Several reviews on the issue have concluded that the *quality* of QoL research in AF is suboptimal. There are many criteria by which one might evaluate the quality of studies aiming to quantify QoL. The following eight criteria may be useful when planning new studies as well as when evaluating the existing literature.

Criteria to be fulfilled when planning or evaluating quality of life studies

1. Having a conceptual definition of QoL.
2. Identifying what dimensions of QoL are measured.
3. Specifying the rationale for choice of measures selected.
4. Using at least one measure that is general in focus – generic instrument.
5. At least one measure that is specific to the population of interest – i.e. disease-specific.
6. Selecting measures with evidence for reliability and validity and reporting appropriately.
7. If appropriate, collecting data at several points in the treatment process to consider any change over time.
8. Asking patients to give an overall rating of QoL.

As described in Chapter 5 the range of complaints at presentation by the patients with AF is wide and related to the age of the patient as well as the type of AF, i.e. paroxysmal, persistent or permanent. Furthermore at least a quarter of the patients have silent AF with no obvious symptoms. QoL in AF cannot be appropriately evaluated without keeping these differences in mind. A few previous studies of QoL in patients with paroxysmal, persistent and permanent AF are shown below. They have used to some extent validated QoL measurements although none of the studies meet the above-mentioned criteria.

Quality of life in paroxysmal atrial fibrillation and persistent atrial fibrillation

In a cross-sectional study by Dorian et al[10] QoL in 152 relatively young (58±12 years) patients with paroxysmal or persistent AF referred to tertiary care, was compared with a group of healthy individuals, and four cardiac control groups:

1. A group of stable post percutaneous coronary intervention (PCI) patients created for the study;

2. Post-PCI patients from a previous published study;[11]
3. Postmyocardial infarction patients published in the SF-36 data manual;[12] and
4. Heart failure patients published in the SF-36 data manual.[12]

QoL was assessed using the following five instruments:

1. *The Medical Outcome Study Short-Form Health Survey, SF-36*[13] provides standardized scores ranging from 0 to 100 to measure eight health domains including role-physical domain, role-emotional domain, physical functioning, social functioning, mental health, vitality, bodily pain, and general health perceptions. Finally a physical component summary score and a mental component summary score is calculated using the scores obtained in the physical and mental domains respectively. Higher score represents better QoL (Tables 10.1 and 10.2).[10–12,14] The questionnaire has been used and validated in a diverse spectrum of cardiac populations including patients with implantable cardioverter defibrillator (ICD).
2. *Goldman Specific Activity Scale*[15] is a functional status scale for patients with cardiovascular diseases. Evaluation in a small sample of pacemaker patients suggests a good convergent validity and a high test reliability.
3. *The Symptom Checklist: Frequency and Severity*[16] (16 items) quantifies both symptom frequency and severity of symptoms related to arrhythmias. The initial investigation of content validity was in an AF population.
4. *Illness Intrusiveness Rating Scale*[17] was developed to measure the degree of life disruption in social, emotional, physical, affective and spiritual spheres caused by chronic illness.
5. *The University of Toronto Atrial Fibrillation Severity Scale*[10,18] is a 14 item disease-specific scale developed to capture subjective and objective ratings of AF

disease burden, including frequency, duration and severity of episodes.

Both the disease-specific and generic QoL was significantly worse in AF patients compared to healthy controls. The impairment was similar on most scales to the impairment seen in the four different cardiac control groups, in which all had a greater degree of structural heart disease (Table 10.1). Furthermore, there was a relatively poor correlation of QoL scores with 'objective' indices i.e. left ventricular ejection fraction, left atrial dimension, New York Heart Association functional class, AF frequency, and AF duration. Dorian et al[10] conclude that QoL in patients with paroxysmal or persistent AF is significantly impaired and commensurate with patients with significant cardiac disease. The poor correlation of QoL scores with left ventricular ejection fraction and NYHA class is in accordance with prior studies.[19,20]

However, it must be emphasized that the patients were symptomatic and referred to tertiary care. Nearly half of the patients (44.6%) had been to the emergency room at least once in the previous year, and 51% had been hospitalized for their AF at least once in the previous year. The impaired QoL as indicated in this study does not necessarily represent the AF patient group

in a primary or even secondary care center. This is a limitation which is seen also in other studies on QoL in AF and which must be borne in mind before the findings are accepted as representative in clinical practice. In addition, the cross-sectional design is a limitation; a longitudinal study would have provided more reliable data by compensating for spontaneous variation in QoL.[21]

The Canadian Trial of Atrial Fibrillation[22] was a double-blinded, prospective, multicenter study of the effect of amiodarone versus sotalol or propafenone in preventing AF recurrence in patients with a history of symptomatic paroxysmal or persistent AF. QoL was a secondary endpoint in this study and was assessed at baseline, before initiation of drug therapy, and after 3 and 12 months of the study using the following validated instruments:

- *The Medical Outcomes Study Short Form Health Survey* (SF-36);[13]
- *The Duke Activity Status Index*[23] is a self-administered 12-item questionnaire that provides a global measure of functional capacity;
- *Symptom Checklist: Frequency and Severity;*[16]
- *The University of Toronto Atrial Fibrillation Severity Scale;*[10,18]

Table 10.1 QoL scores across AF and five control groups. Higher scores represent better QoL (From Dorian et al[10])

Stages SF-36 scale	AF patients	(1)PCI patients	(2)PCI patients	(3)CHF patients	(4)Post MI patients	Healthy controls
General health	54±21	51±23	65±22*	47±24*	59±19	78±17*
Physical functioning	68±27	60±29	76±25	48±31*	70±26	88±19*
Role physical	47±42	47±45	71±39*	34±40*	51±39	89±28*
Vitality	47±21	48±26	60±20*	44±24	58±19*	71±14*
Mental health	68±18	74±18	75±16*	75±21*	76±16*	81±11*
Role emotional	65±41	64±44	83±35*	64±43	73±38	92±25*
Social functioning	71±28	74±29	87±21*	71±33	85±21*	92±14*
Bodily pain	69±19	68±17	73±27	63±31	73±25	77±15

Data presented as raw mean ± SD

*$p < 0.001$, compared to with AF patients

(1) PCI patients = patients 6 months after percutaneous coronary intervention

(2) PCI patients = patients after percutaneous coronary intervention from Krumholz et al[11]

(3) CHF patients = congestive heart failure patients, from Ware JE Jr[12]

(4) Post-MI patients = patients with recent myocardial infarction, from Ware JE Jr[12]

- *The Barsky Somatosensory Amplification Scale*[24] is a 10-item validated measure of somatization (tendency to amplify benign bodily sensations) that has been used in a wide variety of cardiac populations including patients with paroxysmal AF. This instrument was only administered at baseline.

A total of 264 patients returned complete baseline and 3 months questionnaires; and 170 had complete baseline, 3 month and 12 month data. The mean age of the study group was 65±10 years and the majority of patients had a normal ejection fraction, were NYHA class I and had a low incidence of comorbid illnesses. At baseline, patients with AF had significantly worse QoL compared with healthy controls from a population survey.[25] QoL improved after 3 months antiarrhythmic treatment compared to baseline. The magnitude of this improvement was independent of the specific drug used (amiodaron, sotalol or propafenone) to maintain sinus rhythm, whether cardioversion was required to restore sinus rhythm or whether the pattern of AF was predominantly paroxysmal or persistent. There were no significant changes in any QoL variable from the 3-month to the 12-month assessment. Patients with no recurrence of AF in the first 3 months of the study had greater improvements in QoL than those who did have recurrence of AF. Based of this finding the authors hypothesize that the improvement in QoL over the first 3 months may be a result of the restoration and maintenance of sinus rhythm by the antiarrhythmic drugs themselves. Unfortunately there was no control group included in the study, which makes it impossible to determine if the greater improvement in patients without the recurrence was the result of the antiarrhythmic drugs or other unknown factors.

In addition, a substudy[26] on the 170 patients who completed questionnaires at baseline, 3 months, and at 12 months have shown that women had significantly more impaired QoL than men, specifically on domains related to physical rather than emotional functioning. As an important clinical consequence the authors suggests that women are notably more debilitated than men, and hence, may derive a greater benefit from therapy than men. A major limitation in this substudy was that women were significantly older than men and a greater proportion had hypertension. Furthermore, women may very well have had a greater disease burden that the authors were unable to capture with the available data.

In a cross-sectional study by van den Berg et al[27] QoL in 73 (54±13.4 years) outclinic patients with paroxysmal AF was compared with QoL in a control group of 180 persons taken from a random population of 1063 healthy adults. QoL was measured by The Medical Outcomes Study Short Form Health Survey (SF-36); symptoms during paroxysms of AF were assessed retrospectively by a semiquantitative questionnaire using a five-point scale. In addition, autonomic function was tested using a battery of four tests: deep breathing, isometric handgrip, standing up and head-up tilting. Patients with AF had statistically significantly lower scores on all SF-36 subscales, with the exception of the pain subscale. Scores in four subscales were markedly lower ($p < 0.001$): physical role functioning, role-emotional domain, vitality and general health perceptions. Furthermore the autonomic variables were independent predictors of QoL in the latter four subscales, depressed vagal functioning being predictive of low scores. In other words symptoms during paroxysms of AF and a depressed vagal function were significantly predictive of an impaired QoL.

However, there are some limitations in the design and in the interpretation of the study, which should be borne in mind. First the study is cross-sectional and performed in a tertiary referral center with highly selected patients. It is not clear how many of the patients were in AF while completing the questionnaire and only one validated QoL instrument was used. Second, as mentioned in a commentary by Lewalter and Lüderitz[28] we face the classic 'chicken/egg dilemma' when interpreting the role of the autonomic nervous system in AF. Defects in the autonomic nervous system may not only lead to AF, but it reacts on the occurrence, and can also be modified by AF itself via changes in hemodynamics.

Quality of life in permanent atrial fibrillation

Howes et al[14] compared 52 ambulatory active stable patients with permanent AF to a group of 48 age-matched healthy subjects in sinus rhythm (76±6.4 years). QoL was assessed by: The Medical Outcomes Study Short Form Health Survey (SF-36), physical activity was assessed by the *Yale Physical Activity Survey*,[29] which is a validated self-report instrument that estimates the amount of time an individual spends performing physical activities. The Charlson Weighted Index of Comorbidity[30] was used to quantify the degree of comorbid conditions. Furthermore each person underwent physiological testing that included a Modified Bruce Protocol exercise tolerance test.

The AF group demonstrated a higher level of comorbidity than the reference group. Furthermore the AF patients reached the maximal heart rate during exercise more often than those in sinus rhythm, however the exercise duration was similar in both groups. The Yale Physical Activity Survey and both the Physical and Mental components of the SF-36 did not reveal any deterioration in QoL in the AF group (Table 10.2). These data suggest there is a subset of elderly, well-compensated patients with permanent AF being treated with a strategy of anticoagulation and rate control who report similar levels of QoL as subjects in sinus rhythm. A major limitation in this study was the use of only one QoL measure, a disease-specific instrument may have been able to distinguish differences in QoL that the generic SF-36 was unable to identify.

A number of studies have assessed QoL in patients undergoing radiofrequency catheter ablation of the His bundle (or the atrioventricular node) and implantation of various pacemakers (DDD-R, VVI, VVI-R). In a recent study by Levy et al[31] 36 patients with a mixed fast and slow ventricular response rate to their permanent AF were randomized to either rate control alone (atrioventricular modifying drugs plus VVI pacing) or rhythm regulation (His bundle ablation plus VVI-R). Outcomes assessed at

Table 10.2 QoL in permanent AF compared to control group (From Howes et al[14])

SF-36 scores	AF group	Control group	P values[1]
No. of points.	52	48	
Physical functioning	67.5±27.9	76.4±26.7	0.35
Role physical	59.6±39.6	72.4±37.6	0.31
Bodily pain	75.1±26.8	77.9±24.0	0.77
General health	64.5±28.8	67.7±20.1	0.88
Vitality	56.1±29.1	64.2±21.8	0.30
Social functioning	77.2±28.8	89.3±21.1	0.07
Role emotional	82.1±32.6	94.4±19.9	0.04
Mental health	79.2±17.1	80.3±18.9	0.73
Physical component summary	43.0±11.0	45.9±10.4	0.58
Mental component summary	52.5±9.6	55.3±8.4	0.24

Data presented as raw mean ± SD
[1]P value adjusted for Charlson comorbidity index between AF group and control group

baseline, 1, 3, 6, and at 12 months included cardiopulmonary exercise testing and QoL. The QoL was assessed using the following two instruments:

1. Modified *Karolinska Questionnaire (KQ)* which is a 16-item cardiac specific questionnaire that has been validated for pacemaker patients.[32] Patients are asked to grade their response between 0 (no symptoms) and 10 (severe symptoms) to a series of questions on: chest pain, palpitations, dizziness, shortness of breath, general health and activity level.

2. *The Nottingham health profile (NHP)* is a general QoL instrument validated for cardiac patients. It is divided into two parts. The first consists of six dimensions: physical mobility, pain, sleep, energy, social isolation, and emotional reaction. A score is then calculated for each dimension and the six individual scores from each dimension can be added to give a total score (0–600), a higher score means a greater limitation. The second part lists seven aspects of life that may be affected by the patients' health: occupation, ability to perform jobs around the home, social life, home relationships, sex life, hobbies and holidays. Patients answer yes or no to whether their health interferes with these activities.

Both patient groups had significant improvement in exercise duration, total KQ scores and total NHP part 1 scores at all follow-ups. For intergroup comparison there was no significant difference in any baseline result or between groups in follow-up. For part 2 of the NHP there was no significant change from baseline in either group at any time or any difference between groups. Levy et al[31] conclude that in these patients improved rate control will lead to a significant improvement in exercise duration and QoL. A conclusion identical to conclusions drawn in other studies evaluating QoL in AF patients treated with pacemaker implantation. The study illustrates some of the methodological problems involved in QoL

assessment of pacemaker patients. Among these are, small sample size, lack of a control group, lack of blinding, and highly selected patients who prior to the intervention have been burdened by severe symptoms caused by tachyarrhythmia and by side-effects to antiarrhythmic drugs.[32] Often it is not clear to which degree the improvement in QoL can be attributed to the His bundle ablation or to the discontinuation of antiarrhythmic drugs or indeed to the pacemaker implantation itself. In spite of these limitations the studies unanimously indicate a substantial impairment of QoL in this group of AF patients and a beneficial effect on QoL after pacemaker treatment.

Quality of life in silent atrial fibrillation

Silent AF is likely to be associated with morbidity and mortality rates similar to those in symptomatic AF, but the effects on QoL have not yet been established.[33] Intuitively it could be expected that asymptomatic patients would have a QoL identical to age-matched normal subjects. At present only one study has been published on QoL in patients with silent AF. Savelieva et al[33] studied 38 patients with silent AF from a group of 154 patients with paroxysmal (60.5%) or persistent (39.5%) AF. The control group consisted of 49 age-matched subjects (54±14 years) without documented cardiovascular or serious systemic disease. QoL was assessed by:

- *The Medical Outcomes Study Short Form Health Survey* (SF-36);[13]
- *Goldman Specific Activity Scale;*[15]
- *Symptom Checklist: Frequency and Severity.*[16]

In addition, global life satisfaction was evaluated using a visual analog scale ranging from 1 (worst possible life) to 10 (best possible life).

Patients with AF had substantially impaired QoL compared with the healthy control group and symptomatic patients reported significantly lower scores on all SF-36 scales as well as in total functional capacity and global life satisfaction compared to 'asymptomatic' (silent) patients. Furthermore, most SF-36 scale scores and total functional capacity did not differ much between the healthy control group and patients with silent AF. However, the latter had significantly lower scores in general health ($p < 0.003$) and global life satisfaction (Table 10.3). This study suggest that the effects of silent AF on isolated physical, social and emotional aspects may be subtle, but the overall perception of well-being may be significantly decreased in these patients. The authors conclude that QoL should be assessed and treatment for the improvement of QoL should be considered in patients with silent AF. However, before this finding is transferred to clinical practice it should be emphasized that this is the only study published on QoL in patients with silent AF, the design was cross-sectional, the patients were highly selected, and the number of patients with silent AF was small. Finally it is not clear from the paper whether the control group is gender-matched (see above regarding women and sex in AF).

QUALITY OF LIFE IN MIXED POPULATIONS OF PATIENTS WITH ATRIAL FIBRILLATION

International study on quality of life in atrial fibrillation

This international prospective multicenter study was designed to examine the primary hypothesis that AF has a negative impact on patient perceived QoL compared to an age and sex matched control group. The design was multidimensional using validated generic measures and specifically constructed disease-specific scales.[21,34] Patients completed the following instruments at baseline and at 3, 6 and 12 months:

- *The Medical Outcomes Study Short Form Health Survey* (SF-36);[13]
- *Symptom Checklist: Frequency and Severity*;[16]
- *Goldman Specific Activity Scale*;[15]
- *The Illness Intrusiveness Scale* is a 13-item scale designed for patients with chronic illnesses.

Table 10.3 Comparison of QoL in patients with silent, symptomatic and all atrial fibrillation, and healthy subjects (From Saveliera et al[34])

QoL scale	Control group	Silent AF	Symptomatic AF	All AF patients
No. of patients	49	38	116	154
General health (SF-36)	78±18	63±17*	51±21*†	55±21*
(1)Symptom burden	10±6	11±5	26±8*†	22±10*
(1)Symptom severity	8±5	9±3	22±6*†	19±8*
(2)Total functional capacity	93±11	90±11	71±20*†	75±20*
Global life satisfaction	8.0±1.2	7.3±1.6*	5.9±1.9*†	6.2±1.9*

Data presented as raw mean ± SD; *$p < 0.003$ compared with controls; †$p < 0.005$ compared with silent AF.
(1)Symptom Checklist, Frequency and Severity
(2)Goldman Specific Activity Scale

This scale has been validated in several different disease states.

In addition patients will complete the following instruments at baseline only:

- *The Life Orientation Test* (13 items), which is a measure of optimism, has been shown to have a good internal consistency in past studies and it has good discriminant validity with respect to related constructs;
- The Barsky Somatosensory Amplification Scale.[24]

Finally a summary score will be used to classify the patient's clinical burden of AF as mild, moderate, or severe. The 'clinical disease burden score' will reflect objective and subjective portions of the clinical disease burden and severity obtained from the subject. The physician or study coordinator will record objective assessments, and these variables will be combined with the patients' self-reported items to provide a matrix of disease severity and a summary score, the *'Atrial Fibrillation Severity Score'*.

At first glance the number of instruments used may seem overwhelming but it is hoped that this multidimensional approach may help to identify the types of instruments that may be useful in assessing QoL in AF in future studies.

Preliminary results from 160 patients (69% male, mean age 59±12 years) with paroxysmal, n=85; persistent, n=50; and permanent, n=25 AF have shown that patients with paroxysmal AF who often have frequent and highly symptomatic recurrences seem to have a significantly lower QoL than those with persistent or permanent AF when using the 'atrial fibrillation severity score'.[35] However, when a similar group of 160 patients was assessed using the SF-36 no significant differences in QoL were noted across the AF subgroups except for vitality and social functioning.[36] These are results that emphasize the need for disease-specific QoL instruments. The long-term impact of AF on QoL has been assessed in 175 patients at baseline and at 3, 6 and 12-months. At baseline the scores on the SF-36 demonstrated health dysfunction for patients with AF compared with reference ranges for this instrument. There was no change in the scores for the SF-36 subscales over the 12 months follow-up, indicating that traditional therapy does not appear to greatly improve QoL in AF patients over time.[37] Finally a substudy on 147 patients showed that the overall QoL in SF-36 was significantly worse in women indicating that the impact of AF on QoL is greater in women.[38]

Atrial fibrillation follow-up: investigation of rhythm management (AFFIRM)

AFFIRM was a prospective randomized evaluation of treatment of atrial fibrillation by one of two strategies: ventricular rate control and anticoagulation versus rhythm control and anticoagulation. It was expected that some patients would not be able to maintain sinus rhythm in the long term, so this study was actually an evaluation of a strategy that initially allows patients to remain in AF versus a strategy that initially attempts to restore sinus rhythm. From 1995 to 1999, 4060 patients with AF were randomized and followed for an average of 3.5 years (minimum 2 years) with a primary endpoint of total mortality. QoL was a secondary endpoint in this study and was assessed at baseline, at intervals during the first year of follow-up and annually using the following validated instruments:

- *The Medical Outcomes Study Short Form Health Survey* (SF-36);[13]
- *Quality of Life Index – Cardiac Version II*[39] considers four dimensions of QoL. Characteristic for this instrument is that the scoring schema adjusts satisfaction scores according to importance as indicated by the individual responders;
- *The Ladder of Life* is being used to allow patients to rate their life currently, 5 years ago, and 5 years in the future

using a 10-point scale ranging from worst possible to best possible;

- Symptom Checklist: Frequency and Severity.[16]

At the most global level the patients rated their health by choosing one of five options ranging from poor to excellent.[40] This large-scale study examined minimally symptomatic patients with AF (who are responsive to antiarrhytmic treatment) and may provide important knowledge of QoL in the AF patients most frequently seen in the real world of daily cardiology.

Preliminary results on baseline characteristics have shown that most patients (93%) had symptoms with their AF.[41]. Over two-thirds had been in AF for more than 48 h, 42% for more than 30 days. In 7% of the patients the qualifying episode of AF was less than 6 h, and 7% had been in continuous AF for more than 6 months.[41] In a substudy, baseline QoL was evaluated in 710 patients of whom 51% were in AF at randomization. While differences in QoL scores were not evident between patients with first versus recurrent AF, there were differences in QoL scores by age on three of the subscales in SF-36 as well as total QoL Index Scores. Furthermore, QoL measurements differed by gender, with women tending to report lower SF-36 scores on all eight subscales and higher scores in the disease-specific instrument Symptom Checklist: Frequency and Severity[42] – which is in accordance with the findings in The Canadian Trial of Atrial Fibrillation[26] as well as in the International Study on Quality of Life in AF.[38]

CONCLUSION

There is an increasing awareness that QoL is important and QoL has become a key issue in a growing number of clinical trials. However, despite the fact that AF is a very common disorder with profound impact in terms of morbidity and mortality, the currently available data from adequately designed studies are sparse. From the studies reviewed, the available data show that QoL is impaired in patients with AF. Furthermore, the data indicate a pronounced variation in the extent of QoL impairment between different groups of AF patients. QoL in patients with AF may be conceived as a continuum with severely impaired, often younger, patients with paroxysmal or persistent AF at one extreme and the marginally impaired elderly patient with permanent AF at the other. Since both may need anticoagulation and rate or rhythm control therapy according to standard criteria the challenge in clinical practice is to reduce symptoms and improve QoL. According to the reviewed studies above one could hypothesize future criteria for therapy selection such as:

- patients with silent AF should be treated to improve QoL and the relief of previously unrecognized symptoms;
- more intensive therapy for some women due to a greater negative QoL burden imposed by AF;
- selection of therapy according to the patients' autonomic characteristics.

However, a prerequisite for the clinician to employ additional criteria will be the development of valid, responsive, clinically relevant, and practical QoL instruments appropriate for clinical practice. As the knowledge on QoL in patients with AF accumulates, the need for such instruments becomes increasingly urgent.

References

1. Slevin ML. Quality of life: philosophical question or clinical reality? BMJ 1992; 305:466–469.
2. Jung W, Lüderitz B. Quality of life in patients with atrial fibrillation. J Cardiovasc Electrophysiol 1998; 9:S177–186.
3. Fitzpatrick R, Fletcher A, Gore S, et al. Quality of life measures in health care. I: Applications and issues in assessment. Br Med J 1992; 305:1074–1077.
4. Lüderitz B, Jung W. Quality of life in patients with atrial fibrillation. Arch Intern Med 2000; 160:1749–1757.
5. Testa MA, Simonson DC. Assesment of quality-of-life outcomes. N Engl J Med 1996; 334:835–840.
6. Gill TM, Feinstein AR. A critical appraisal of the quality of quality-of-life measurements. JAMA 1994; 272:619–626.

7. Sanders C, Egger M, Donovan J, et al. Reporting on quality of life in randomised controlled trials: bibliographic study. Br Med J 1998; 317:1191–1194.

8. Fletcher A, Gore S, Jones D, et al. Quality of life measures in health care. II: Design, analysis, and interpretation. Br Med J 1992; 305:1145–1148.

9. Higginson IJ, Carr AJ. Measuring quality of life: Using quality of life measures in the clinical setting. Br Med J 2001; 322:1297–1300.

10. Dorian P, Jung W, Newman D, et al. The impairment of health-related quality of life in patients with intermittent atrial fibrillation: implications for the assessment of investigational therapy. J Am Coll Cardiol 2000; 36:1303–1309.

11. Krumholz HM, Cohen DJ, Williams C, et al. Health after coronary stenting or balloon angioplasty: results from the Stent Restenosis Study. Am Heart J 1997; 134:337–344.

12. Ware JE Jr. SF-36 health survey: manual and interpretation guide. Boston: The Health Institute, New England Medical Center;1993.

13. McHorney CA, Ware JE Jr, Lu JF, et al. The MOS 36-item Short-Form Health Survey (SF-36): III. Tests of data quality, scaling assumptions, and reliability across diverse patient groups. Med Care 1994; 32:40–66.

14. Howes CJ, Reid MC, Brandt C, et al. Exercise tolerance and quality of life in elderly patients with chronic atrial fibrillation. J Cardiovasc Pharmacol Ther 2001; 6:23–29.

15. Goldman L, Hashimoto B, Cook EF, et al. Comparative reproducibility and validity of systems for assessing cardiovascular functional class: advantages of a new specific activity scale. Circulation 1981; 64:1227–1234.

16. Bubien RS, Knotts-Dolson SM, Plumb VJ, et al. Effect of radiofrequency catheter ablation on health-related quality of life and activities of daily living in patients with recurrent arrhythmias. Circulation 1996; 94:1585–1591.

17. Devins GM. Illness intrusiveness and the psychosocial impact of lifestyle disruptions in chronic life-threatening disease. Adv Ren Replace Ther 1994; 1:251–263.

18. Maglio C, Sra J, Paquette M, et al. Measuring quality of life and symptom severity in patients with atrial fibrillation. Pacing Clin Electrophysiol 1998; 21:839(Abstract).

19. Gorkin L, Norvell NK, Rosen RC, et al. Assessment of quality of life as observed from the baseline data of the studies of left ventricular dysfunction (SOLVD) trial quality-of-life substudy. Am J Cardiol 1993; 71:1069–1073.

20. Ganiats TG, Browner DK, Dittrich HC. Comparison of Quality of Well-Being scale and NYHA functional status classification in patients with atrial fibrillation. New York Heart Association. Am Heart J 1998; 135:819–824.

21. Lüderitz B, Jung W. Quality of life in atrial fibrillation. J Interv Card Electrophysiol 2000; 4:201–209.

22. Dorian P, Paquette M, Newman D, et al. Quality of life improves with treatment in the Canadian Trial of Atrial Fibrillation. Am Heart J 2002; 143:984–990.

23. Hlatky MA, Boineau RE, Higginbotham MB, et al. A brief self-administered questionnaire to determine functional capacity (the Duke Activity Status Index). Am J Cardiol 1989; 64:651–654.

24. Barsky AJ, Goodson JD, Lane RS, et al. The amplification of somatic symptoms. Psychosom Med 1988; 50:510–519.

25. Ware JE Jr, Sherbourne CD. The MOS 36-item short-form health survey (SF-36). I. Conceptual framework and item selection. Med Care 1992; 30:473–483.

26. Paquette M, Roy D, Talajic M, et al. Role of gender and personality on quality-of-life impairment in intermittent atrial fibrillation. Am J Cardiol 2000; 86:764–768.

27. van den Berg MP, Hassink RJ, Tuinenburg AE, et al. Quality of life in patients with paroxysmal atrial fibrillation and its predictors: importance of the autonomic nervous system. Eur Heart J 2001; 22:247–253.

28. Lewalter T, Lüderitz B. Quality of life in atrial fibrillation: relevance of the autonomic nervous system. Eur Heart J 2001; 22:196–197.

29. Dipietro L, Caspersen CJ, Ostfeld AM, et al. A survey for assessing physical activity among older adults. Med Sci Sports Exerc 1993; 25:628–642.

30. Charlson ME, Pompei P, Ales KL, et al. A new method of classifying prognostic comorbidity in longitudinal studies: development and validation. J Chronic Dis 1987; 40:373–383.

31. Levy T, Walker S, Mason M, et al. Importance of rate control or rate regulation for improving exercise capacity and quality of life in patients with permanent atrial fibrillation and normal left ventricular function: a randomised controlled study. Heart 2001; 85:171–178.

32. Linde C. How to evaluate quality-of-life in pacemaker patients: problems and pitfalls. Pacing Clin Electrophysiol 1996; 19:391–397.

33. Savelieva I, Paquette M, Dorian P, et al. Quality of life in patients with silent atrial fibrillation. Heart 2001; 85:216–217.

34. Jung W, Lüderitz B. Quality of life in patients with atrial fibrillation. J Cardiovasc Electrophysiol 1998; 9(suppl 8):S177–186.

35. Jung W, Herwig S, Camm AJ, et al. for the Incontrol Quality of Life Investigators. Are there differences in quality of life measures depending on clinical type of atrial fibrillation? Pacing Clin Electrophysiol 1998; 21:890 (Abstract).

36. Jung W, Herwig S, Camm AJ, et al. for the Incontrol Quality of Life Investigators. Impact of atrial fibrillation on quality of life: a prospective, multicenter study. Pacing Clin Electrophysiol 1998; 21:981 (Abstract).

37. Jung W, Herwig S, Newman D, et al. for the Incontrol Quality of Life Investigators. Impact of atrial fibrillation on quality of life: a prospective,

multicenter study. J Am Coll Cardiol 1999; 33:104A (Abstract).

38. Bygrave AJ, Waktare JEP, Camm AJ. Gender differences in 'quality of life' in atrial fibrillation. J Am Coll Cardiol 1999; 33:104A (Abstract).

39. Ferrans CE, Powers MJ. Quality of life index: development and psychometric properties. Adv Nurs Sci 1985; 8:15–24.

40. Atrial fibrillation follow-up investigation of rhythm management — the AFFIRM study design. The Planning and Steering Committees of the AFFIRM study for the NHLBI AFFIRM investigators. Am J Cardiol 1997; 79:1198–1202.

41. Wyse DG and the AFFIRM investigators. Baseline characteristics of patients with atrial fibrillation - the AFFIRM study. Circulation 2000; AHA, november (Abstract).

42. Jenkins LS, Eleanor S, Brodsky M, et al AFFIRM investigators. Quality of life in patients with atrial fibrillation: baseline data from AFFIRM. Circulation 2000; AHA, november (Abstract).

INVESTIGATIONS

Non-invasive diagnosis of cardiac arrhythmias

Aleksandras Laucevičius PhD FESC FACC
Vilnius University Hospital, Vilnius, Lithuania

Incidence and prevalence of arrhythmias - particularly AF and VT - are currently increasing with a steep age gradient

Introduction

There are several widely used methods for the non-invasive diagnosis and risk assessment of arrhythmias:

- ambulatory electrocardiogram (AECG);
- arrhythmias risk assessment by signal-averaged electrocardiogram (SAECG);
- heart rate variability in predicting of arrhythmic events;
- repolarization alternans for stratification of cardiovascular risk;
- transesophageal atrial pacing and electrophysiology.

AMBULATORY ELECTROCARDIOGRAM

Continuous AECG

The ambulatory electrocardiogram (AECG) allows continuous (24 or 48 h) recording and analysis of the ECG. AECG permits recognition of rhythm or conduction disturbances and ischemic events occurring during the daily activities. Two or three channels of ECG information (24–48 h recordings) are stored on a tape cassette, microcassette or compact disk. Patient-activated event markers allow easy correlation between ECG waveforms and the patient's diary entries. The data recorded is digitized and analyzed with a playback unit connected to personal computer (PC). Computer analysis includes recognition of myocardial ischemia, arrhythmias, conduction disturbances and pacemaker analysis. Special digital recorders are available for late potential and heart rate variability analysis.

In-hospital long-term ECG telemetry monitoring provides continuous ECG monitoring in the coronary or intermediate care unit in patients who are seriously ill, or have life-threatening cardiac arrhythmias. Telemetry systems accommodate two channels of ECG data, thereby permitting analysis of both cardiac arrhythmias and ST segment changes. The continuously looping stored telemetry signal is presented in hourly full-disclosure format to permit a review of all continuous events that occurred during the previous 12 to 24 h.

American College of Cardiology/ American Heart Association (ACC/AHA) Task Force[1] presents main indications for the use of AECG:

- assessment of symptoms that may be related to disturbances of heart rhythm;
- assessment of risk in patients without symptoms of arrhythmias;
- efficacy of antiarrhythmic therapy;
- assessment of pacemaker and implantable cardioverter-defibrillator (ICD) function.

Assessment of symptoms that may be related to disturbances of heart rhythm

It is the most widely used indication for the AECG (Table 11.1).[1–3]

The AECG has to be precisely time-related with respect to the occurring symptoms. Establishment of the onset and resolution of the arrhythmia or conduction disturbance, qualitative and quantitative characteristics of various ECG morphologies are important. The causal causes of arrhythmias could be verified in up to 15% of cases during AECG in one study.[2] The value of AECG monitoring in the diagnostic evaluation of syncope is relatively low.[1] The uses of AECG monitoring in patients with syncope are presented in the 'Guidelines on management (diagnosis and treatment) of syncope' of European Society of Cardiology (Table 11.2).[3]

AECG in syncope is performed only after the thorough clinical evaluation and usually is followed by invasive electrophysiological (EP) testing. Extension of the monitoring time up to 3 days increases the sensitivity of the method by 50% and for up to 5–21 days (mean 9 days) by 75%.[4,5]

Examples – Figs 11.1 and 11.2.

Table 11.1 Indications for ambulatory ECG monitoring to assess symptoms possibly related to rhythm disturbances (ACC/AHA classes*)

Class I
Patients with unexplained syncope, near syncope, or episodic dizziness in whom the cause is not obvious
Patients with unexplained recurrent palpitation

Class IIb
Patients with episodic shortness of breath, chest pain, or fatigue that is not otherwise explained
Patients with neurological events when transient atrial fibrillation or flutter is suspected
Patients with symptoms such as syncope, near syncope, episodic dizziness or palpitation in whom a probable cause other than an arrhythmia has been identified but in whom symptoms persist despite treatment of this other cause

Class III
Patients with symptoms such as syncope, near syncope, episodic dizziness or palpitation in whom other causes have been identified by history, physical examination, or laboratory tests
Patients with cerebrovascular accidents, without other evidence of arrhythmia

*Explanation of ACC/AHA classes
Class I: Conditions for which there is evidence and/or general agreement that a given procedure or treatment is useful and effective.

Class II: Conditions for which there is conflicting evidence and/or a divergence of opinion about the usefulness/efficacy of a procedure or treatment.

Class IIa. Weight of evidence/opinion is in favor of usefulness/efficacy.

Class IIb. Usefulness/efficacy less well established by evidence/opinion.

Class III: Conditions for which there is evidence and/or general agreement that the procedure/treatment is not useful and in some cases may be harmful.

Table 11.2 The role of AECG in syncope

Indications
Class I:
Holter monitoring is indicated in patients with structural heart disease and frequent (or even infrequent) symptoms when there is a high pretest probability of identifying an arrhythmia responsible for syncope
When the mechanism of syncope remains unclear after full evaluation
External or implantable loop recorders are recommended when there is a high pretest probability of identifying an arrhythmia responsible for syncope.

Diagnosis
Class I:
ECG monitoring is diagnostic when a correlation between syncope and an electrocardiographic abnormality (brady- or tachyarrhythmia) is detected
ECG monitoring excludes an arrhythmic cause when there is a correlation between syncope and sinus rhythm
In the absence of such correlations additional testing is recommended with the possible exception of:
–ventricular pauses longer than 3 s when awake
–periods of Mobitz II or third-degree atrioventricular block when awake
–rapid paroxysmal ventricular tachycardia

Assessment of risk in patients without symptoms of arrhythmias

AECG monitoring has been increasingly used to identify patients, both with and without symptoms, at risk for arrhythmias (Table 11.3)[1]

Postmyocardial infarction (post-MI) patients with complex ventricular arrhythmia have threefold – and those with

AECG in a patient with syncope

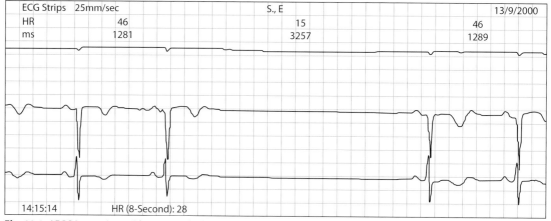

Fig. 11.1 AECG in a patient with syncope discloses the asystolic pauses exceeding 3 s.

AECG in a patient with transient palpitations

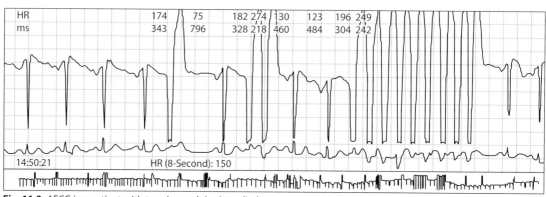

Fig. 11.2 AECG in a patient with transient palpitations discloses non-sustained ventricular tachycardia.

Table 11.3 Indications for AECG arrhythmia detection to assess risk for future cardiac events in patients without symptoms from arrhythmia

Class I
None

Class IIb
Post-MI patients with LV dysfunction (EF 40% or less)
Patients with CHF
Patients with idiopathic hypertrophic cardiomyopathy

Class III
Patients who have sustained myocardial contusion
Systemic hypertensive patients with LV hypertrophy
Post-MI patients with normal LV function
Preoperative arrhythmia evaluation of patients for non-cardiac surgery
Patients with sleep apnea
Patients with valvular heart disease

ventricular tachycardia or early-ectopic beats, up to fivefold – increased mortality compared with the subjects without ventricular arrhythmias.[6] The prognosis for patients with ventricular arrhythmias and decreased left ventricular (LV) ejection fraction (EF) is poorer than with only decreased LV EF.[7] AECG monitoring in two-thirds of patients with hypertrophic cardiomyopathy[8,9] and in up to 90% of patients with dilated cardiomyopathy[10,11,12] revealed frequent and complex ventricular arrhythmias.

Example – Fig. 11.3.

Effect of antiarrhythmic therapy

AECG has been widely used to assess the effects of antiarrhythmic therapy by statistical analysis of the incidence and morphology of the arrhythmias before and after the treatment (Table 11. 4).[1]

Antiarrhythmic therapy is efficacious when mean frequency is supressed by 70–90% and all repetitive forms of ventricular ectopy disappear.[12] Abolishing of repetitive ventricular activity during antiarrhythmic therapy assessed by AECG in conjunction with the exercise testing, predicts long-term survival in the

Sustained ventricular arrhythmia in a patient after MI

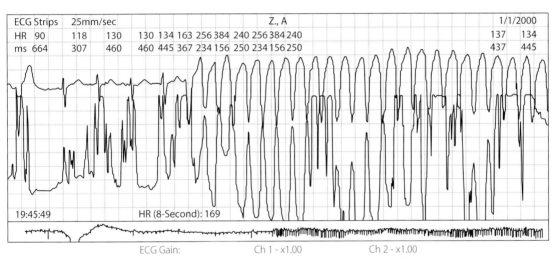

Fig. 11.3 Sustained ventricular arrhythmia (ventricular tachycardia) is discovered by AECG in a patient after MI.

Table 11.4 Indications for AECG to assess antiarrhythmic therapy

Class I
To assess antiarrhythmic drug response in individuals in whom baseline frequency of arrhythmia has been characterized as reproducible and of sufficient frequency to permit analysis

Class IIa
To detect proarrhythmic responses to antiarrhythmic therapy in patients at high risk

Class IIb
To assess rate control during atrial fibrillation
To document recurrent or asymptomatic non-sustained arrhythmias during therapy in the outpatient setting

Class III
None

patients.[13] The AECG is as important as invasive EP testing in assessing the efficacy of antiarrhythmic drug therapy in patients with a high density of spontaneous runs of non-sustained ventricular tachycardia.[14]

Evaluation of pacemaker and implantable cardioverter-defibrillator

The use of AECG is useful in the patients after implantation of pacemaker in order to start the antiarrhythmic therapy as well as to detect ICD or pacemaker malfunction (Table 11.5)[1]

Example – Fig. 11.4.

Intermittent AECG

Intermittent AECG is widely used in the patients with transient and rare symptoms that could not be detected by continuous 24–48 h AECG. External or implantable event recorders are carried over a long period of time and the ECG is recorded intermittently when the symptoms are occurring.[15] These continuous memory devices with the loop storage (retrospective and prospective time) of a 4–5 min ECG are excellent for documenting transient episodes of arrhythmias disclosing their onset and offset.[16]

Table 11.5 Indications for AECG monitoring to assess pacemaker and ICD malfunction

Class I
Evaluation of frequent symptoms of palpitation, syncope or near syncope to assess device function to exclude myopotential inhibition and pacemaker-mediated tachycardia and to assist in the programming of enhanced features such as rate responsivity and automatic mode switching
Evaluation of suspected component failure or malfunction when device interrogation is not definitive in establishing a diagnosis
To assess the response to adjunctive pharmacological therapy in patients with frequent symptoms on (ICD) therapy

Class IIb
Evaluation of immediate postoperative pacemaker function after pacemaker or ICD implantation as an alternative or adjunct to continuous telemetric monitoring
Evaluation of the rate of supraventricular arrhythmias in patients with ICDs

Class III
Assessment of ICD/pacemaker malfunctions when device interrogation, ECG, or other available data (chest radiograph and so forth) are sufficient to establish an underlying cause/diagnosis
Routine follow-up in asymptomatic patients

Holter ECG strip disclosing pacemaker malfunction

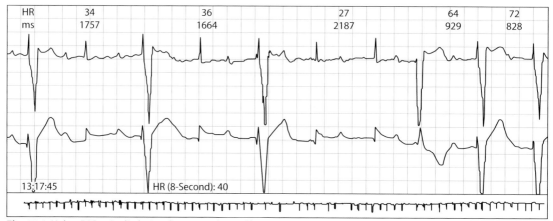

Fig. 11.4 Holter ECG strip disclosing the pacemaker malfunction.

Transtelephonic electrocardiographic devices are capable of direct transmission of an ECG as an audio signal by telephone.[16] These ECG signals are received at a base station equipped with a demodulator and an ECG strip chart recorder. The transtelephonic monitoring device could be the wrist recorder activated by contact of the index finger and thumb, or hand contact to the opposite wrist.

Transtelephonic ECG is now the part of the official recommendations for pacemaker follow-up policy of the North American Society for Pacing and Electrocardiography.[17]

AECG and transtelephonic ECG are complementary.

Intermittent ECG monitoring is recommended:

- in patients with recurrent or unexplained syncope, who have undergone previous clinical and ambulatory ECG examination without occurrence of symptoms or disclosure of an etiological ECG abnormality;[18]
- in the follow-up of patients treated with antiarrhythmic drugs for the evaluation

of drug efficacy over a long period of time.[16]

An implantable loop recorder is a device that can record the ECG for over 1 year, storing events when the device is activated automatically by a rapid rate or manually with magnet application. This device is helpful in the evaluation of patients with unexplained syncope.

Example – Fig. 11.5.

ARRHYTHMIA RISK ASSESSMENT BY SIGNAL-AVERAGED ELECTROCARDIOGRAM

Signal-averaged ECG in patients at risk of ventricular tachycardia

Signal-averaged (SA) ECG is a computerized method of analyzing surface ECG that has been used over the past 20

ECG event-recording for 1 month in patient with palpitations and syncope

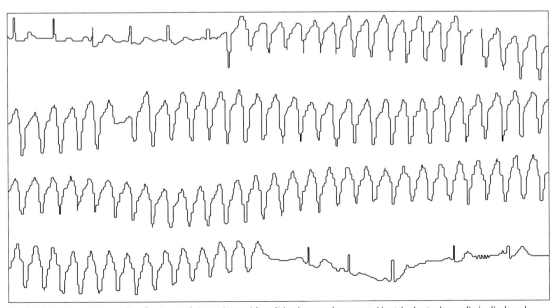

Fig. 11.5 ECG event-recording for 1 month in patient with palpitations and syncope. Ventricular tachycardia is disclosed.

years to identify the patients at high risk of ventricular tachycardia (VT). The technique introduced by Simson and Breithardt[19,20] in 1981 identifies electrical signals at the end of the QRS complex, termed late potentials (LP) representing delayed conduction through diseased myocardium and, thus, a potential substrate for re-entrant VT.

The presence of LP is measured on orthogonal Frank XYZ or standard 12-lead ECG by assessing the total duration of the filtered QRS complex (FQRSD), the low-amplitude signal duration at the end of the filtered QRS complex (LASD), and the root mean square voltage of the terminal 40 ms of the filtered QRS complex (RMSV). These values are dependent on the type of filtering and the leads used. Normal criteria with the use of a Butterworth filter and bipolar orthogonal XYZ leads are as follows: FQRSD of 114 ms; LASD of 38 ms; and RMSV of 20 mV.[21] In the most devices time domain analysis to detect the LP in the terminal QRS complex is used. A sequence of time domain signals can be represented in the frequency domain mode by using Fourier transformation. The detection of LP is unreliable in the ventricular conduction disturbance with prolonged QRS complex.[22]

Over the past two decades there has been much criticism of SAECG – and the clinical use and the indications of SAECG for risk stratification have markedly decreased. SAECG is combined nowadays with other tests (repolarization alternans, heart rate variability, AECG and assessment of LV function) when used for stratification of the cardiovascular risk.

The American College of Cardiology has published guidelines for the clinical use of the SAECG (Table 11.6).[23]

Signal-averaged ECG after myocardial infarction

SAECG has been used extensively in patients after MI in an attempt to establish those at risk for sudden death or VT. Analysis of several studies revealed a positive predictive value of 14% and a negative predictive value of 96% for SAECG in identifying the patients at high risk for VT and sudden death.[24–27]

Table 11.6 American College of Cardiology expert consensus document on the use of SA ECG

SA ECG of established value
1. Stratification of risk of development of sustained ventricular arrhythmias in patients recovering from myocardial infarction who are in sinus rhythm without ECG evidence of bundle branch block or intraventricular conduction delay (QRS complex > 120 ms)
2. Identification of patients with ischemic heart disease and unexplained syncope who are likely to have inducible sustained ventricular tachycardia

SA ECG clinically valuable, but further supportive evidence is desirable
1. Stratification of risk development of sustained ventricular arrhythmias in patients with non-ischemic cardiomyopathy
2. Assessment of success of operation for sustained ventricular tachycardia

SA ECG promising but currently unproven
1. Detection of acute rejection of heart transplants
2. Assessment of efficacy of proarrhythmic effects of antiarrhythmic drug therapy in patients with ventricular arrhythmias
3. Assessment of success of pharmacological, mechanical or surgical interventions to restore coronary artery blood flow

SAECG not indicated
1. Patients with ischemic heart disease and documented sustained ventricular tachycardia
2. Stratification of risk of development of sustained ventricular arrhythmias in asymptomatic patients without detectable heart disease

---

The frequency of LP is reduced after reperfusion therapy with fibrinolytic agents or with acute percutaneous transluminal coronary angioplasty. SAECG has a positive predictive accuracy of 12% in patients receiving fibrinolytic therapy compared with 38% in patients not receiving fibrinolytic therapy.[28] The identification of the patients at high risk for an arrhythmic event after fibrinolytic therapy on the basis of the presence of LP alone is unreliable and the strongest predictive factors are a history of MI, a closed infarct related artery, and EF.[29] Patients with positive LP, reduced LV EF < 40%, and presence of non-sustained VT by AECG monitoring have a 50% risk for an arrhythmic event. Only the combination of all these prognostic tests may be helpful in identifying post-MI patients at highest risk of sudden cardiac death and VT who would benefit most from antiarrhythmic therapy.

Signal-averaged ECG in syncope due to ventricular tachycardia

SAECG has low sensitivity and specificity when used as a single technique for identifying patients with syncope and high probability of VT induced at EP testing.[30–32] However, when other predictors of VT (a history of prior MI, reduced ventricular function) are added to positive LP, the probability of VT induced during EP study increases significantly. A negative LP result in these patients does not exclude the need for invasive EP testing.

Example – Fig. 11.6.

Prediction of atrial fibrillation with P wave averaging

The use of SAECG for the P wave analysis started in 1991[32–34] but still continues to be a research technique. P wave averaging

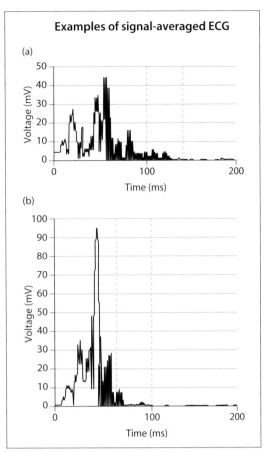

Examples of signal-averaged ECG

(a)

(b)

Fig. 11.6 Examples of SAECG: (a) with positive LP finding VT; (b) negative LP in a healthy adult.

procedure is usually translated from the ventricular LP recordings, adapting the same techniques and lead systems for new applications. We are using three bipolar thoracal leads for P wave averaging. The leads form a closed triangle for the estimation of a summarized vector using following formula:

$$V = |s| A_1 + |s| A_2 + |s| A_3,$$

where V is summarized vector, s - lead vector sign, A_1, A_2, A_3 - ASL leads.

P wave duration, atrial conduction intervals: right atrium, right-to-left atrium and left atrium can be estimated using our system.[34,35]

P wave averaging can be used for prediction of the developing of the atrial fibrillation (AF).[36] P wave duration >140 ms predicted AF with a positive predictive accuracy of 37% and negative predictive accuracy of 87%.[37] The technique has also been shown to predict patients with paroxysmal AF who progress to chronic AF. In a study of 122 patients with paroxysmal AF with 14 developing chronic AF, a P-wave duration >145 ms and RMSV of the terminal 30 ms <3 mV predicted patients who would develop chronic AF. The SAECG was found to be superior to echocardiographically-estimated left atrial size in predicting AF.[38] By using a P wave acquisition method that triggers off the QRS, filtering with a least squares fit with a bandwidth filter of 29–250 Hz (window width of 100 ms) provided the strongest association with AF.[39]

Examples – Figs 11.7 and 11.8.

HEART RATE VARIABILITY – CURRENT STATUS AND CLINICAL APPLICATIONS

Heart rate variability (HRV) in healthy subjects is quantified using a threshold value of 50 ms difference from the preceding RR interval (NN50).[40] Low values or absence of HRV, as measured by the standard deviation of the RR intervals in sinus rhythm in patients after MI, with heart failure, spontaneous arrhythmias and diabetic patients, increase the risk of arrhythmic events and sudden cardiac death. The measurement of HRV is based on the assumption that increased sympathetic and reduced parasympathetic activity trigger and sustain malignant ventricular arrhythmias and reduces the threshold for ventricular fibrillation.

Methodological aspects

HRV can be measured by two methods:[41]

1. time domain;
2. frequency domain.

Usually measured parameters of HRV are:

- standard deviation of NN (normal to normal RR) intervals over a 24 h period (SDNN);

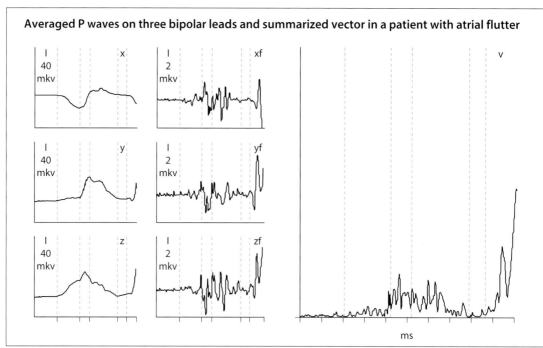

Averaged P waves on three bipolar leads and summarized vector in a patient with atrial flutter

Fig. 11.7 Averaged P waves on three bipolar leads (left half) and summarized vector (right half) in a patient with atrial flutter. P wave duration = 146 ms (prolonged). Atrial conduction intervals: RA 53 ms (36%), IA 25 ms (17%) and LA 68 ms (46%) (prolonged).

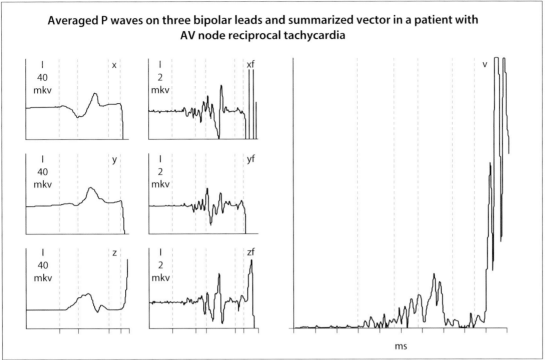

Averaged P waves on three bipolar leads and summarized vector in a patient with AV node reciprocal tachycardia

Fig. 11.8 Averaged P waves on three bipolar leads (left half) and summarized vector (right half) in a patient with AV node reciprocal tachycardia. P wave and atrial conduction intervals are normal: P wave duration 116 ms; atrial conduction intervals: RA 44 ms (37%), IA 30 ms (25%) and LA 42 ms (36%).

- standard deviation of the average NN intervals for the 288 five min intervals in a 24 h continuous ECG recording (SDANN);
- HRV triangular index;
- total power (frequencies between 0.0033 and 0.40 Hz), ultralow frequency (ULF) power, very low frequency (VLF) power, low frequency (LF) power, high frequency (HF) power, the ratio of LF/HF, and power law regression parameters.

HF power is in the range of 0.15–0.40 Hz and reflects the modulation of efferent parasympathetic (vagal) activity, LF power, in the frequency range of 0.04–0.15 Hz , reflects modulation of both efferent parasympathetic (vagal) and efferent sympathetic nervous system activity.

The Task Force on Heart Rate Variability of the European Society of Cardiology and the North American Society of Pacing and Electrophysiology recommend the use of the power spectral analysis in 5 min ECG recordings.[41]

Clinical use of HRV

At present time the measurement of HRV is more a research technique than a routine clinical tool.[42]

It is used in :

- stratification for the cardiac death and arrhythmic events after acute MI;
- prediction of arrhythmic events with HRV in cardiomyopathy and heart failure;
- HRV measurements in spontaneous ventricular and atrial arrhythmias;
- detection and quantification of autonomic neuropathy in patients with diabetes mellitus.

Main indications for measurement of HRV are stated in the Task Force on Heart Rate Variability and the Task Force of the

American College of Cardiology/American Heart Association (ACC/AHA).[41,43]

HRV for risk stratification for cardiac death and arrhythmic events after acute myocardial infarction

In 1996 an ACC/AHA Task Force published recommendations on the use of AECG and HRV in patients with an acute MI.[44] The ACC/AHA recommendedation is that HRV be used as a prognostic index of predisposition for sudden death or ventricular failure only in combination with AECG, SAECG, LV EF with stress testing as a class II b indication.

Stability over time of HRV parameters was shown in two groups of patients with chronic coronary heart disease and ventricular arrhythmias: a random sample of patients with sustained ventricular arrhythmias; and a random sample of patients in the placebo group with non-sustained ventricular arrhythmias.[45] Measures of HRV are reduced by 25% 2–3 weeks after MI.[46] The first study to show the usefulness of HRV for predicting long-term outcome after a MI involved 808 patients who underwent ambulatory monitoring within 11 days of an acute MI.[47] The time domain measurement of HRV, SDNN, was calculated for the 24 h period and a value of 50 ms was chosen arbitrarily to divide the group into those with a low or high value. After a 31-month follow-up, the mortality rate of patients with SDNN < 50 ms was 34% compared to 12% in those with a SDNN ≥ 50 ms (relative risk of 2.8). SDNN predicted mortality independently of other risk predictors such as left ventricular EF or ventricular arrhythmias.

In one study a 24 h AECG recording was performed 6 or 7 days after MI in 416 patients.[48] RR variability was quantified by triangular interpolation of the frequency distribution of normal RR intervals (TINN). TINN is a measure of low frequency fluctuations of RR intervals and is strongly correlated with SDNN, SDANN, total power and ULF power. During an average follow-up of 20 months, the risk of experiencing a cardiac death was about seven times higher in those with a TINN < 20 ms compared to those with a TINN > or =20 ms. TINN did not predict recurrent MI.

The ability of the TINN to predict arrhythmic events (sustained ventricular arrhythmias or arrhythmic death) was evaluated in 416 patients with acute MI.[48] The presence of late potentials on the SAECG to the TINN doubled the positive predictive accuracy which doubled again when the presence of repetitive ventricular premature complexes was considered. The best multivariate predictor for arrhythmic events, with a positive predictive accuracy of 58%, was the triad of TINN < 20 ms, a positive signal averaged ECG, and repetitive ventricular premature complexes present in the same AECG recording that was used to calculate TINN.

Correlations between time or frequency domain measures of RR variability and previously identified postinfarction risk factors such as left ventricular EF and ventricular arrhythmias are remarkably weak.[47] This lack of correlation suggests that measures of RR variability will improve the identification of patients at high risk after MI.

Cut-off points for prediction of mortality in patients after MI have been estimated by measuring parameters of HRV (Table 11.7).[49]

Prediction of arrhythmic events with HRV in cardiomyopathy and heart failure

There are limited data that HRV may be of predictive value in dilated cardiomyopathy and congestive heart failure in general. In one study of patients with dilated cardiomyopathy the measures of HRV were reduced compared to controls and reduced HRV was associated with disease severity measures such as the New York Heart Association (NYHA) functional class, left ventricular diastolic dimension, reduced LV

Table 11.7 Optimal cutpoints for predication of all-cause mortality after MI by frequency domain measures of heart period variability (From Zipes[49])

Variable	Optimal cutpoints	
	At discharge 2 weeks after MI	After recovery from MI
Ultra low frequency power (ms^2)	1600	5000
Very low frequency power (ms^2)	180	600
Low frequency power (ms^2)	35	120
High frequency power (ms^2)	20	35
Total power (ms^2)	2000	6000
Low frequency/high frequency ratio	0.95	1.6

EF and peak O_2 consumption.[44] At 12 months, patients with an SDNN of less than 50 ms had a lower survival rate free of progressive heart failure than those with a higher value.

In another study with the larger group of patients after a follow-up of 482 days, SDNN was found to be an independent predictor of all-cause mortality and the most powerful predictor of death from progressive heart failure.[50] Reduced SDNN <100 ms was predictive of arrhythmic events and sudden cardiac death in one more study.[51]

HRV in spontaneous ventricular and atrial arrhythmias

Spontaneous ventricular tachycardia:

Increased sympathetic activity, manifested as an increase in heart rate, precedes the onset of sustained VT in the majority of patients in whom the initiation of the VT has been recorded.[52] In one study of patients with spontaneous VT recorded on an AECG, all patients had an increase in heart rate 15 min prior to VT onset.[53] However, 68% had a decrease in total power, LF power and LF/HF ratio 15 min prior to VT, and these patients had a higher baseline level of these parameters during the 2 h before VT. The remaining patients who had a lower baseline level of total power, LF power and LF/HF ratio had an increase in these parameters prior to VT. These data suggest that change in the

dynamics of RR intervals, rather than the direction of change, facilitates VT induction in most patients.

Atrial fibrillation: Though the presence of AF precludes the use of standard RR variability analysis, analysis of the variability and irregularity of the ventricular response interval (VRI) may provide useful information.[54] After a follow-up of 33 months, reductions in all VRI variability and irregularity measures were associated with an increased risk of cardiac death, but not fatal stroke.

HRV can predict early recurrence of AF after cardioversion during amiodarone therapy.[55] The recurrence rate at 2 weeks in those with an LF/HF ratio ≥ 2, an indicator of increased sympathetic and reduced vagal activity, was significantly higher than in patients with a ratio < 2 (73 versus 9%); a value of ≥ 2 predicted recurrence with a sensitivity and specificity of 76 and 90%, respectively. This ratio was not predictive of late recurrences of the arrhythmia.

HRV in detection and quantification of autonomic neuropathy in patients with diabetes mellitus

Diabetes can cause severe autonomic dysfunction that can be responsible for sudden cardiac death. Although traditional measures of autonomic function are able to document the presence of neuropathy, in general they are only abnormal when there

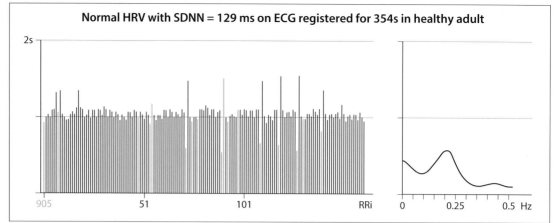

Fig. 11.9 Normal HRV with SDNN = 129 ms on ECG registered for 354 s. in healthy adult.

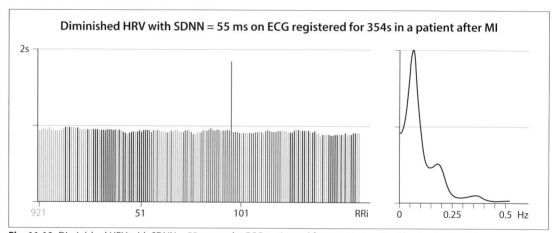

Fig. 11.10 Diminished HRV with SDNN = 55 ms on the ECG registered for 354 s in a patient having had an MI.

is severe symptomatology. HRV in deep breathing is used for reflex cardiovascular testing in these patients.

Examples – Figs 11.9 and 11.10.

REPOLARIZATION ALTERNANS FOR STRATIFICATION OF CARDIOVASCULAR PATIENTS

The heterogeneous repolarization of the alternate beats is assessed on the T to P segment of the surface ECG and is called repolarization alternans (RPA). Techniques for its measurement have been approved for the non-invasive prediction of ventricular arrhythmias and sudden cardiac death. Visual inspection of the ECG sometimes enables detection of only macrovolt RPA of 50–100 mV.[56] After the development of a computerized interbeat spectral decomposition technique it was realized that RPA occurs much more often than can be estimated by visual inspection – it may be of the microvolt level.[57–59] RPA discriminates well between patients with ventricular tachycardia (VT) or ventricular fibrillation (VF) and those without.[60]

Methodological aspects

RPA analysis these days is based on Fourier spectral decomposition or sometimes, time domain analysis.[61] Regardless of the analytical method used, ECG data are first collected from the 12 standard leads of a surface ECG, although orthogonal Frank XYZ leads may be used.[57]

RPA detection is rate dependent with the optimal rate being between 100 and 120 beats per minute (bpm) achieved during bicycle ergometry or atrial pacing. It was demonstrated that exercise produced equivalent results to atrial pacing.[62]

The most often used parameter for detecting RPA is the T wave alternans ratio (TWAR), which represents the difference between alternating and non-alternating periodicity.[57]

Clinical uses of RPA

RPA is a non-invasive method for identifying patients at high risk of sustained ventricular tachyarrhythmias and sudden cardiac death.

The measurement of RPA seems to be useful in several patient populations:

- patients undergoing invasive EP testing for the induction of VT/VF;
- patients after MI;
- patients with congestive heart failure;
- patients with hypertrophic cardiomyopathy;
- patients in whom a proarrhythmic effect of cardiovascular drugs is suspected.

RPA in patients undergoing invasive EP study for the induction of sustained VT/VF

In one study the efficacy of RPA in predicting arrhythmic events was assessed in patients undergoing EP testing.[63] The level of RPA was measured during atrial pacing at 100 bpm and it was compared with two clinical endpoints:

1. the inducibility of sustained VT or VF during programmed stimulation (EP study); and
2. arrhythmia-free survival.[63]

It was shown that RPA predicts EP testing results with a sensitivity of 81% and specificity of 84%. Free survival sensitivity was of 89% and specificity of 89%. These results were each highly significant ($p < 0.001$). Patients with low level of RPA had 95% arrhythmia-free survival rate at 20 months, whereas those patients who were RPA positive had only 20% arrhythmia-free survival rate. The results were almost identical to invasive EP testing. The results of another study were very similar – RPA sensitivity and specificity for induction of VT was 88 and 78%, respectively.[64]

A cut-point of TWAR > 2.5 during atrial pacing for predicting inducible ventricular arrhythmias is accepted in most studies.[56,63] In other series, a TWAR > 3 successfully identified patients at risk for inducible VT.[60–64] The mean absolute voltage difference of alternation Valt=2.6 mV across the JT interval obtained with atrial pacing to 120 bpm, may also be used for predicting of VT induction.[65]

The accuracy of RPA to predict outcome appears to be at least as favorable as that for invasive EP testing.[66,67]

In one study RPA, SAECG and EP study as predictors of events during follow-up were compared.[68] The primary endpoint was 'ventricular tachyarrhythmic events' defined as resuscitated VT, VF and sudden death and the second was 'resuscitated VT, VF and total mortality'. RPA was more informative than SAECG for predicting an arrhythmic event. The relative risk for predicting an event (sudden death, sustained ventricular tachyarrhythmia or appropriate implantable defibrillator therapy) was 10.9 for RPA, 7.1 for EP testing, and 4.5 for signal averaged ECG.

Measurement of RPA could be used for estimation of survival in patients when ventricular arrhythmias could not be provoked during the invasive EP study. In one study the actuarial survival without arrhythmia was significantly lower in patients with positive RPA testing by atrial pacing, compared to those without RPA induced (19 versus 94%).[57] RPA measured during exercise testing is also predictive of outcome, and in one study of 148 patients, the 1 year event-free survival was lower in those with, compared to those without, RPA (82 versus 98%, relative risk 10.6).[69]

After the implantation of an ICD, patients with positive RPA results experienced more inducible ventricular arrhythmias, cardiac arrest, ICD discharge or death compared to those without RPA (33 versus 13%, relative risk 3.5).[70]

RPA for risk assessment after myocardial infarction

Positive RPA is more frequent in the early period after MI, its incidence becoming lower during the follow-up period. Comparing RPA and SAECG in the patients with a recent MI, 49% were RPA positive and in 21% late potentials were present.[71] After a follow-up of 15 months, the sensitivity and negative predictive value of RPA for predicting arrhythmic events were 93 and 98%, respectively, whereas the positive predictive value was 28%; when RPA and late potentials were combined, the positive predictive value was 50%.

RPA in patients with congestive heart failure (CHF)

The highest risk for sudden cardiac death is in patients with the lowest left ventricular EF. Results from the Marburg Cardiomyopathy Study (MACAS) of patients with non-ischemic dilated cardiomyopathy showed that those with an LV EF below 30% were more likely to demonstrate positive RPA compared to those with a higher LV EF (59 versus 37%).[72]

During follow-up of patients with CHF, no recent MI, with no prior history of VT/VF RPA but not SA ECG, HRV or QT dispersion was the only significant predictor of resuscitated VT/VF and sudden death. No patient with negative RPA testing had an event within 24 months of follow-up, providing a sensitivity of 100%. The positive predictive value was 23%.[73]

In a preliminary study 52% of patients with a non-ischemic dilated cardiomyopathy had positive RPA measurement; these patients experienced a higher incidence of VT or VF at 6 months (21 versus 0% in those without RPA).[74]

RPA in hypertrophic cardiomyopathy

Evidence is growing that positive RPA in patients with hypertrophic cardiomyopathy predicts arrhythmic events. In one study RPA was present in 71% of those at high risk for an arrhythmia (prior VT, non-sustained VT, abnormal paced electrograms or a family history); none of the low risk patients or control subjects had RPA.[75] All patients with sustained VT or abnormal ventricular electrograms were RPA positive.

RPA and proarrhythmic effect of cardiovascular drugs

It was shown that treatment with procainamide or beta-blockers is reducing the sensitivity of RPA.[76,77] Macrovolt RPA seen on surface ECG could be related to the repolarization dispersion and proarrhythmia associated with amiodarone, procainamide, quinidine and other antiarrhythmic drugs.[78–81]

Examples – Figs 11.11, 11.12 and 11.13.

TRANSESOPHAGEAL ATRIAL PACING AND ELECTROPHYSIOLOGY

The anatomical vicinity of the esophagus to the posterior wall of the left atrium enables the recording of atrial electrograms and atrial pacing from esophagus.[82] Transesophageal electrophysiological study (TEEPS) includes recordings of the atrial electrograms and transesophageal atrial pacing (TAP). TAP was introduced to the

Macrovolt RPA

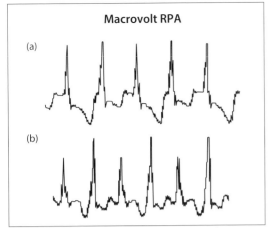

Fig. 11.11 Macrovolt RPA: (a) concordant; and (b) discordant T wave alternans.

Spectral assessment of microvolt RPA from 128 beats

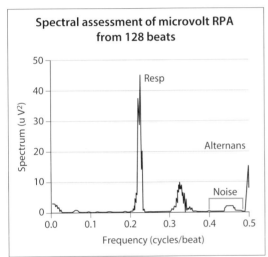

Fig. 11.12 Spectral assessment of microvolt RPA from 128 beats (From Smith et al[57]).

clinical practice by Burack and Furman in 1962.[83] It is widely used these days in many institutions all over the world. TEEPS is an easily repeatable technique, it does not need X-ray control. Technical improvements made have improved the tolerance to TAP.[84–86] TEEPS can be performed on outpatient basis or during a short hospitalization period. It markedly reduces the costs of patient investigation and can be a good substitution for invasive EP.

Electrical alternans occurring during repolarization

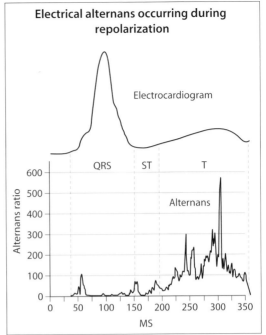

Fig. 11.13 Electrical alternans occurring during the repolarization (From Rosenbaum et al[63]) © 1994 Massachusetts Medical Society.

Technique of transesophageal electrophysiological study

The pharynx is sprayed with local anesthetic and four to six pollar catheters are introduced through the mouth and swallowed by the patient. The largest and sharpest atrial electrogram is found with the catheter in the esophagus in the vicinity of the left atrium (usually 28–40 cm from tooth). Recording of a 12-lead surface ECG and from two transesophageal leads is performed using a computerized system (Cordelectro or Bard systems). Pacing impulses of 10 or 20 ms width and amplitude range of 7.5–20 volts are applied. Patients can be sedated intravenously before TAP if necessary.

TAP consists of programmed left atrial pacing:

- extrastimuli applied during sinus rhythm as well as on the top of overdrive pacing with cycle length of 600 and 460 ms;

- incremental atrial pacing up to 220 bpm;
- rapid left atrial pacing 200 (+20) – 300 bpm.

Sinus node parameters

Sinoatrial conduction time (SACT) with extrastimulus during sinus rhythm and sinus node recovery time (SNRT) 30 s and 60 s after overdrive pacing with cycle length of 600 ms and 460 ms are measured. Atrioventricular 1:1 conduction is estimated during incremental atrial pacing; refractory periods of atria and AV conduction are measured by extrastimulus technique.

Indications for the use of TEEPS

The main clinical indications for the use of TEEPS are:

1. interpretation of complex cardiac arrhythmias and revealing of the low amplitude electrical heart signals;
2. assessment of sinus node function and AV conduction;
3. EP testing and termination of supraventricular tachycardias;
4. stress testing in coronary artery disease.

Clinical uses of TEEPS

Interpretation of complex cardiac arrhythmias and revealing of the low amplitude electrical heart signals

Complex arrhythmias that can not be explained by the surface ECG can be interpreted by the means of an esophageal lead.[87] An esophageal atrial lead can also be used for the revealing of low amplitude electrical cardiac signals: His-bundle potential, late potentials.[88,89]

Examples – Figs 11.14, 11.15 and 11.16.

Assessment of sinus node function and AV conduction

TAP is widely used in everyday clinical practice for the assessment of sinus and atrioventricular node function.[90–92] It can be repeated during follow-up period easily and safely. Several parameters could be estimated: SACT by isolated extrastimulus during sinus rhythm technique; SNRT measured 30 s and 60 s after overdrive pacing with cycle length of 600 ms and 460 ms; 1:1 atrioventricular conduction by incremental atrial pacing.

Example – Fig. 11.17.

Atrial Wenckebach phenomenon

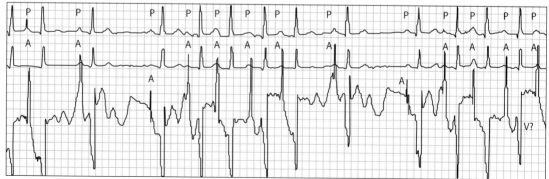

Fig. 11.14 Esophageal lead (lower tracing) reveals an intermittent disorder of atrial conduction – atrial Wenckebach phenomenon.

Beat-to-beat recording of His bundle potential (H) on the amplified esophageal ECG

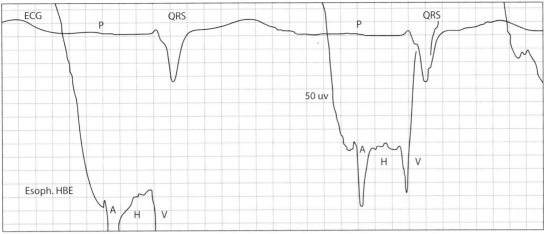

Fig. 11.15 Beat-to-beat recording of His bundle potential (H) on the amplified esophageal ECG.

Beat-to-beat recording of late potentials (LP) on the amplified esophageal ECG

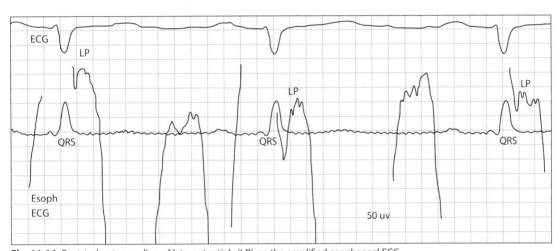

Fig. 11.16 Beat-to-beat recording of late potentials (LP) on the amplified esophageal ECG.

Electrophysiological testing and termination of supraventricular tachycardias

TAP is widely used for conversion of AV node tachycardia, atrial flutter to sinus rhythm.[90,91] The low-output, short-duration TAP was used for the conversion of 31 patients with paroxysmal atrial flutter: 16 patients (52%) were converted directly to sinus rhythm and 12 (38%) to AF. TAP was ineffective in three (10%) patients.[93]

The efficacy and reliability of TAP for induction of supraventricular paroxysmal tachycardia (SPT) is well established.[94–98] SPT was induced in 744 (94.9%) cases: all 710 (100.0%) for patients with documented SPT and for 34 (63.0%) of those without (previously) documented SPT. In all cases the mechanism of re-entry of SPT was determined. In 379 (50.9%) cases SPT was

TAP 80bpm in a patient with sick sinus syndrome

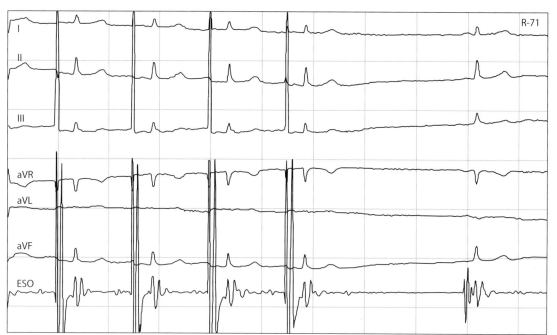

Fig. 11.17 TAP 80 bpm in a patient with sick sinus syndrome with SNRT = 1740 ms. Lower tracing is transesophageal ECG.

Termination of AV nodal tachycardia by applying a burst of TAP

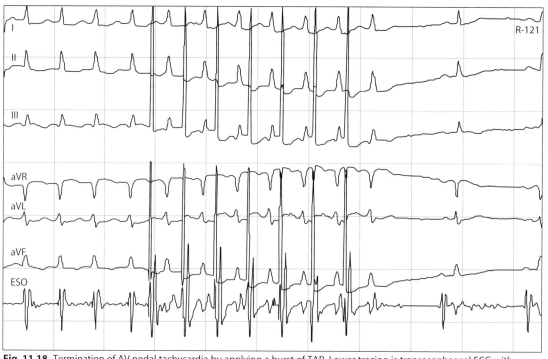

Fig. 11.18 Termination of AV nodal tachycardia by applying a burst of TAP. Lower tracing is transesophageal ECG with retrograde A wave inside V wave.

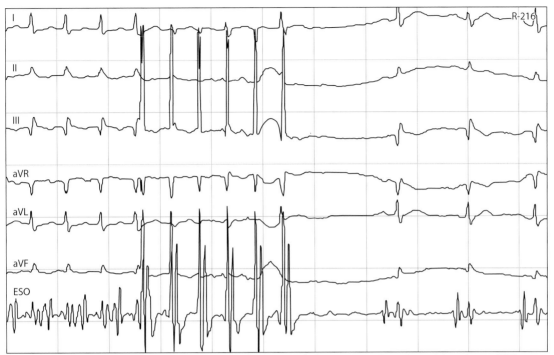

Fig. 11.19 Termination of atrioventricular tachycardia due to concealed accessory pathway by applying a burst of TAP. Lower tracing is transesophageal ECG with A wave after V wave.

due to re-entry in AV node, in 365 (49.1%), SPT with accessory pathways.[97]

TAP is used for follow-up of antiarrhythmic therapy or after ablation procedures.[98–100] Atrio-nodal re-entrant tachycardia (ANRT) was induced in 4 of 34 patients (12%) after the successful radio frequency slow pathway of AV node and accessory pathway ablation.[98] In all of them successful slow pathway ablation was performed during the second session. There was no more arrhythmia recurrence in these patients. It was stated that TAP is a simple means of assessing the medium-term (average 9 months) results of RF ablation of ANRT.[99] The induction of ANRT using isoproterenol and TAP was possible in two of five patients with palpitations and in 3 of 25 asymptomatic patients. TAP was used as a routine early (1–2 days) control study in 84 patients after SVT ablation (including 36 with ANRT).[100] ANRT was induced in two patients (2.5%). In one patient with Wolff-Parkinson-White

(WPW) syndrome the SVT was non-inducible with TAP but the retrograde conduction via AP recurred during the 2-month follow-up period.

Examples – Figs 11.18, 11.19 and 11.20.

References

1. Crawford MH, Bernstein SJ, Deedwania PC, et al. ACC/AHA guidelines for ambulatory electrocardiography: Executive summary and recommendations. A report of the American College of Cardiology/American Heart Association task force on practice guidelines (Committee to revise the guidelines for ambulatory electrocardiography) developed in collaboration with the North American Society for Pacing and Electrophysiology. Circulation 1999; 100:886–893.
2. Zeldis SM, Levine BJ, Michaelson EL, et al. Cardiovascular complaint. Correlation with cardiac arrhythmias on 24 hour electrocardiographic monitoring. Chest 1980; 78:456–461.
3. Brignole M, Alboni P, Bergfeldt L, et al. Guidelines on management (diagnosis and treatment) of

Assessment of antegrade conduction in Wolff-Parkinson-White syndrome in two patients

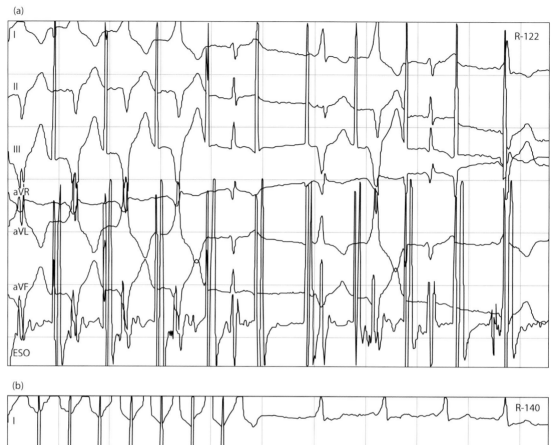

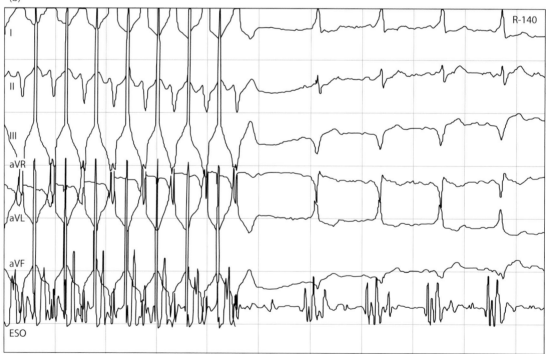

Fig. 11.20 Assessment of antegrade conduction in Wolff-Parkinson-White syndrome in two patients. (a) accessory pathway is blocked at the rate of incremental pacing 120 bpm; (b) 1:1 conduction through accessory pathway at pacing rate of 200 bpm – potentially dangerous antegrade conduction.

syncope: Task force report. Eur Heart J 2001; 22:1256–1306.

4. Gibson TC, Heitzman MR. Diagnostic efficacy of 24 hour electrocardiographic monitoring for syncope. Am J Cardiol 1984; 53:1013–1017.

5. Bass EB, Curtis EI, Arena VC, et al. The duration of Holter monitoring in patients with syncope: is 24 hour enough? Arch Intern Med 1990; 150:1073–1078.

6. The Coronary Drug Project Research Group. Prognostic importance of premature beats following myocardial infarction. JAMA 1973; 223:1116–1124.

7. Bigger JT, Fleiss JL, Kleiger RE, et al. The relationships among ventricular arrhythmias, left ventricular dysfunction, and mortality in the 2 years after myocardial infarction. Circulation 1984; 69:250–258.

8. Maron BJ, Savage DD, Wolfson JK, et al. Prognostic significance of 24 hour ambulatory electrocardiographic monitoring in patients with hypertrophic cardiomyopathy: a prospective study. Am J Cardiol 1981; 48(2):252–257.

9. McKenna WJ, England D, Dio YL, et al. Arrhythmia in hypertrophic cardiomyopathy: Influence on prognosis. Br Heart J 1981; 46:168–172.

10. Huang SK, Messer JV, Denes P. Significance of ventricular tachycardia in idiopathic dilated cardiomyopathy: observations in 35 patients. Am J Cardiol 1983; 51:507–512.

11. Meinertz T, Hofmann T, Kasper W, et al. Significance of ventricular arrhythmias in idiopathic dilated cardiomyopathy. Am J Cardiol 1984; 53(7):902–907.

12. Pratt CM, Delclos G, Wierman AM, et al. The changing baseline of complex ventricular arrhythmias. A new consideration in assessing long-term antiarrhythmic drug therapy. N Engl J Med 1985; 313:1444–1449.

13. Hohnloser SH, Raeder EA, Podrid PJ, et al. Predictors of antiarrhythmic drug efficacy in patients with malignant ventricular tachyarrhythmias. Am Heart J 1987; 114:1–7.

14. Mason JW, for the ESVEM Investigators. A comparison of electrophysiologic testing with Holter monitoring to predict antiarrhythmic drug efficacy for ventricular tachyarrhythmias. N Engl J Med 1993; 329:445–451.

15. Brown AP, Dawkins KD, Davies JG. Detection of arrhythmias: use of a patient-activated ambulatory electrocardiogram device with a solid-state memory loop. Br Heart J 1987; 58:251–253.

16. Zimetbaum PJ, Josephson ME. The evolving role of ambulatory arrhythmia monitoring in general clinical practice. Ann Intern Med 1999; 130:848–856.

17. Levine PA, Belott PH, Bilitch M, et al. Recommendations of the NASPE Policy Conference on Pacemaker Programmability and Follow-up. Pacing Clin Electrophysiol 1983; 6:1222–1223.

18. Linzer M, Prystowsky EN, Brunetti LL, et al. Recurrent syncope of unknown origin diagnosed by ambulatory continuous loop recording. Am Heart J 1988; 116:1632–1634.

19. Simson MB. Use of signals in the terminal QRS complex to identify patients with ventricular tachycardia after myocardial infarction. Circulation 1981; 64:235–241.

20. Breithardt G, Becker R, Seipel L, et al. Noninvasive detection of late potentials in man a new marker for ventricular tachycardia. Eur Heart J 1981;2:1–11.

21. Gomes JA, Winters SL, Stewart D, et al. Optimal band-pass filters for time-domain analysis of the signal-averaged electrocardiogram. Am J Cardiol 1987; 60:1290–1298.

22. Buckingham TA, Thessen CC, Stevens LL, et al. Effect of conduction defects on the signal averaged electrocardiographic determination of late potentials. Am J Cardiol 1988; 61:1265–1271.

23. Cain ME, Anderson JL, Arnsdorf MF, et al. Signal-averaged electrocardiography: ACC Expert Consensus Document. J Am Coll Cardiol 1996; 27:238–249.

24. Steinberg JS, Regan A, Sciacca RR, et al. Predicting arrhythmic events after acute myocardial infarction using the signal-averaged electrocardiogram. Am J Cardiol 1992; 69:13–21.

25. Hammill SC. Ambulatory and signal-averaged electrocardiography. In: Topol EJ, ed. Comprehensive cardiovascular medicine. Philadelphia: Lippincott-Raven; 1998:1751–1776.

26. Breithardt G, Schwartzmaier J, Borggrefe M, et al. Prognostic significance of late ventricular potentials after acute myocardial infarction. Eur Heart J 1983; 4:487–495.

27. Breithardt G, Borggrefe M, Karbenn U, et al. Prevalence of late potentials in patients with and without ventricular tachycardia: Correlation with angiographic findings. Am J Cardiol 1982; 49:1932–1937.

28. Malik M, Kulakowski P, Odemuyiwa O, et al. Effect of thrombolytic therapy on the predictive value of signal-averaged electrocardiography after acute myocardial infarction. Am J Cardiol 1992; 70:21–25.

29. Kawalsky DL, Garratt KN, Hammill SC, et al. Effect of infarct related artery patency and late potentials on late mortality after acute myocardial infarction. Mayo Clin Proc 1997; 72:414–421.

30. Steinberg JS, Prystowsky E, Freedman RA, et al. Use of the signal-averaged electrocardiogram for predicting inducible ventricular tachycardia in patients with unexplained syncope: Relation to clinical variables in a multivariate analysis. J Am Coll Cardiol 1994; 23:99–106.

31. Hammill SC. Value and limitations of noninvasive assessment of syncope. In: Klein GA, ed. Cardiology clinics. Vol 15. Philadelphia: WB Saunders; 1997:195–218.

32. Fukunami M, Yamada T, Ohmori M, et al.

Detection of patients at risk for paroxysmal atrial fibrillation during sinus rhythm by p-wave-triggered signal-averaged electrocardiogram. Circulation 1991; 83:162–169.

33. Stafford PJ, Turner I, Vincent R. Quantitative analysis of signal-averaged p-waves in idiopathic paroxysmal atrial fibrillation. Am J Cardiol 1991; 68:751–758.

34. Cerniauskas R, Juskevicius K, Laucevičius A, et al. Late potentials analyzer. Annual Report of the Recognition Processes Department, Vilnius, 1991, pp.75–89.

35. Laucevičius A, Aidietis A, Cerniauskas R, et al. The signal averaged P wave electrocardiogram – methodological problems and perspective. Semin Cardiol 1998; 4:114–119.

36. Abe Y, Fukunami M, Yamada T, et al. Prediction of transition to chronic atrial fibrillation in patients with paroxysmal atrial fibrillation by signal-averaged electrocardiography: a prospective study. Circulation 1997; 96:2612–2616.

37. Steinberg JS, Zelenkofske S, Wong SC, et al. Value of the P-wave signal-averaged ECG for predicting atrial fibrillation after cardiac surgery. Circulation 1993; 88:2618–2622.

38. Guidera SA, Steinberg JS. The signal-averaged P wave duration: a rapid and noninvasive marker of risk of atrial fibrillation. J Am Coll Cardiol 1993; 21:1645–1651.

39. Ehler FA, Korenstein D, Steinberg JS. Evaluation of P wave signal-averaged electrocardiographic filtering and analysis methods. Am Heart J 1997; 134:985–993.

40. Ewing DJ, Neilson JM, Travis P. New method for assessing cardiac parasympathetic activity using 24 hour electrocardiograms. Br Heart J 1984; 52:396–402.

41. Task Force of the European Society of Cardiology and the North American Society of Pacing and Electrophysiology. Heart rate variability. Standards of measurement, physiologic interpretation, and clinical use. Circulation 1996; 93:1043–1065.

42. Huikuri HV, Makikallio T, Airaksinen KEJ, et al. Measurement of heart rate variability: a clinical tool or a research toy? J Am Coll Cardiol 1999; 34:1878–1883.

43. Crawford MH, Bernstein SJ, Deedwania PC, et al. ACC/AHA guidelines for ambulatory electrocardiography: Executive summary and recommendations. A report of the American College of Cardiology/American Heart Association task force on practice guidelines (Committee to revise the guidelines for ambulatory electrocardiography) developed in collaboration with the North American Society for Pacing and Electrophysiology. Circulation 1999; 100:886–893.

44. Yi G, Goldman JH, Keeling PJ, et al. Heart rate variability in idiopathic dilated cardiomyopathy: Relation to disease severity and prognosis. Heart 1997; 77:108–114.

45. Bigger JT, Fleiss JL, Rolnitzky LM, et al. Stability over time of heart period variability in patients with chronic coronary heart disease and ventricular arrhythmias. The CAPS and ESVEM Investigators. Am J Cardiol 1992; 69:718–723.

46. Bigger JT Jr, Fleiss JL, Rolnitzky LM, et al. Time course of recovery of heart period variability after myocardial infarction. J Am Coll Cardiol 1991; 18:1643–1649.

47. Kleiger RE, Miller JP, Bigger, JT Jr, et al. and the Multicenter Postinfarction Research Group. Decreased heart rate variability and its association with increased mortality after acute myocardial infarction. Am J Cardiol 1987; 59:256–262.

48. Farrell TG, Bashir Y, Cripps T, et al. Risk stratification for arrhythmic events based on heart rate variability, ambulatory electrocardiographic variables and the signal averaged electrocardiogram. J Am Coll Cardiol 1991; 18:687–697.

49. Zipes DP, Jalife J, eds. Cardiac electrophysiology from cell to bedside. 2nd edn. Philadelphia: WB Saunders; 1995:1151–1170.

50. Nolan J, Batin PD, Andrews R, et al. Prospective study of heart rate variability and mortality in chronic heart failure: Results of the United Kingdom Heart Failure Evaluation and Assessment of Risk Trial (UK-Heart). Circulation 1998; 98:1510–1516.

51. Fauchier L, Babuty D, Cosnay P, et al. Prognostic value of heart rate variability for sudden death and major arrhythmic events in patients with idiopathic dilated cardiomyopathy. J Am Coll Cardiol 1999; 33:1203–1207.

52. Nemec J, Hammill SC, Shen WK. Increase in heart rate precedes episodes of ventricular tachycardia and ventricular fibrillation in patients with implantable cardioverter defibrillators: Analysis of spontaneous ventricular tachycardia database. Pacing Clin Electrophysiol 1999; 22:1729–1738.

53. Shusterman V, Aysin B, Weiss R, et al. Dynamics of low-frequency R-R interval oscillations preceding spontaneous ventricular tachycardia. Am Heart J 2000; 139:126–133.

54. Yamada A, Hayano J, Sakata S, et al. Reduced ventricular response irregularity is associated with increased mortality in patients with chronic atrial fibrillation. Circulation 2000; 102:300–306.

55. Lombardi F, Colombo A, Basilico B, et al. Heart rate variability and early recurrence of atrial fibrillation after electrical cardioversion. J Am Coll Cardiol 2001; 37:157–162.

56. Lewis T. Notes upon alternation of the heart. Q J Med 1910; 4:141.

57. Smith JM, Clancy EA, Valeri CR, et al. Electrical alternans and cardiac electrical instability. Circulation 1988; 77:110–121.

58. Smith JM, Blue B, Clancy EA, et al. Subtle alternating electrocardiographic morphology as an indicator of decreased cardiac electrical stability. Comput Cardiol 1985; 12:109–112.

59. Pastore, JM, Girouard, SD, Laurita, KR, et al. Mechanism linking T-wave alternans to the genesis of cardiac fibrillation. Circulation 1999; 99:1385–1394.

60. Rosenbaum DS, Albrecht P, Cohen RJ. Predicting sudden cardiac death from T wave alternans of the surface electrocardiogram: promise and pitfalls. J Cardiovasc Electrophysiol 1996; 7:1095–1111.

61. Adam DR, Smith JM, Akselrod S, et al. Fluctuations in T-wave morphology and susceptibility to ventricular fibrillation. J Electrocardiol 1984; 17:209.

62. Hohnloser SH, Klingenheben T, Zabal M, Li YG, Albrect P, Cohen RJ. T-wave alternans during exercise and atrial pacing in humans. J Cardiovasc Electrophysiol 1997; 8:987–993.

63. Rosenbaum DS, Jackson LE, Smith JM, et al. Electrical alternans and vulnerability to ventricular arrhythmias. N Engl J Med 1994; 330:235–241.

64. Narayan SM, Smith JM. Differing rate dependence and temporal distribution of repolarization alternans in patients with and without ventricular tachycardia. J Cardiovasc Electrophysiol 1999; 10:61–71.

65. Narayan SM, Smith JM. Exploiting rate-related hysteresis in repolarization alternans to improve risk stratification for ventricular tachycardia. J Am Coll Cardiol 2000; 35:1485–1492.

66. Buxton AE, Lee KL, Fisher JD, et al. A randomized study of the prevention of sudden death in patients with coronary artery disease. Multicenter Unsustained Tachycardia Trial Investigators. N Engl J Med 1999; 341:1882–1890.

67. Armoundas AA, Osaka M, Mela T, et al. T-wave alternans and dispersion of the QT interval as risk stratification markers in patients susceptible to sustained ventricular arrhythmias. Am J Cardiol 1998; 82:1127–1129.

68. Gold MR, Bloomfield DM, Anderson KP, et al. A comparison of T-wave alternans, signal averaged electrocardiography and programmed ventricular stimulation for arrhythmia risk stratification. J Am Coll Cardiol 2000; 36:2247–2253.

69. Gold M. T wave alternans predicts arrhythmia vulnerability in patients undergoing electrophysiology study (abstract). Circulation 1998; 98:I–647.

70. MacMurdy KS, Shorofsky SR, Olsovsky MR, et al. T wave alternans predicts arrhythmia vulnerability in patients with ischemic cardiomyopathy (abstract). PACE 1999; 22(4) Part II:767.

71. Ikeda T, Sakata T, Takami M, et al. Combined assessment of T-wave alternans and late potentials used to predict arrhythmic events after myocardial infarction. A prospective study. J Am Coll Cardiol 2000; 35:722–730.

72. Grimm W, Glaveris C, Hoffmann J, et al. Noninvasive arrhythmia risk stratification in idiopathic dilated cardiomyopathy: design and first results of the Marburg Cardiomyopathy Study. Pacing Clin Electrophysiol 1998; 21:2551–2556.

73. Klingenheben T, Cohen RJ, Peetermans JA, et al. Predictive value of T wave alternans in patients with congestive heart failure (abstract). Circulation 1998; 98(suppl):I–864.

74. Klingenheben T, Credner SC, Bender B, et al. Exercise induced microvolt level T wave alternans identifies patients with non-ischemic dilated cardiomyopathy at high risk of ventricular tachyarrhythmic events (abstract). Pacing Clin Electrophysiol 1999; 22:860.

75. Momiyama Y, Hartikainen J, Nagayoshi H, et al. Exercise-induced T wave alternans as a marker of high risk in patients with hypertrophic cardiomyopathy. Jpn Circ J 1997; 61:650–656.

76. Kavesh NG, Shorofsky SR, Sarang SE, et al. The effect of procainamide on T wave alternans. J Cardiovasc Electrophysiol 1999; 10:649–654.

77. Kirk MM, Cooklin M, Shorofsky SR, et al. Beta adrenergic blockade decreases T wave alternans (abstract). J Am Coll Cardiol 1999; 33:108A.

78. Houltz B, Darpo B, Edvardsson N, et al. Electrocardiographic and clinical predictors of torsades de pointes induced by almokalant infusion in patients with chronic atrial fibrillation or flutter: a prospective study. Pacing Clin Electrophysiol 1998; 21:1044–1057.

79. Surawicz B, Fisch C. Cardiac alternans: diverse mechanisms and clinical manifestations. J Am Coll Cardiol 1992; 20:483–499.

80. Bardaji A, Vidal F, Richart C. T wave alternans associated with amiodarone. J Electrocardiol 1993; 26:155–157.

81. Habbab MA, el-Sherif N. TU alternans, long QTU, and torsade de pointes: clinical and experimental observations. Pacing Clin Electrophysiol 1992; 15:916–931.

82. Binkley P, Bush CA, Kolibash AL, et al. The anatomic relationship of the esophageal lead to the left atrium. PACE 1982; 5: 583–389.

83. Burack B, Furman S. Transesophageal cardiac pacing. Am J Cardiol 1969; 23:469–472

84. Stopczych MS, Prochaczek F, Galecka J. The new achievements in transesophageal diagnostic cardiac stimulation.(Abstract). Cardiologia 1989; 34 (suppl 5):29.

85. Volkmann H, Kuhnert H, Dannberg G, et al. Electrophysiologische Diagnostik mit Hilfe transosophagealer Stimulation und Ableitung. Teil 2: Tachycardie rhythmusstorungen. Herzschrittmacher 1987; 7: 127–140.

86. Volkmann H, Taubert FP, Kuhnert H, et al. Prognostische Bedeutung der seriellen phannakologisch-elektrophysiologischen Testung bei supraventrikularen Tachyckardien. Z. Klin.Med 1988; 43, 4: 281–285.

87. Gallagher JJ, Smith WN, Kassel J, et al. Use of esophageal lead in the diagnosis of mechanism of reciprocating tachycardia. PACE 1980; 3:440–448.

88. Hombach V, Behrenbeck DW, Hilger HH. Oesophagosternal and oesophagoapical leads for registration of surface Hisbundle potentials. Z Kardiol 1977; 66:565–571.

89. Laucevičius A, Matulionis A, Ivaskevicius J, et al. Esophageal beat-to-beat recordings of low amplitude electrical heart signals. Klinische medizin 1986; 41:267–271.

90. Stopczyk MJ, Pieniak M, Sadowski Z, et al. Transesophageal atrial pacing as a simple diagnostic and therapeutic procedure. In: Kadefors R, Magnusson RI, Petersen I, eds. The Third International Conference on Medical Physics, Including Medical Engineering. Goeteborg, Sweden: The Third ICMP Executive Committee; 1972:40–45.

91. Swiatecka G, Lubinski A, Raczak G, et al. Transesophageal programmed atrial pacing as a method of selecting patients with sick sinus syndrome for permanent atrial pacing. PACE 1988; 11:1655–1661.

92. Trusz-Gluza M. Wlasciwosci elektrofizjologiczne serca w zespole chorego wezla zatokowego. Pol Tyg Lek 1985; 44:1243–1250.

93. Ajisaka H, Hiraki T, Ikeda H, et al. Direct conversion of atrial flutter to sinus rhythm with low-output, short-duration transesophageal atrial pacing. Clin Cardiol 1997; 20(9):762–766.

94. Brembilla-Perrot B, Spatz F, Khaldi E, et al. Value of esophageal pacing in evaluation of supraventricular tachycardia. Am J Cardiol 1990; 65:322–330.

95. D'Este D, Pasqual A, Bertaglia M, et al. Evaluation of atrial vulnerability with transoesophageal stimulation in patients with atrioventriclar junctional reentrant tachycardia. Comparison with patients with ventricular pre-excitation and with normal subjects. Eur Heart J 1995; 16:1632–1636.

96. Pongiglione G, Saul JP, Dunnigan A, et al. Role of transesophageal pacing in evaluation of palpitations in children and adolescents. Am J Cardiol 1988; 62:566–570, 2–6.

97. Giedrimiene DA, Lukoseviciute AJ, Transesophageal cardiac pacing for induction and control of supraventricular paroxysmal tachycardia for patients with follow-up antiarrhythmic therapy. Heart Web 1996; 2: Article No. 96110031.

98. Kozluk E, Michalkiewicz D, Franciszek Walczak F, et al. Transesophageal atrial pacing in patients with suspected arrhythmia recurrence after its nonpharmacologic treatment. Heart Web 1999; 4:article No. 99020010.

99. Deharo JC, Moustaghfir A, Macaluso G, et al. Utilisation de l'exploration oesophagiene pour le suivi a moyen terme apres ablation par radiofrequence des tachycardies par reentree intranodale. Arch Mal Coeur 1996; 89:1375–1379.

100. Pytkowski M, Sterlinski M, Kowalewski M, et al. Utility of transoesophageal atrial pacing to estimate the results of catheter ablation of supraventricular tachycardias. (Abstract). Arch Mal Coeur 1998; 91(special III):294.

CLINICAL PHARMACOLOGY

Current and novel drugs for cardiac arrhythmias

Melanie Hümmelgen MD
Universitätsklinikum Hamburg-Eppendorf, Hamburg,
Germany

Thomas Meinertz MD
Universitätsklinikum Hamburg-Eppendorf, Hamburg,
Germany

Most antiarrhythmic agents
share a narrow therapeutic
range and there is a lack of
markers that can accurately
predict efficacy of an
antiarrhythmic agent against
a specific arrhythmia

Introduction

With antiarrhythmic drugs arrhythmias can be suppressed or even, paradoxically, exacerbated. Such unpredictable responses are caused by factors determined by plasma and tissue concentrations of drugs and metabolites and factors determined by cellular and organ responses to those concentrations. The study of drug concentrations following drug administration is termed pharmacokinetics, the study of variability in response to those concentrations *pharmacodynamics*. Antiarrhythmic agents share a narrow therapeutic range, e.g. a doubling of an effective dose or plasma concentration often produces dangerous cardiac side-effects while a diminuation of dose respective plasma concentration by e.g. of 50% can result in treatment failure. Furthermore there is a lack of markers that can accurately predict efficacy of an antiarrhythmic agent against a specific arrhythmia.

Therefore it is important that the treating consultant does not rely on one piece of information about an antiarrhythmiac agent but that he always takes all available information into consideration including pharmacokinetics, pharmacodynamics, potential adverse effects, circumstances of potential proarrhythmia and actual recommendations on the clinical use and dose regime of specific antiarrhythmic agents.

CLASS I ANTI-ARRHYTHMIC AGENTS

Under the modified Singh-Vaughan Williams classification sodium channel blocking drugs are class I, with subdivision into classes IA (prolongation of conduction and repolarization), IB (no effect on conduction and shortening of repolarization), and IC (prolongation of conduction but little effect on repolarization).

In general class IB agents display rapid binding and unbinding kinetics, those of IC drugs are slow, and those of the IA drugs are intermediate.

Quinidine

Pharmacokinetics

See Table 12.1.

Pharmacodynamics

Quinidine affects depolarization and repolarization by blocking sodium and potassium channels, respectively. Quinidine's net electrophysiological effects result from a complex interaction of its individual actions on various inward and outward currents. For example it blocks the fast sodium current (I_{Na}). This effect is greater at faster rates and under ischemic conditions. In addition it blocks alpha 1- and alpha 2-adrenergic receptors. Vagolytic effects occur through muscarinic receptor block.

On the surface electrocardiogram, QRS duration is directly related to plasma level, whereas the effect on the QT interval is not. Sometimes marked prolongation of the QT interval or prominent U waves can be seen even at low plasma concentrations and should alert for possible proarrhythmia.

Adverse effects

Gastrointestinal side-effects, most commonly abdominal cramping and diarrhea, occur in one-third of the patients. Furthermore rash, thrombocytopenia and Coombs-positive hemolytic anemia can occur as relatively rare complications.

Proarrhythmia

Quinidine syncope which is most frequently due to ventricular tachycardia (usually from the torsade de pointes type) has a reported incidence of 0.5–4.4%. Quinidine-induced ventricular fibrillation

Table 12.1 Pharmacokinetics

	Bioavailability (%)	Protein binding (%)	Time to peak concentration (hr)	Elimination $T\frac{1}{2}$ (hr)	Therapeutic range (µcg/ml)	Elimination route
Quinidine	70–85	70–95	1–4	6–8	2–5	Hepatic
Disopyramide	85	Concentration dependent	2	4–8	2–5	Both[†]
Lidocaine	-	50–80	-	1–4	1.5–5.0	Hepatic
Mexiletine	90	70	2–4	8–16	0.75–2.0	Hepatic
Phenytoin	55–90	90	8–12	24	10–20	Hepatic
Flecainide	95	30–40	2–4	12–27	0.2–1.0	Both[†]
Propafenone	5–50	95	2–3	2–10 (EM) 10–32 (PM)	0.2–1.0*	Hepatic

EM, early metabolizers; PM, poor metabolizers
*Plasma levels for guiding propafenone therapy may not be useful
[†]Hepatic and renal

is clustered as an early event with a median occurrence at 3 days for all class IA drugs.[1]

Because quinidine's vagolytic effect can enhance conduction through the atrioventricular node, the ventricular response during atrial fibrillation or flutter may increase. This can be particularly dangerous during atrial flutter, when slowing of the atrial rate and faster AV nodal conduction can combine to create 1:1 atrioventricular (AV) response. Therefore antiarrhythmic treatment with quinidine should be combined with an AV nodal blocking agent whenever possible.

The proarrhythmic potential of antiarrhythmic drugs argues for in-hospital continuous electrographic monitoring during their initiation in most cases. This is particularly so with class I drugs, where proarrhythmia appears to be – at least in some patients – not necessarily related to the arrhythmia being treated or the presence of underlying diseases or predisposing factors. When the QTc prolongs to more than 500 ms, quinidine should be discontinued in an attempt to prevent proarrhythmia. Hypokalemia

facilitates induction of the typical quinidine-induced proarrhythmia (torsade de pointes tachycardia) and should be treated before initiation of quinidine therapy.

Clinical use

Because of the potential proarrhythmic effect of quinidine this drug should no longer be used for the treatment of ventricular arrhythmias. It is currently indicated that quinidine should be used to prevent attacks of paroxysmal atrial fibrillation and recurrence of atrial fibrillation following cardioversion. One year after beginning quinidine therapy for atrial fibrillation following cardioversion about 50% of patients remain in sinus rhythm, compared with 25% of those treated with placebo.[2]

Dosing

For chronic treatment only long-acting preparations that allow dosing intervals of

8 or 12 h should be used. Using these sustained release preparations the drug should be administered up to maximum daily dose of about 1200 mg.

Disopyramide

Pharmacokinetics

See Table 12.1.

Pharmacodynamics

Use-dependent block of I_{Na} develops with binding predominantly to the activated state of the channel. The recovery kinetics of I_{Na} is longer than it was observed with other class IA agents and is more comparable to that of class IC drugs. Block of I_K, I_{KI}, I_{Ca} and I_{to} currents has been shown. The anticholinergic effect of disopyramide occurs due to block of cardiac, intestinal smooth muscle and exocrine gland muscarinic receptors.

Adverse effects

Anticholinergic side-effects occur in one-third of patients with patients reporting a dry mouth, blurred vision, constipation and urinary retention. Predisposing factors appear to be advanced age, malnutrition and chronic renal failure. Disopyramide is a negative inotrope. This effect is directly related to plasma concentration and is seen predominantly in those patients with underlying left ventricular dysfunction. Disopyramide should be avoided in patients with ventricular systolic dysfunction and/or a history of systolic congestive heart failure.[3]

Proarrhythmia

As with other drugs that prolong repolarization, disopyramide can cause ventricular fibrillation or torsade de pointes tachycardia, although its propensity appears to be less than that of quinidine.[4]

Clinical use

Disopyramide is effective in the treatment of atrial arrhythmias [prevention of atrial fibrillation in paroxysmal atrial fibrillation and following direct current (DC) cardioversion].

Dosing

For chronic treatment disopyramide should be given in a controlled release preparation 200–300 mg every 12 h.

Lidocaine (lignocaine)

Pharmacokinetics

See Table 12.1.

Pharmacodynamics

Lidocaine (lignocaine) blocks the I_{Na} current with binding predominantly to the inactivated state. Because of the rapid binding and unbinding kinetics conduction slowing is evident only at fast heart rate or in diseased tissue with partially depolarized membranes. Both normal and abnormal automaticity are suppressed in Purkinje fibers and ventricular muscle.

Adverse effects

Central nervous system side-effects predominate, including perioral numbness, paresthesias, diplopia, hyperacusis, slurred speech, altered consciousness, seizures and respiratory arrest. Typically, lidocaine (lignocaine) does not alter hemodynamics.

Proarrhythmia

Clinically relevant proarrhythmia is very rare.

Clinical use

Because of its ease of administration and rapid onset of action, lidocaine (lignocaine) is a drug of first choice for the acute treatment of sustained ventricular tachycardia. In the hospital setting of acute myocardial infarction (MI) lidocaine (lignocaine) reduces the occurrence of ventricular fibrillation, but does not improve prognosis.[5] Thus, prophylactic lidocaine (lignocaine) use during acute MI is not warranted in most cases.

Dosing

A number of administration protocols have been proposed. In principle these protocols include one or up to three bolus doses and at the same time start with a maintenance infusion. An initial intravenous loading bolus of 1.5 mg/kg can be administered over 5–10 min and then a maintenance infusion of 2–4 mg/min can begin. In some patients an additional bolus of 1 mg/kg must be given 20–30 min following the first bolus in order to avoid subtherapeutic plasma concentrations. In patients with overt heart failure a reduction in both bolus and maintenance infusions is mandatory because both the volume of distribution and the clearance are reduced.

Mexiletine

Pharmacokinetics

See Table 12.1

Pharmacodynamics

The cardiac electrophysiological effects of mexiletine are very similar to those of lidocaine (lignocaine).

Adverse effects

Gastrointestinal and central nervous system side-effects are the most prominent and are related to dose and plasma concentration. These side-effects are usually dose-limiting factors. Similar to lidocaine (lignocaine) mexiletine has little effect on heart rate, blood pressure and cardiovascular hemodynamics.

Proarrhythmia

Proarrhythmia is rare and has been reported to occur in 1.3% in patients being treated for ventricular tachycardia or ventricular fibrillation.[4]

Dosing

The typical dose is 200–300 mg every 8 h or in a slow release preparation twice daily.

Flecainide

Pharmacokinetics

See Table 12.1

Pharmacodynamics

Flecainide displays potent sodium channel block with slow binding and unbinding kinetics. In addition it blocks the I_K, and the slow inward calcium currents. Prolongation of atrial refractoriness is probably the mechanism of termination atrial fibrillation.[6]

Adverse effects

When used in a proper way extracardiac side-effects rarely occur. Possible negative effects include central nervous system adverse reactions such as a blurred vision, headaches and ataxia.
Flecainide has negative inotropic effects similar to those of disopyramide. Exacerbation of congestive heart failure occurred in 16% of patients with a history of congestive heart failure and in 6% of those without such a history.[7] Its use is therefore not recommended for patients with a medium or severe ventricular systolic dysfunction and/or a history of congestive heart failure.

Proarrhythmia

In the cardiac arrhythmias suppression trial which tested the hypothesis that suppression of ventricular ectopy after MI reduces the incidence of sudden death, patients treated with flecainide or encainide compared with placebo[8] showed a higher mortality rate. In this study proarrhythmia was not just an early event during therapy but occurred also during long-term follow-up. Predictors of proarrhythmia are reduced left ventricular function and the presence of ischemia. Because of the significant use-dependent effects of the drug, proarrhythmia sometimes occurs with exertion.[9] A characteristic issue of flecainide induced proarrhythmia is incessant ventricular tachycardia.

Ventricular proarrhythmia from flecainide is rare in treatment of paroxysmal atrial fibrillation or following DC cardioversion for atrial fibrillation. Only a few cases of serious proarrhythmias have been reported in patients with no or minimal structural heart disease.[9]

Clinical use

Flecainide is effective and useful for the treatment of many supraventricular arrhythmias, e.g. in paroxysmal atrial fibrillation or following DC cardioversion for atrial fibrillation. When used for the treatment of symptomatic ventricular arrhythmias [e.g. right ventricular outflow tract tachycardia (RVOT)] it should be limited to patients with no or minimal structural heart disease.

Dosing

Flecainide therapy should be initiated with 100 mg every 12 h or in older patients or those with reduced renal clearance with 50 mg every 8 h. The dose should not be increased more often than every 3 days. The dose can be increased up to a total of 300 mg daily.

A single 200 mg or if necessary 300 mg oral loading dose can be successful in converting recent-onset atrial fibrillation in patients with no or minimal structural heart disease.

In order to prevent proarrhythmic effects the QRS duration should be monitored and it should not increase more than 20% compared with baseline. The intravenous dose for the treatment of atrial fibrillation is 2 mg/kg (maximum dose 150 mg) given over at least 10 min.

Propafenone

Pharmacokinetics (see Table 12.1)

Although propafenone is well absorbed its bioavailability is unpredictable because of high first-pass metabolism. Propafenone exhibits non-linear, dose-dependent kinetics in patients who are extensive metabolizers because of a saturable metabolic pathway (probably 5-hydroxylation); thus, the dose-concentration relationship is not linear in these patients and the bioavailability increases dramatically with doses above 600 mg/day. The primary metabolic pathway is hepatic through saturable mechanism to 5-hydroxy-propafenone. In approximately 7% of whites, lacking the needed enzyme, markedly higher concentrations of propafenone are found even at low doses. These so called 'poor metabolizers' are much more susceptible to therapeutic and toxic effects of the drug.

Pharmacodynamics

Propafenone blocks effectivly the I_{Na} current in a use-dependent manner with slow binding and unbinding kinetics. Its two major metabolites also block I_{Na}. Potassium channel block by propafenone has been demonstrated for different potassium currents and also for the L-type calcium channels. In addition propafenone demonstrates non-selective beta-adrenergic block.

Adverse effects

Nausea, a feeling of dizziness, and a metallic taste are the most common side-effects. Furthermore blurred vision, paresthesias and constipation as well as exacerbation of asthma are seen in rare cases. Central nervous system side-effects appear to be related to the propafenone plasma concentration and are more frequent in poor metabolizers. Approximately 10–25% of patients discontinue therapy with propafenone because of side-effects.

Propafenone has a negative inotropic effect, at least partially due to its beta-adrenergic and calcium channel blocking activity. However, a decrease in LV ejection fraction can be seen in patients with compromised left ventricular function only. This negative inotropic property seems to be less pronounced than that of disopyramide and flecainide.

Proarrhythmia

The incidence of serious proarrhythmia with propafenone treatment of ventricular arrhythmias is approximately 5%.[4] These arrhythmias include polymorphic ventricular tachycardia, in rare cases torsade de pointes tachycardia, ventricular fibrillation and also incessant ventricular tachycardia. When treating atrial arrhythmias propafenone can sometimes cause atrial flutter with 1:1 atrial to ventricular conduction when AV nodal block is inadequate. Ventricular arrhythmia occurring with propafenone therapy during treatment of supraventricular arrhythmias is a rare event in patients with no or minimal structural heart disease.

Clinical use

Propafenone is effective against a wide range of supraventricular arrhythmias. Recurrence of atrial fibrillation following DC cardioversion is controlled during chronic therapy in 40–65% of patients.[10,11] Propafenone should be used only for the treatment of symptomatic ventricular arrhythmias in patients with no or minimal structural heart disease. The spectrum of indications and contraindications are similar to that of flecainide.

Dosing

Long-term dosing of propafenone is 150–300 mg every 8 h or use of the long-term controlled release preparation twice daily within the same dose range.

A single 600 mg oral loading dose can be successful in converting recent-onset atrial fibrillation. Similar to flecainide the QRS duration should be monitored and it should not increase more than 20% compared with baseline.

CLASS III ANTIARRHYTHMIC DRUGS

All available class III antiarrhythmic drugs prolong the action potential duration by inhibiting potassium currents. The potassium currents identified in human heart cells that could be the target of class III drugs are listed in Table 12.2 along with their tissue localization and examples of class III agents known to block them. A variety of pure class III compounds, including d-sotalol and dofetilide, are highly selective blockers of I_{Kr}. These drugs prolong the action potential duration and refractoriness and are effective in treating re-entrant arrhythmias.[12] On the other hand their actions are more pronounced at slower heart rates ('reverse use dependence'),[13] a phenomenon that tends to limit efficacy[14] and increases the risk of arrhythmogenic early afterdepolarizations that underly torsade de pointes arrhythmias.[15] Several class III agents including amiodarone and the experimental drugs ambasilide and azimilide are relatively non-selective potassium channel blockers. These agents appear to have fewer reverse use-dependent effects on action potential duration which may make them more secure and more effective for certain arrhythmias.

In the clinical situation class III agents appear to be more effective than class I drugs in treating re-entrant ventricular

Table 12.2 Potassium currents in human heart cells

Current	Expression	Molecular equivalent	Effect of blockade	Blockers
I_{to}	$A^{9,10}$, V^{11}	Kv4.3	Delay early repolarization	Ambasilide
I_{Kr}	A^{16}, $V^{17,18}$	HERG	Increased APD (A,V)	Sotalol Amiodarone
I_{Ks}	A^{16}, V^{18}	minK/K_vLQT1	Increased APD (A,V))	Amiodarone
I_{Kur}	$A^{25,26}$	Kvl.5	Increased APD (A only)	Ambasilide
I_{Kl}	A^{30}, V^{30}	Kir2.1^{31}, 2.2, 2.3	Delayed terminal repolarization	Amiodarone

A, atria; V, ventricles; APD action potential duration

tachycardia and, although relatively effective in preventing atrial fibrillation recurrence, they are less effective than class I agents in terminating atrial fibrillation. It should be taken into account that most available class III drugs are not pure class III agents. Amiodarone has actions of all four antiarrhythmic classes and sotalol has the actions of at least two of them.

Amiodarone

Amiodarone was initially developed as an antianginal agent, and subsequently was found to have antiarrhythmic properties. The drug has an unusual chemical structure that includes two iodide moieties and confers great lipid solubility.

Pharmacokinetics

One of the unique aspect of amiodarone pharmacology is its unusual pharmacokinetics. It is a highly lipid soluble with concentrations in fat approximately 1000-fold higher than plasma after 7 days of administration. Consequently the drug's volume of distribution is enormous – in the range of 5000 L.[16] Because of the very long time required for sufficient loading to saturate body lipids, drug concentrations build up slowly with repeated dosing. Furthermore

the very large lipid stores act as a massive drug reservoir when dosing is discontinued. This results in a very long elimination half-life (in the order of about 30–50 days) after termination of long-term therapy.[16] Amiodarone undergoes hepatic biotransformation, primarily by conversion to desethylamiodarone. Desethylamiodarone accumulates slowly during long-term amiodarone therapy with concentrations reaching 80% of those of the parent compound after several months.[17] This metabolite shows antiarrhythmic activity and can contribute to the changing electrophysiological effects after initiation of amiodarone therapy.

Pharmacodynamics

The other unique feature of amiodarone is that it has the actions of all four antiarrhythmic classes and it has a changing pattern of electrophysiological actions with continuous administration: the drug has been considered as a class III agent despite having the actions of all four antiarrhythmic classes.[18] Amiodarone reduces V_{max} and I_{Na} in a fashion suggestive of an inactivated-state blocker with rapid unbinding at diastolic potentials (class IB-like). It produces non-competitive antagonism of adrenergic effects (a class II antiarrhythmic action). The potential duration-prolonging action, along with the similarity between the effects of amiodarone and of thyroidectomy[19] have led to the notion that the drug's class III properties are due to antagonism of thyroid effects on the heart. Recent studies suggest that chronic amiodarone administration prolongs action potential duration in guinea pig ventricular myocytes by inhibiting three potassium currents, whereas hypothyroidism affects only I_{Ks}.[20] These results suggest that a part of amiodarone's class III properties can be attributed to an inhibition of thyroid effects on the heart. Finally amiodarone also blocks the calcium inward current in a time- and frequency-dependent way (class IV action).[21,22]

The changing pattern of its electrophysiological actions with continued administrations may explain why the various effects of amiodarone on patients develop with different time patterns.

The effects on calcium-dependent tissues (sinuatrial and AV nodes) develop more rapidly compared to the effect on repolarization parameters such as the QT interval and ventricular refractoriness. During steady-state, all clinical electrophysiological consequences of amiodarone are a reflection of its class I, II, III and IV properties. All electrocardiographic intervals and clinical electrophysiological variables are prolonged with chronic administration.[18]

Adverse effects

Amiodarone is associated with a wide range of adverse effects outside the cardiovascular system. There is an abundance of literature on these effects. For the purpose of this presentation only the most important effects can be summarized.

Pulmonary toxicity is of particular concern because of its potentially grave impacts. Typical features include an interstitial pattern on chest radiographs and a restrictive pattern on a pulmonary function test. The clinical picture may resemble interstitial pneumonitis and

respond, in some cases, to steroid therapy. Although pneumonitis rarely occurs at doses lower than 400 mg/day, it can occur at the early stage of therapy and also with lower doses.[23]

Central nervous system toxicity is relatively common and can include anxiety, tremor, headache and peripheral neuropathy.[24,25]

Ocular side-effects occur frequently and are dose related.[26] The most frequent ocular side-effects are corneal microdeposits. In the majority of cases there is subclinical toxicity on examination, symptomatic ocular side-effects being relatively rare.[27] Typical symptoms were photophobia, blurred vision and an impression of colored haloes around lights.

Gastrointestinal side-effects include small appetite, nausea and reversible liver function abnormalities.

Cutaneous photosensitivity is common. Avoiding exposure to the sun is recommended for all patients taking the drug. A cosmetically disturbing blue–gray discoloration occurs in a few of the patients treated with high doses for a long time.

Thyroid function abnormalities are relatively common (for detailed review see Harjai and Licata).[28] Amiodarone can affect thyroid metabolism at a wide variety of stages. As a clinical consequence patients may experience clinical hypothyroidism as well as hyperthyroidism. The incidence of both types of thyroid dysfunction differ significantly between geographical regions. Also clinical disturbance of thyroid function has to be differentiated from abnormalities in the laboratory values.

Drug interactions with amiodarone occur with a variety of agents concomitantly used with amiodarone. Among these were digitoxin and coumarin oral anticoagulants.

Proarrhythmia

There is evidence from the literature that amiodarone is less likely to cause proarrhythmias than other class I and class III antiarrhythmic agents. Amiodarone is associated with a lower mortality rate in atrial fibrillation patients compared with other drugs used for the maintenance of sinus rhythm.[29] In addition the drug has been used safely in patients with a history of drug-induced torsade de pointes.[30] In the Canadian Amiodarone Myocardial Infarction Arrhythmia Trial (CAMIAT) and in the European Myocardial Infarction Amiodarone Trial (EMIAT) studies suspected proarrhythmia occurred in less than 1% of amiodarone-treated patients, a rate that is very low and even less than the prevalence of suspected proarrhythmia in placebo groups. On the other hand bradycardia as proarrhythmic effect occurs in a number of patients treated with amiodarone on a long-term run. Amiodarones with their combination of class I–IV actions produce a pattern of bradycardic side-effects such as sinus bradycardia and excessive slowing of ventricular rates during atrial fibrillation.

Clinical use

Amiodarone is widely perceived to be a uniquely effective antiarrhythmic compound. Data that have become available recently from several large-scale clinical trials support this impression while at the same time point to some limitations in its clinical usefulness.

Amiodarone is effective for the prevention of potentially lethal arrhythmias in patients resuscitated from cardiac arrest.[31] However, amiodarone is less effective in reducing mortality than implantable cardioverter-defibrillator (ICD) therapy.[32] Amiodarone has been found to prevent sudden cardiac death and thereby reduce mortality in other risk groups, particular patients with recent MI and congestive heart failure. Two recent meta-analyses based on randomized, controlled trials concluded that amiodarone reduces the mortality in these patient groups by 17–19 %.[33,34] Individual trials produced sometimes conflicting results.

Two large-scale, randomized, double-blinded, placebo-controlled, post-MI trials (CAMIAT and EMIAT) showed statistically significant reductions (by approximately 35%) in presumed arrhythmic death rate by amiodarone, although neither found a significant decrease in all-cause mortality.[35,36]

The relative value of amiodarone compared to conventional antiarrhythmic therapy for the maintenance of sinus rhythm following cardioversion was evaluated recently in a randomized, controlled trial, the Canadian Trial of Atrial Fibrillation (CTAF). In this study amiodarone was clearly superior to the class antiarrhythmic IC agent, propafenone and to the class III agent, sotalol.[37]

From this it can be concluded that amiodarone is the best choice for medical therapy in patients at high risk of malignant ventricle tachyarrhythmias, particularly when ICD implantation is inappropriate or impossible. Intravenous amiodarone is superior to other antiarrhythmic agents in the clinical emergency situation of drug-refractory ventricular tachycardia and for facilitating resuscitation in cardiac arrest due to DC shock-resistant VF.

Amiodarone is the drug of choice in drug-resistant atrial fibrillation (paroxysmal or following cardioversion) and can be regarded as the drug of first choice in those with valvular heart disease or with depressed left ventricular dysfunction.

Sotalol

Sotalol was first developed as a beta-adrenergic receptor antagonist. Later it was described by Kaumann and Olson[38] as an agent which prolonged the action potential duration being the basis of the drug's antiarrhythmic property. This 'new' mechanism was subsequently designated a third class of antiarrhythmic action in the classic paper by Singh and

Vaughan Williams,[39] giving rise to the term class III drug. Like amiodarone, sotalol is not a pure class III compound, but has both class III and beta-blocking actions.

Pharmacokinetics

Sotalol is very well absorbed after oral administration and is eliminated largely unchanged in the urine. Sotalol doses should therefore be reduced in patients with renal dysfunction but also for older patients. The plasma elimination half-life averages 15 h, hence oral dosing does not have to be given more than twice a day, and many patients are well controlled with a single morning dose. Oral daily dosages vary from 80 to 640 mg/day. Doses exeeding 320 mg/day have an increased risk of torsade de pointes.[40]

Pharmacodynamics

Sotalol is a competitive beta-adrenergic receptor antagonist. Virtually all of the beta-blocking activity resides in the L-isomer which is over 50 times as potent as beta-blocker as the D-isomer.[41] On the other hand both isomers exert a similar prolonging action on the action potential duration. The beta-blocking actions of racemic sotalol are manifest at lower concentrations than the class III properties.[42,43] Thus, smaller doses (80 mg/day or less) produce partial beta-blockade with little class III action, and class III properties become prominent at doses over 160 mg/day. The electrophysiological effect of sotalol in humans is as would be expected from a combination of class II and III actions – a slowing of the heart rate, prolongation of the AV conduction and prolongation of the atrial and ventricular refractoriness.

There is evidence that sotalol's reverse use-dependent action may limit its efficacy for atrial fibrillation termination. Sotalol class III properties result from block of I_K.[44]

Adverse effects

Sotalol is a non-selective, competitive beta-adrenergic receptor antagonist which has all adverse effects produced by beta-blockers.

Proarrhythmia

Potential cardiovascular adverse effects of beta-blockade included sinus node dysfunction, AV block and impaired left ventricular function. The most worrisome potential cardiovascular adverse effect is the induction of torsade de pointes tachycardia. This complication is dose related, with an incidence of approximately 1% in patients taking between 160 and 240 mg/day, compared with 5–7% at 480–640 mg/day.[45] Concomitant therapy with thiazide diuretics and hypokalemia increases the risk of torsade de pointes with sotalol[46] as does renal failure. As with quinidine, torsade de pointes tachycardia can be seen, although rarely, in patients on low doses of sotalol.

Clinical use

For indications well treated by pure class II drugs there is little reason to choose sotalol over a pure class II agent (beta-blocking agents). Sotalol is particularly useful for long-term therapy of atrial fibrillation, because it prevents atrial fibrillation recurrences and slows the ventricular response rate should atrial fibrillation reoccur. It should be noted however, that even with low doses of sotalol this drug may produce torsade de pointes tachycardia in rare cases especially if the above-mentioned circumstances (hypokalemia, renal dysfunction) come into play. Sotalol is relatively ineffective in terminating atrial fibrillation. Because of its potential proarrhythmic activity at high doses, sotalol should not be used in patients for the treatment of symptomatic ventricular arrhythmias unless a defibrillator is already implanted.

Dosing

The dosage should be up-titrated in each individual patient starting with a dose of 80 mg twice daily up to a dose of 160 mg twice daily. The dose should be increased in steps of at least 3 days. Dosages higher than 320 mg/day should be used only in exceptional cases.

CLASS II ANTIARRHYTHMIC DRUGS

Beta-blocking-agents

A number of beta-blockers have had their antiarrhythmic actions characterized to varying extents and are in common clinical use. Their major pharmacodynamic and pharmacokinetic properties are repeatedly summarized in the literature.[47,48] Some of these properties are of direct clinical relevance.

Pharmacokinetics

See Table 12.1.

Pharmacodynamics

The major action of beta-blockers is mediated via their property for competitively blocking cardiac beta 1-receptors. Thus, they are likely to be most effective in those arrhythmias in which an imbalance between sympathetic and parasympathetic drive plays an important role in their genesis and perpetuation. As it is the case for most major therapeutic indications for beta-antagonists, the beneficial effect of these agents is class rather than agent specific. A distinction should be made when this class of agents appears to exert a primary role in controlling symptomatic cardiac arrhythmias, when their effect is utilized for the prevention of such arrhythmias, and when their use is associated with prolongation of survival by prevention of the onset of life-threatening ventricular arrhythmias. Whenever used for the treatment in context with arrhythmias, these different indications should be taken into account.

Adverse effects

The adverse effects of beta-blocking agents used for the treatment of arrhythmias correspond to those observed when beta-blockers were used for other treatment indications.

Proarrhythmia

Clinically relevant proarrhythmias has not been described for beta-blocking agents. There is however no doubt that in patients with a diseased conduction system, beta-blockers can produce bradycardic effects at the sinus- and AV node-level.

Clinical use

Impact on mortality in survivors of acute myocardial infarction: Beta-blockers reduce the incidence of ventricular fibrillation and death in patients with MI at the time of diagnosis outwith hospital[49] as well during a hospital stay[50] and following discharge from the hospital.[50] Under these circumstances there is an 18–39% reduction in sudden cardiac death and total mortality in the first year following the event.[50,51] Mortality is also reduced over the first 10 days when the drug is given in an initial intravenous dose followed by oral therapy[50,51] and when these agents are given in conjunction with thrombolytic agents during the early stages of acute MI.

The preventive effect of beta-blockers in patients following MI is well known and has been confirmed in a relatively large number of trials. The reduction of mortality was evident irrespective of age, sex, race, site of infarction or the comparative risk profile of the patients. However, the benefit was greater in those at highest risk of sudden death. The degree of benefit also correlated positively with the degree of bradycardia produced by individual agents.

Prophylactic use of beta-blockers in congestive heart failure: Patients with heart failure irrespective of etiology show significantly increased activity of the sympathetic nervous system. A number of small trials supported the assumption that beta-blockade may have a potential to reduce mortality in these patients. Recently three large randomized trials have been published showing that beta-blocking agents have the potential to reduce mortality in these patients. This reduction in total mortality was in the range of 20–30% and it was assumed that a major part of this reduction in mortality was due to the prevention of sudden cardiac death.

Beta-blockade in survivors of cardiac arrest: There are no randomized or systematic studies that have been carried out to determine the role of beta-blockade in survivors of sudden cardiac death. However, beta-blockers prolonged survival significantly when compared with the group not given beta-blockers. The limitations of these retrospective observations are clearly evident. Furthermore it should be emphasized that there is increasing evidence that favors the role of ICD in prolonging survival in patients with aborted cardiac arrest.

Long QT interval syndrome: Beta-blockade has been the cornerstone of therapy for this congenital disorder. It is possible that in this syndrome, sympathetic excitation may induce non-uniform shortening of repolarization with a tendency for less dispersion of the overall QT interval. Beta-blockers are highly effective in preventing sudden death in the long QT interval syndrome. However, in patients at very high risk of sudden cardiac death, implantation of an ICD is mandatory.

Beta-blockade in sustained monomorphic ventricular tachycardia: It has been found that in a subset of patients with clinically documented monomorphic ventricular tachycardia, the administration of isoproterenol may facilitate induction of ventricular tachycardia by programmed electrical stimulation. Beta-blockers may be effective in producing a long-term control in such catecholamine-sensitive ventricular tachycardias.[52] It appears that although beta-blockers are most effective in those forms of ventricular tachycardia that are due to augmented automaticity, they may also play a role in those that arise on the basis of re-entry or triggered automaticity. The role of beta-blockers in those types of ventricular tachycardia has been studied by Steinbeck and associates.[53] During 2-year follow-up period, almost an identical number of cases of arrhythmia recurrences or sudden death occurred in the group with guided therapy (guided by programmed electrical stimulation) versus those treated with empirical beta-blockade. These data suggest that beta-blockade may be a significant therapeutic approach for the treatment of symptomatic sustained ventricular tachycardia/ventricular fibrillation.

Beta-blockers and ICDs

First: Beta-blockers can reduce the number of ICD discharges by preventing the development of ventricular tachycardia/ventricular fibrillation.

Second: Beta-blockers slow the rate of ventricular tachycardia.

Third: Beta-blockers can prevent sinus tachycardia as well as high ventricular rates during supraventricular arrhythmias and thereby reduce the number of inadequate ICD interventions.

Atrial flutter and fibrillation

Beta-blockade has no significant impact on effective conversion of atrial flutter or fibrillation to sinus rhythm when given over the short term or long term. By contrast, beta-blockers appear to maintain the stability of sinus rhythm after electrical cardioversion.[54]

Beta-blockers in atrial fibrillation following cardiac surgery: In the last decade the reported incidence of atrial fibrillation following cardiac surgery has varied between 17 and 33%.[55] It is known that the occurrence of atrial fibrillation after open heart surgery increases the overall hospital costs. Beta-blockers induce a broad range of beneficial effects in the time period following cardiac surgery. These beneficial effects have been shown in 18 randomized studies: the mean event rate in the controls was 34% compared with 8.7% in the beta-blocker treatment group. Only 3 of the 18 studies were placebo controlled and double blinded; in all of these beta-blocker studies nearly all patients received preoperative beta-blockade. Thus, the data suggest that a period of preoperative prophylaxes ideally followed by an overlapping regimen as a continuing therapy might constitute the most effective approach to the prevention of atrial fibrillation following cardiac surgery.

Dosing of beta-blockers

There are some general rules for the treatment of arrhythmias with beta-blocking agents. As a general rule beta-blocking therapy should be started with relatively low doses and the dose should be increased slowly up to the effective dose. Using such a procedure the tolerance against beta-blockers can be markedly increased. In general, heart rate reduction during exercise can be regarded as a good clinical indicator for the adequacy of beta-blockade. For the purpose of antiarrhythmic therapy, beta-blockers with beta 1-selectivity without intrinsic sympathomimetic activity are recommended. The types of beta-blocker preferred are those that can be given once a day.

ADENOSINE AND DIGOXIN

Adenosine

Adenosine is an endogenous nucleoside that is an important biochemical intermediate, a local physiological regulator in many organs, and a pharmacological agent with a number of clinical uses.

Pharmacokinetics

Once it is injected into the bloodstream, adenosine is rapidly cleared by cellular uptake and enzymic metabolism. Adenosine has a half-life of elimination in blood of about 0.5–5 sec. A given dose of adenosine administered through a peripheral cannula has therefore already been substantially eliminated before it reaches the heart, and the direct effects of the dose are seen only during its first passage through the circulation. Because adenosine is cleared so rapidly, relatively minor differences in site or speed of injection and in circulation time may influence the patients' response to any given dose.

Clinically relevant drug interactions may be seen with dipyridamole, which potentiates adenosine's effect by blocking cellular uptake, and with methylxanthines, which are adenosine A_1 and A_2 receptor antagonists.

Pharmacodynamics

The primary direct action of adenosine is the activation of an outward potassium current (I_{KAdo}), which is present in the atrium and the sinus and AV node but not present in ventricular myocytes. Inhibition of the pacemaker current (I_f) in sinuatrial and AV nodal cells is also a direct effect of adenosine in atrial myocytes.

DiMarco and co-workers[56] systematically studied the effects of bolus infusions of adenosine in humans. They observed that rapid intravenous infusion of adenosine in patients undergoing electrophysiological study resulted in a transient (less than 10 s) sinus slowing, with or without AV nodal block, followed by a short (15–45 s) period of sinus tachycardia. If adenosine was administered during atrial pacing, typical Wenckebach-type prolongations in the atrio-His (A-H) interval were observed.

Adverse effects

About 30–50% of treated patients report dose related, typically brief and mild side-effects such as facial flushing, chest pain and dyspnea following adenosine administration. Furthermore adenosine increases respiratory drive by chemoreceptor activation.

Proarrhythmia

Frequent atrial or premature ventricular beats that are produced by an unknown mechanism are often seen at the time of termination of paroxysmal supraventricular tachycardia by adenosine. These beats may actually contribute to the termination of the arrhythmia. More serious forms of proarrhythmias have also been reported: a few seconds of sinus bradycardia, sinus arrest or AV block are commonly noted when adenosine terminates paroxysmal supraventricular tachycardia. In patients at risk for bradycardia-dependent arrhythmias, polymorphic ventricular tachycardia has been reported with and without long QT intervals.[57]

Clinical use

Numerous studies have confirmed the efficacy of adenosine in terminating paroxysmal supraventricular tachycardia. In AV nodal re-entry tachycardia the usual site of block is during antegrade conduction over the slow AV nodal pathway. In one large, randomized controlled study paroxysmal supraventricular tachycardia conversion rates of 35%, 62%, 80% and 91% were reported after sequential adenosine doses of 3, 6, 9 and 12 mg, respectively.[58] In those clinical studies that placed no upper limit on dosage, essentially all episodes of paroxysmal supraventricular tachycardia requiring AV nodal conduction have been suspended, at least briefly. The dosage required for tachycardias caused by AV nodal re-entry seems to be the same as the treatment of tachycardias caused by atrioventricular re-entry.

Adenosine is also effective in pediatric patients.[59,60]

Several trials have compared the efficacy of adenosine with that of Verapamil.[61–63] These comparative efficacy data suggest that in most cases either adenosine or Verapamil is an appropriate first choice for terminating paroxysmal supraventricular tachycardia. Adenosine would be preferred in patients with severe left ventricular dysfunction, in patients who had recently received an intravenous beta-blocker, and in neonates. A calcium channel blocker would be preferred in patients receiving drugs known to interfere with adenosine's actions or metabolism and in patients with active bronchoconstriction. In patients in whom the diagnosis of paroxysmal supraventricular tachycardia is suspected but uncertain, adenosine has less depressant effects on blood pressure should the arrhythmia persist. However, adenosine can provoke a variety of arrhythmias, and its indiscriminate use for diagnostic purposes should be discouraged.

Dosing

The effective dose (single bolus dose) is in the range of 6–12 mg.

Digoxin

Pharmacokinetics

The oral bioavailability of digoxin is between 60 and 80%. It is eliminated through renal excretion, and its elimination half-life is between 24 and 48 h in patients with normal renal function. The desired serum concentration range during steady state is 0.8–2.0 ng/ml.

Pharmacodynamics

The major antiarrhythmic effects of digoxin are mediated by central and peripheral actions to augment vagal tone. Although direct actions on the AV node and atria have been demonstrated, these actions are seen only at concentrations above those used clinically. In the AV node, conduction is slowed and the effective refractory period is prolonged. Sinus node automaticity is unaffected or minimally slowed in most individuals, but occasional patients with sinus node dysfunction will show marked bradycardia.

Adverse effects and proarrhythmia

Non-cardiac manifestations of digoxin toxicity are anorexia, nausea and vomiting, headache, malaise and changes in vision, including scotoma, halo vision and altered color perception.

Cardiac toxicity may be caused by several factors: exaggerated effects on the AV or sinus node, leading to bradycardia and increased ventricular automaticity. Almost any arrhythmia has been documented in patients with high digoxin levels. Several arrhythmias are more specific for digoxin toxicity. These are the development of either high-grade AV block with an accelerated junctional rhythm or bidirectional ventricular tachycardia. These arrhythmias strongly suggest digoxin toxicity. Atrial tachycardia with block was formerly thought to be diagnostic for digoxin toxicity but more recent studies suggest that digoxin is only one of many causes of this arrhythmia.

Clinical use

The major role of digoxin as an antiarrhythmic drug is for control of ventricular rate during atrial tachyarrhythmias. Because digoxin exerts its beneficial effects by augmenting background parasympathetic tone, it has only limited value during exercise, physiological stress or other situations with increased sympathetic tone.

Among patients with new-onset atrial fibrillation and rapid ventricular rate who were given either intravenous or oral digoxin, effective rate control is delayed for at least 4–12 h. Calcium channel blockers or beta-adrenergic blockers will provide more rapid and reliable rate control.

Patients with paroxysmal episodes of atrial fibrillation are only ineffectively controlled by digoxin. Furthermore digoxin is ineffective in controlling ventricular rates in these patients. Patients with chronic continuous atrial fibrillation are the primary candidates for digoxin therapy. In those patients therapy to control ventricular rates has the following goals: to avoid symptoms due to excessive tachycardia, to avoid continuous heart rate elevations that may produce a tachycardia-induced cardiomyopathy and to allow an appropriate increase in heart rate with graded exercise. Based on data from asymptomatic subjects, Pitcher and associates[64] concluded that daytime pauses of up to 2.8 s and nocturnal pauses of up to 4.0 s should be considered normal.

Dosing

During steady-state the digoxin dose should be titrated up to the desired clinical effects within a daily dose range of 0.2–0.4 mg. In order to achieve a desired effect acutely a total dose up to 0.6 mg can be given.

NEW ANTIARRHYTHMIC DRUGS

There is a need for antiarrhythmic agents which are more effective and less toxic than those currently in use. The outstanding clinical efficacy of amiodarone in treating a wide variety of arrhythmias has led to a search for new class III drugs with a better safety profile. This development has evolved in two directions: amiodarone analogs and agents that block one or more components of the delayed rectifier potassium current.

Almost all drugs of this generation are closer to sotalol than to amiodarone in their chemical and electrophysiological characteristics. Chemically they can be grouped based on the fact that they contain a methanesulfonamide moiety. The developer of amiodarone has maintained a program to find analogs of amiodarone (e.g. drodenarone) that would have more desirable safety profiles and improved pharmacokinetic characteristics.

At least nine potassium channels have been identified. Most antiarrhythmic drugs that prolong repolarization have overlapping specificity for different groups of channels.[65] A great effort has been made in developing agents that are selective for more discrete ion currents that contribute to repolarization. In atrial tissue, the candidate currents are the transient outward current (I_{TO}) and the ultrarapid component of I_K (I_{KUR}). In the ventricles, the major repolarizing currents are I_K (composed of slow and rapid component, I_{KS} and I_{KR}) and the outwardly rectifying component of I_{K1}. Out of these currents drug development has focused on drugs to block I_{KR} or I_{KS}. Yet, at this point, there is no evidence that a selective effect of either of these components provides any clinical advantage.

Ibutilide

Ibutilide has recently been introduced in the USA as an intravenous agent for the termination of re-entrant atrial tachyarrhythmias.

Pharmacokinetics

Ibutilide, a methanesulfonamide derivative, is available only as an intravenous preparation. The drug is usually given as 10 min infusions with an initial dose of 1 mg followed if necessary by a second dose of 0.5–1 mg.[66] The drug is eliminated primarily by hepatic biotransformation with a mean elimination half-life of 6 h (range 2–12 h).

Pharmacodynamics

Ibutilide mechanism of ionic action involves the potentiation of a late inward current and the inhibition of I_{KR}. The precise contribution of I_{KR} blockade versus inward current enhancement to ibutilide's electrophysiological actions is uncertain. In canine models ibutilide shows antiarrhythmic efficacy against both atrial flutter and atrial fibrillation. Ibutilide increases the QT and QTc intervals in humans, without altering PR or QRS durations.

Adverse effects/proarrhythmia

The most significant potential adverse effect of ibutilide is the induction of polymorphic ventricular tachycardia in association with excess QT prolongation (torsade de pointes tachycardia). In an extensive, randomized, double-blinded trial, polymorphic ventricular tachycardia occurred in 15 of 180 (8.3%) ibutilide-treated and none of 86 placebo-treated patients.[67] Heart failure, female gender, non-white race, and slower heart rate were associated with a greater risk of polymorphic ventricular tachycardia. Apart from the risk of proarrhythmia short-term treatment with intravenous ibutilide seems generally well tolerated.

Clinical use

Ibutilide is used as an intravenous agent for the termination of atrial flutter and atrial fibrillation. Termination efficacy is dose related, and is maximal at 0.015 mg/kg.[67] The drug was more effective in terminating atrial flutter (63%) than atrial fibrillation (31%). Ibutilide facilitates pacing-induced conversion of atrial flutter in patients failing to convert with intravenous drug therapy alone. Ibutilide is valuable for rapid and effective treatment of atrial flutter in the emergency ward and obviates the need for DC cardioversion for many patients. Its efficacy for atrial fibrillation termination is inferior to that of class I drugs.

Dosing

Ibutilide is available as intravenous preparation. It is usually administered as a 10 min infusion, with an initial dose of 1 mg followed by a second dose of 0.5–1 mg if necessary.

Dofetilide

Dofetilide was developed for the treatment of life-threatening ventricular arrhythmias and for the prevention of recurrent atrial fibrillation of flutter. Like ibutilide it belongs to the class of methanesulfonamide compounds.

Pharmacokinetics

Dofetilide is completely absorbed after oral administration, its bioavailability nearly complete. Elimination is relatively evenly divided between renal and hepatic. The elimination half-life is usually approximately 8 h and therefore the dosing interval is 8–12 h.

Pharmcodynamics

Dofetilide blocks the rapidly activating component of the delayed rectifier potassium current (I_{KR}). At these concentrations, it does not block I_{KS} or the inward rectifier current. It has been found to prolong the QT and QTc interval with little if any effect on QT dispersion.[68] Dofetilide has no effects on conduction parameters, sinus cycle length or sinus node recovery time.[69]

Adverse effects/proarrhythmia

Early experience with dofetilide in large clinical trials showed an occurence of torsade de pointes tachycardia of up to 2.8%. After adjustment of the dosage according to renal function the incidence fell to 2.9%. The majority of these torsade de pointes cases occurred within the first 3 days following the start of a dofetilide therapy. A number of patients with torsade de pointes tachycardia had to be resuscitated and some patients died. Thus the incidence of serious adverse arrhythmic events associated with dofetilide appears to be comparable to other drugs such as sotalol.

Clinical use

Dofetilde has been developed for the treatment of supraventricular arrhythmias and of ventricular tachycardia and for the prevention of sudden cardiac death. Atrial fibrillation can be successfully converted to sinus rhythm with intravenous or oral dofetilide in at least 50% of the patients treated. Dofetilide seems to be even more effective in converting atrial flutter to sinus rhythm. The overall safety and efficacy of dofetilide was investigated in two groups of high-risk patients: in those following acute MI having an reduced left ventricular function; and those with heart failure (DIAMOND trials). These were randomized placebo-controlled trials. Each of these two studies enrolled 700 patients who were randomized to receive dofetilide or a matching placebo. Patients were titrated to a target dose of 500 µg twice daily. All patients were continuously monitored by telemetry for the first 3 days of the study to detect possible arrhythmic events and to ensure resuscitation in case of serious arrhythmias. Follow-up was ensured for a minimum period of 12 month. The overall 1 year mortality rate for randomized patients was 28% and 22% in both studies. This was within the expected range but dofetilide did not reduce the mortality in both patient populations.

There was however evidence that there was a lower incidence of new episodes of atrial fibrillation in the treated group. Those with atrial fibrillation at entry (25% of patients) had a higher incidence of conversion if they were in the dofetilide treatment group.

These results give reason to conclude that dofetilide is indicated in symptomatic life-threatening, ventricular arrhythmia if treatment of symptoms is required. Furthermore dofetilide is effective in the treatment and prevention of atrial flutter and atrial fibrillation.

Dosing

The usual daily dose during oral long-term treatment is 500 µg twice daily. During the first days of the treatment phase all patients should be permanently monitored by telemetry.

The effective intravenous dose is 4–8 µg/kg as a bolus dose given over 5 min.

Azimilide

Azimilide blocks both the slowly (I_{KS}) and the rapidly activating (I_{KR}) components of the delayed rectifier potassium current, which distinguishes it from most other potassium channel blockers such as sotalol, dofetilide or ibutilide. Yet the drug is not approved for treatment of arrhythmias.

Pharmacokinetics

Azimilide is completely absorbed. Because of its relatively long elimination half-life (4–5 days) once daily administration of the drug is recommended. Dose adjustment seems to be not required for age, gender, hepatic or renal function. The mean daily oral dose is 125 mg/day.

Pharmacodynamics

Preclinical and clinical studies indicate that azimilide prolongs cardiac refractory period in a dose-dependent manner, as manifested by increases in action potential duration, QTc interval and effective refractory period.

Adverse effects

The most relevant adverse effect of the drug is neutropenia which occurs in about 1% of the patients receiving the drug. Agrannulocytoses is a rare event and can probably be avoided by carefully checking the white blood count in the first 8 weeks of therapy.

Proarrhythmia

As has to expected from the mechanism of action, torsade de pointes tachycardia can occur as a proarrhythmic event. Compared to sotalol, ibutilide and dofetilide, such a proarrhythmic activity seems to occur less frequently. It has been observed in about 1% of the patients treated for atrial fibrillation or atrial flutter and in about 0.3% of a postinfarct population with an ejection fraction of 15–35%.

Clinical use

Azimilide is effective in preventing attacks of atrial fibrillation in patients with the paroxysmal form of this arrhythmia. Furthermore, this drug can prevent recurrence of atrial fibrillation following DC cardioversion. Up to now there has been a lack of comparative studies with other antiarrhythmic agents. In the azimilide postinfarction survival evaluation (ALIVE) trial the potential of azimilide for improving survival in patients at high risk of sudden cardiac death was studied. The major entry criteria for the study included patients with a left ventricular ejection fractions below 35% who have had a recent MI. The trial consisted of three groups – patients receiving 75 mg azimilide orally each day, patients receiving 100 mg each day and those receiving placebo. The authors found that azimilide did not increase the mortality in those randomized to active treatment, and that azimilide does not cause any harm to patients at high risk following MI. On the other hand, there was no evidence for a beneficial effect of azimilide on prognosis in this patient population. Therefore azimilide is indicated in patients with life-threatening, symptomatic ventricular arrhythmias, e.g. following implantation of an ICD. Furthermore azimilide produces beneficial effects in preventing atrial fibrillation in patients with the paroxysmal form of this arrhythmia or following DC cardioversion.

Dosing

The recommended dose range is 75, 100 or 125 mg, once a day.

References

1. Minardo JD, Heger JJ, Miles WM, et al. Clinical characteristics of patients with ventricular fibrillation during antiarrhythmic drug therapy. N Engl J Med 1988, 319:257–262.
2. Coplen SE, Antman EM, Berlin JA, et al. Efficacy and safety of quinidine therapy for maintenance of sinus rhythm after cardioversion. A metaanalysis of randomized control trials. Circulation 1990, 82:1106–1116.
3. Podrid PJ, Schoenberger A, Lown B. Congestive heart failure caused by oral disopyramide. N Engl J Med 1980; 302:614–617.
4. Stanton MS, Prystowsky EN, Fineberg NS, et al. Arrhythmogenic effects of antiarrhythmic drugs: a study of 506 patients treated for ventricular tachycardia or fibrillation. J Am Coll Cardiol 1989; 14:209–215.
5. Lie KI, Wellens HIJ, Van Capelle FJ, et al. Lidocaine in the prevention of primary ventricular fibrillation: a double-blind randomized study of 212 consecutive patients. N Engl J Med 1974; 291:1324–1326.
6. Wang Z, Page P, Nattel S. Mechanism of flecainide's antiarrhythmic action in experimental atrial fibrillation. Circ Res 1992; 71:271–287.
7. Josephson MA, Ikeda N, Singh BN. Effects of flecainide in ventricular function: Clinical and experimental correlations. Am J Cardiol 1984; 53:95B–100B.
8. Echt DS, Liebson PR, Mitchell LB, et al. Mortality and morbidity in patients receiving encainide, flecainide, or placebo: The Cardiac Arrhythmia Suppression Trial. N Engl J Med 1991; 324:781–788.
9. Falk RH. Flecainide-induced ventricular tachycardia and fibrillation in patients treated for atrial fribrillation. Ann Intern Med 1989; 111:107–111.
10. Hammill SC, Wood DI, Gersh BJ, et al. Propafenone for paroxysmal atrial fibrillation. Am J Cardiol 1988; 61:473–474.
11. Antman EM, Beamer AD, Cantillon C, et al. Long-term oral propafenone therapy for suppression of refractory symptomatic atrial fibrillation and atrial flutter. J Am Coll Cardiol 1988; 12:1005–1011.
12. Nattel S. Antiarrhythmic drug classification: A critical appraisal of their history, present status, and clinical relevance. Drugs 1991; 41:672–701.
13. Hondeghem LM, Snyders DJ. Class III antiarrhthmic agents have a lot of potential but a long way to go: reduced effectiveness and dangers of reverse use dependence. Circulation 1990; 81:686–690.
14. Wang J, Bourne GW, Wang Z, et al. Comparative mechanisms of antiarrhythmic drug action in experimental atrial fibrillation: The importance of use-dependent effects on refractoriness. Circulation 1993; 88:1030–1044.
15. Nattel S, Quantz MA. Pharmacological response of quinidine induced early afterdepolarisations in canine cardiac Purkinje fibres: Insights into underlying ionic mechanisms. Cardiovasc Res 1988; 22:808–817.
16. Holt DW, Tucker GT, Jackson PR, et al. Amiodarone pharmacokinetics. Am Heart J 1983; 106:840–847.
17. Heger JJ, Prystowsky EN, Zipes DP. Relationships between amiodarone dosage, drug concentrations, and adverse side effects. Am Heart J 1983; 106:931–935.
18. Nattel S, Taljic M, Fermini B, et al. Amiodarone: pharmacology, clinical actions, and relationships between them. J Cardiovasc Electrophysiol 1992; 3:266–280.
19. Singh BN, Vaughan Williams EM. The effect of amiodarone, a new anti-anginal drug, on cardiac muscle. Br J Pharmacol 1970; 39:657–667.
20. Bosch RF, Li G-R, Gaspo R, et al. Ionic mechanisms of electrophysiologic effects of chronic amiodarone therapy and hypothyroidism: Does amiodarone act via cardiac hypothyroidism [abstract]? Circulation 1996, 94:I–161.
21. Nattel S, Talajic M, Quantz M, et al: Frequency-dependent effects of amiodarone on atrioventricular nodal function and slow-channel action potentials: Evidence for calcium channel-blocking activity. Circulation 1987; 76:442–449.
22. Nishimura M, Follmer CH, Singer DH. Amiodarone blocks calcium current in single guinea pig ventricular myocytes. J Pharmacol Exp Ther 1989; 251:650–659.
23. Polkey MI, Wilson POG, Rees PJ. Amiodarone pneumonitis: No safe dose. Respir Med 1995; 89:233–235.

24. Charness ME, Morady F, Scheinman MM. Frequent neurologic toxicity associated with amiodarone therapy. Neurology 1984; 34:669–671.

25. Anderson NE, Lynch NM, O´Brien KP. Disabling neurological complications of amiodarone. Aust NZ J Med 1985; 15:300–304.

26. Kaplan LJ, Cappaert WE. Amiodarone-induced corneal deposits. Ann Ophthalmol 1984; 16:762–766.

27. Ingram DV. Ocular effects on long-term amiodarone therapy. Am Heart J 1983; 106:902–904.

28. Harjai KJ, Licata AA. Effects of amiodarone in thyroid function. Ann Intern Med 1997; 126:63–73.

29. Nattel S, Hadjis T, Talajic M. The treatment of atrial fibrillation. An evaluation of drug therapy, electro therapeutic considerations. Drugs 1994; 48 (3):345–371.

30. Mattioni TA, Zheutlin TA, Sarmiento JJ, et al. Amiodarone in patients with previous drug-mediated torsade de pointes: Long term safety and efficacy. Ann Intern Med 1989; 111:574–580.

31. The CASCADE Investigators. Randomized antiarrhythmic drug therapy in survivors of cardiac arrest (the CASCADE Study). Am J Cardiol 1993; 72:280–287.

32. The Antiarrhythmics Versus Implantable Defibrillators (AVID) Investigators: a comparison of antiarrhythmic-drug therapy with implantable defibrillators in patients resuscitated from near-fatal ventricular arrhythmias. N Engl J Med 1997; 337:1576–1583.

33. McAlister FA, Teo KK. Antiarrhythmic therapies for the prevention of sudden cardiac death. Drugs 1997; 54 (2):235–252.

34. Sim I, McDonald KM, Lavori PW, et al. Quantitative overview of randomized trials of amiodarone to prevent sudden cardiac death. Circulation 1997; 96:2823–2829.

35. Cairns JA, Connolly SJ, Roberts R, et al. for Canadian Amiodarone Myocardial Infarction Arrhythmia Trial Investigators: randomized trial of outcome after myocardial infarction in patients with frequent or repetitive ventricular premature depolarisations. CAMIAT. Lancet 1997; 349:675–682.

36. Julian DG, Camm AJ, Frangin G, et al. for the European Myocardial Infarct Amiodarone Trial Investigators: randomized trial of effect of amiodarone on mortality in patients with left-ventricular dysfunction after recent myocardial infarction. EMIAT. Lancet 1997; 349:667–674.

37. Roy D, Talajic M, Dorian P, et al. The Canadian Trial of Atrial Fibrillation Investigators: amiodarone to prevent recurrence of atrial fibrillation. N Engl J Med 2000; 342:913–920.

38. Kaumann AJ, Olson CB. Temporal relation between long-lasting aftercontractions and action potentials in cat papillary muscles. Science 1968; 161:293–295.

39. Singh BN, Vaughan Williams EM. A third class of anti-arrhythmic action: effects on atrial and ventricular intracellular potentials, and other pharmacological actions on cardiac muscle, of MJ 1999 and AH 3474. Br J Pharmacol 1970; 39:675–687.

40. Antonaccio MJ, Gomoll A. Pharmacology, pharmacodynamics and pharmacokinetics of Sotalol. Am J Cardiol 1990; 65:12A–21A.

41. Kato R, Yabek S, Ikeda N, et al. Electrophysiologic effects of dextro- and levo-isomers of Sotalol in isolated cardiac muscle and their in vivo pharmacokinetics. J Am Coll Cardiol 1986; 7:116–125.

42. Wang T, Bergstrand RH, Thompson KA, et al. Concentration-dependent pharmacologic properties of Sotalol. Am J Cardiol 1986: 57:1160–1165.

43. Nattel S, Feder-Elituv R, Matthews C, et al. Concentration dependence of class III and beta-adrenergic blocking effects of Sotalol in anesthetized dogs. J Am Coll Cardiol 1989; 13:1190–1194.

44. Carmeliet E. Electrophysiologic and voltage clamp analysis of effexts of Sotalol on isolated cardiac muscle and Purkinje fibers. J Pharmacol Exp Ther 1985; 232:817–825.

45. Falk RH. Proarrhythmia in patients treated for atrial fibrillation of flutter. Ann Intern Med 1992; 117:141–150.

46. McKibbin JK, Pocock WA, Barlow JB, et al. Sotalol, hypokalaemia, syncope, and torsade de pointes. Br Heart J 1984; 51:157–162.

47. Opie LH. Pharmacologic options for treatment of ischemic heart disease. In: Smith TW, ed. Cardiovascular therapeutics. Philadelphia: WB Saunders; 1996:22–57.

48. Kelly RA, Smith TW. The pharmacology of heart failure drugs. In: Smith TW, ed. Cardiovascular therapeutics. Philadelphia: WB Saunders; 1996:176–199.

49. Norris RM, Brown MA, Clarke ED, et al. Prevention of ventricular fibrillation during acute myocardial infarction. Lancet 1981; 2:883–886.

50. Yusuf S, Peto R, Lewis J, et al. Beta blockade during and after myocardial infarction: an overview of the randomized trials. Prog Cardiovasc Dis 1985; 27:335–371.

51. Yusuf S, Wittes J, Friedman L. Overview of results of randomized clinical trials in heart disease: I. Treatments following myocardial infarction. JAMA 1988; 260:2088–2093.

52. Meredith JT, Broughton A, Jennings G, et al. Evidence of a selective increase in cardiac sympathetic activity in patients with sustained ventricular arrhythmias. N Engl J Med 1991; 9:618–624.

53. Steinbeck G, Andresen D, Bach P, et al. A comparison of electrophysiologically anti-arrhythmic drug therapy with beta-blocker therapy in patients with symptomatic, sustained ventricular tachyarrhythmias. N Engl J Med 1992; 327:987–992.

54. Kühlkamp V, Schirdewan A, Stangl K, et al. Use of metoprolol CR/XL to maintain sinus rhythm after

cardioversion from persistent atrial fibrillation: a randomized, double-blind placebo-controlled study. J Am Coll Cardiol 2000; 36:139–146.

55. Willems S, Weiss C, Meinertz T. Tachyarrhythmias following coronary artery bypass graft surgery: epidemiology mechanisms and current therapeutic strategies. Thorac Cardiovasc Surgeon 1997; 54:232–237.

56. DiMarco JP, Sellers TD, Berne RM, et al. Adenosine: electrophysiologic effects and therapeutic use for terminating paroxysmal supraventricular tachycardia. Circulation 1983; 68:1254–1263.

57. Smith JR, Goldberger JJ, Kadish AH. Adenosine induced polymorphic ventricular tachycardia in adults without structural heart disease. Pacing Clin Electrophysiol 1997; 20:743–745.

58. DiMarco JP, Miles W, Akhtar M, et al. Adenosine for paroxysmal supraventricular tachycardia: dose ranging and comparison with Verapamil in placebo-controlled, multicenter trials. Ann Intern Med 1990; 113:104–110.

59. Overholt ED, Rheuban KS, Gutgesell HP, et al. Usefulness of adenosine for arrhythmias in infants and children. Am J Cardiol 1988; 61:336–340.

60. Paul T, Pfammatter JP. Adenosine: an effective and safe antiarrhythmic drug in pediatrics. Pediatr Cardiol 1997; 18:118–126.

61. Belhassen B, Glick A, Laniado S. Comparative clinical and electrophysiologic effects of adenosine triphosphate and Verapamil on paroxysmal reciprocating junctional tachycardia. Circulation 1988; 77:795–805.

62. Garratt C, Linker N, Griffith M, et al. Comparison of adenosine and Verapamil for termination of paroxysmal functional tachycardia. Am J Cardiol 1989; 64:1310–1316.

63. Hood MA, Smith WM. Adenosine versus Verapamil in the treatment of supraventricular tachycardia. Am Heart J 1992; 123:1543–1549.

64. Pitcher D, Papouchado M, James MA, et al. Twenty four hour ambulatory electrocardiography in patients with chronic atrial fibrillation. Br Med J 1986; 292:594.

65. Task Force of the Working Group on Arrhythmias of the European Society of Cardiology: the Sicilian gambit: a new approach to the classification of antiarrhythmic drugs based on their actions on arrthythmogenic mechanisms. Circulation 1991; 84(4):1831–1851.

66. Stambler BS, Wood MA, Ellenbogen KA, et al. and the Ibutilide Repeat Dose Study Investigators. Efficacy and safety of repeated intravenous doses of ibutilide for rapid conversion of atrial flutter or fibrillation. Circulation 1996; 94:1613–1621.

67. Ellenbogen KA, Stambler BS, Wood MA, et al. for the Ibutilide Investigators: Efficacy of intravenous ibutilide for rapid termination of atrial fibrillation and atrial flutter. A dose-response study. J Am Coll Cardiol 1996; 28:130–136.

68. Demolis J-L, Funck-Brentano C, Ropers J, et al. Influence of dofetilide on QT-interval duration and dispersion at various heart rates during exercise in humans. Circulation 1996; 94:1592–1599.

69. Sedgwick ML, Rasmussen HS, Cobbe SM. Clinical and electrophysiologic effects of intravenous dofetilide (UK-68, 798), a new class III antiarrhythmic drug in patients with angina pectoris. Am J Cardiol 1992; 69:513–517.

Proarrhythmia – long QT syndrome – torsade de pointes

Thomas Meinertz MD
Universitätsklinikum Hamburg-Eppendorf, Hamburg,
Germany

Melanie Hümmelgen MD
Universitätsklinikum Hamburg-Eppendorf, Hamburg,
Germany

John Godtfredsen MD FESC
Herlev University Hospital, Herlev, Denmark

> **Proarrhythmia must be taken into account whenever antiarrhythmic therapy is planned, both acutely and long term and especially in high risk patients with long QT interval, ventricular hypertrophy or heart failure**

Introduction

The potentially deleterious electrophysiological impact of drugs administered for the stabilization of the heart rhythm have been recognized since the earliest description of the digitalis toxicity. In the early 1920s several authors reported cases of polymorphic ventricular tachycardia and ventricular fibrillation in the course of oral quinidine therapy for atrial tachyarrhythmias. The clinical significance of the proarrhythmia in this clinical setting was re-emphasized in the ground-breaking paper of Selzer and Wray[1] who again reported several cases of ventricular fibrillation to quinidine treatment of atrial fibrillation.

THE SIZE OF THE PROBLEM

Proarrhythmia in both the congenital and acquired long QT syndrome (LQT) has been known for many years in the form of the Jervell, Lange-Nielsen syndrome, the Romano-Ward syndrome and from the once feared so-called 'quinidine syncope'.

Proarrhythmia was for many years neglected, not because it was unknown, but partly because it was overlooked and partly because widespread, long-term antiarrhythmic treatment of benign arrhythmias did not become common until during the 1990s.

If we equate proarrhythmia with torsade de pointes (TdP), its main presentation, then our knowledge about the occurrence in the population is rather sparse. Data from Sweden[2] indicate an incidence of TdP in the general population of about 4/100 000 and this is probably an underestimation. In predisposed patient groups the rate is much higher, for instance in cardiac patients treated with quinidine and sotalol the incidence has been reported as high as 8% and 4.8% respectively. Recent data from the AFFIRM trial's rhythm control arm indicated a rate of TdP of 0.8%, and about one-third of these patients were

treated with sotalol.[3] The congenital LQT syndrome has been characterized electrophysiologically and genetically very thoroughly during the last few decades, but compared to acquired LQT, it is much rarer.

It was not until the end of the 1980s that the potential relationship between increased cardiac mortality and antiarrhythmic drug treatment had been fully established. A meta-analysis of six randomized, controlled trials incorporating 808 patients with chronic atrial fibrillation evaluated quinidine for maintenance of sinus rhythm after cardioversion.[4] Although quinidine was more effective than no antiarrhythmic therapy in preventing the recurrence of atrial fibrillation, the risk of death was approximately three times higher among drug-treated patients. Data from a large randomized trial of patients with ventricular ectopic activity after myocardial infarction did suggest an increased mortality rate of patients treated with antiarrhythmic agents.[5]

Although the cause of death among participants of these studies is speculative; a proarrhythmic drug effect seems to be a likely explanation.

Key points

Typical predisposing factors and conditions in LQT

1. I_{Kr} blocking antiarrhythmic drugs, i.e. quinidine, sotalol (amiodarone), ibutilide
2. Presence of hypo-kalaemia
3. Slow heart rate and long pauses
4. Left ventricular hypertrophy (LVH) and congestive heart failure (CHF) prolong the action potential probably via the electrophysiological mechanism of early afterdepolarization (EAD) induction in an environment with electrical heterogeneity, especially myocardial transmural dispersion of depolarization

CLASSIFICATION OF PROARRHYTHMIA

Antiarrhythmic agents may produce or aggravate arrhythmias at the supraventricular and ventricular level. These tachyarrhythmias have to be considered to be of major clinical significance but bradyarrhythmias can also be regarded as iatrogenically induced rhythm disturbances. Although most of the culprit drugs are specifically antiarrhythmic agents, non-antiarrhythmic agents have also been involved in proarrhythmia.

Definition of proarrhythmia

Proarrhythmia denotes a situation where a drug (usually an antiarrhythmic) is responsible for the precipitation of a potential malignant arrhythmia or electrocardiographic changes known to predispose to a malignant arrhythmia such as a long QT-interval (LQT) in a given patient.

Proarrhythmia thus denotes the undesirable ability of certain drugs to cause life-threatening arrhythmias in predisposed patients

Proarrhythmia may be atrial or ventricular

The reason that proarrhythmia has become of concern is the safety aspect when a common and rather benign arrhythmia is treated with a drug with potential lethal effects, for instance rate or rhythm control with sotalol for atrial fibrillation.

The clinical significance of proarrhythmia is mainly due to the fact, that when recognized it can largely be prevented by avoiding the culprit drugs, by sensible selection of patients, and by initiating antiarrhythmic treatment in individual patients under a safe cover of electrocardiogram (ECG) monitoring.

Proarrhythmia has important clinical consequences regarding:

- the selection of patients for antiarrhythmic treatment
- the selection of specific drugs and co-medication
- the way of initiating antiarrhythmic drug therapy
- the follow-up of patients requiring individual drug information, and
- the recognition of pertinent risk factors

MOLECULAR AND ELECTROPHYSIO-LOGICAL BACKGROUND – A SUMMARY

The clinical antiarrhythmic effect of drugs depends on their specific electrophysiological action. This in turn acts via the conduction system's different ion channels, that are ultimately responsible for the cellular action potential (and hence the ECG). Downregulation of the K-channels seems to be an important feature in, for instance, cardiomyopathy, and age predisposes to an increased QT interval. Women have more often longer QT than men. QT dispersion in the three layers of the myocardium probably also predisposes to the production of arrhythmic substrates. The proarrhythmic effect depends on the same basic mechanisms and may therefore in a way be regarded as a drug side-effect.

DRUG-INDUCED BRADYARRHYTHMIAS

Drug-induced sinus node dysfunction or atrioventricular (AV) block has been clearly documented in patients treated with antiarrhythmic agents.[6–9] These effects can be seen more often with supratherapeutic plasma concentrations and/or in patients with clinically evident conduction disease. It is possible, however, that there are patients with clinically undetected sinus or AV node dysfunction who show the symptoms only when treated with antiarrhythmic agents (Table 13.1).

Sinus node dysfunction can range from sinus bradycardia to sinus arrest or sinoatrial block. Patients with sinus node disease seem to have the highest risk for marked sinus bradycardia or sinus rest especially if they convert from atrial fibrillation to sinus rhythm.

Sinus node dysfunction can be triggered by all antiarrhythmic agents. Since there are no data available from comparative studies

Table 13.1 Drug-induced bradyarrhythmias

A: Exacerbation or induction of sinus node dysfunction
1. Decreased sinus node automaticity, resulting in sinus bradycardia or sinus arrest
2. Sinus node/sinoatrial exit block
3. Exacerbation of sinus node dysfunction in patients with sick sinus syndrome

B: Exacerbation or induction of atrioventricular (AV) block
1. AV node
2. His-Purkinje system

the relative potency of the depressant effect of each antiarrhythmic agent can only be estimated and classified from data given in the literature (in order of decreasing potency at therapeutic blood levels): sotalol, amiodarone, beta blocking agents, verapamil and diltiazem, class IC agents, class IA agents, class IB agents, digitalis.

Drug-induced AV block

Drug-induced AV block may be due to effects on the AV node itself or on the His-Purkinje-system. Both types of effects can be differentiated during electrophysiological testing, the former effect results in the prolongation of the AH interval, the latter in a prolongation of the HV interval.

AV nodal conduction block is preferentially induced by beta adrenergic blockers, calcium channel blockers, class III antiarrhythmic agents and digitalis. This block may range from PQ prolongation in the ECG to complete AV block.

His-Purkinje conduction is preferentially impaired by class IA antiarrhythmic agents. These drugs cause a delay or a block in the His-Purkinje system resulting in the prolongation of the HV interval and potentially complete AV block. This effect is more prominent with IC-compared to class IA drugs and even less pronounced with IB-agents.

Treatment of drug-induced bradycardia or AV block is primarily the

discontinuation of the incriminated antiarrhythmic agents. The use of atropine and/or temporary pacing is only indicated if bradycardia is hemodynamically intolerable.

DRUG-INDUCED TACHYARRHYTHMIAS

Drug-induced supraventricular tachyarrhythmias

Increased frequency/duration of paroxysmal atrial fibrillation or flutter

In patients with paroxysmal atrial fibrillation (PAF), atrial flutter (PAFlu) or atrial tachycardia, antiarrhythmic drugs can increase the frequency and duration of the arrhythmia episodes. This has been shown for digitalis, diltiazem and verapamil. [10–12] It is less clear whether class I agents can also convert previously PAF into persistent (incessant) atrial arrhythmia (Table 13.2). [13]

Acceleration of ventricular response due to enhanced AV node conduction

In patients suffering from PAF, PAFlu or atrial tachycardia, class IA and C drugs can

Table 13.2 Drug-induced supraventricular tachyarrhythmias

Exacerbation or induction of supraventricular arrhythmias
1. Increased frequency/duration of paroxysmal atrial fibrillation or flutter
2. Acceleration of ventricular response due to enhanced AV node conduction
3. Acceleration of ventricular response in atrial flutter due to decreased flutter cycle length and resultant 1:1 AV node conduction
4. Atrial tachycardia with AV block
5. Acceleration of ventricular rate in patients with Wolff-Parkinson-White syndrome and atrial fibrillation
6. Non-paroxysmal AV junction tachycardia
7. Aberrant conduction

enhance AV nodal conduction leading to an accelerated ventricular response. The mechanisms of this effect are heterogeneous. In the case of disopyramide and quinidine the anticholinergic action on the AV node plays a major role. Class IC agents – and to a lesser extent also class IA agents – can convert atrial fibrillation to a more organized rhythm, e.g. atrial flutter – allowing a faster conduction of this atrial activity to the ventricle.[13,14] Such drug-induced atrial flutter may be amenable to catheter ablation.

Recent data[15] also suggest a beneficial role of radiofrequency catheter ablation of the isthmus between the tricuspid annulus and the inferior vena cava in patients who develop atrial flutter after antiarrhythmic therapy for paroxysmal atrial fibrillation. Such a management approach is a good example of 'hybrid therapy' for atrial fibrillation.[16]

Acceleration of ventricular response in atrial flutter due to decreased flutter cycle length

Antiarrhythmic drug therapy (especially with class IC agents or amiodarone) can slow the flutter cycle length and may thereby enhance AV nodal conduction up to 1:1 conduction to the ventricle.

Atrial tachycardia with AV block

Atrial tachycardia with AV block and non-paroxysmal junctional tachycardia are almost typical signs of digitalis intoxication. Factors which predispose patients to digoxin proarrhythmia even within the therapeutic range are: electrolyte disturbances such as hypokalemia, hypomagnesemia, hypercalcemia and hyponatremia, increased adrenergic stimulation, thyroid disease, acid–base imbalance, renal dysfunction, respiratory disease and drug–drug interactions (e.g. between quinidine and digoxin or amiodarone and digitoxin).

Prevalence of drug-induced supraventricular tachyarrhythmias

The literature cited above derives mainly from case reports and studies consisting of patient samples of small size. From these studies the actual occurrence of proarrhythmia cannot be estimated exactly but is probably in the range of 1–10%. A realistic estimate can only be made on the basis of studies of larger patient populations like AFFIRM,[3] Prevention of Atrial Fibrillation After Cardioversion (PAFAC) or Suppression of Paroxysmal Atrial Tachycardias (SOPAT). These studies are under way and not yet published in a final version.

In estimating the actual occurrence of drug-induced supraventricular tachyarrhythmias another fact must also be taken into account: The majority of the proarrhythmic events can occur without showing any clinical symptoms and could be established beyond doubt only by a systematic search process like event or Holter monitoring.

Treatment of drug-induced supraventricular tachyarrhythmias includes immediate removal of the offending agent. Concomitant predisposing factors such as electrolyte imbalances and drug–drug interactions should be corrected. In hemodynamically unstable patients with atrial flutter and 1:1 conduction to the ventricle, immediate direct current (DC) cardioversion is indicated. In order to prevent this type of proarrhythmia treatment with class IC agents should always be combined with a beta-blocking agent.

Drug-induced ventricular tachyarrhythmias

As with most forms of proarrhythmia, it may be difficult to differentiate between changes in the spontaneous variability of those arrhythmias and changes of the arrhythmia pattern as a consequence of a specific drug effect. Therefore if a patient treated with antiarrhythmic agents develops arrhythmias it will be crucial to exclude other causes before attributing this to proarrhythmia. These factors include drug plasma levels of the antiarrhythmic agent, degree of impairment of left ventricular dysfunction, concomitant ischemia, electrolyte imbalance and others.

Proarrhythmic effects at the ventricular level can range from an asymptomatic increase of spontaneous ventricular ectopy to ventricular fibrillation and sudden cardiac death (Tables 13.3 and 13.4).

Increased frequency of ventricular ectopy

The less serious type of ventricular proarrhythmia is a marked increase in baseline ventricular ectopy or short bursts of non-sustained ventricular tachycardia episodes. Such an increase is considered significant – from a statistical point of view – when there is either a four fold increase in hourly ventricular ectopy rate or a

10-fold in the mean hourly frequency of ventricular pairs or bursts of non-sustained ventricular tachycardia. This increase in the density of arrhythmias can be accompanied by clinical symptoms such as palpitations or might be completely asymptomatic.

Although the clinical relevance of this type of proarrhythmic response has not been conclusively proven to be a harbinger of sustained VT, ventricular fibrillation or sudden cardiac death, this proarrhythmia may serve as a warning sign that a chosen antiarrhythmic therapy might produce a harmful effect for the patient. Proarrhythmic effects of this kind have been described for all antiarrhythmic agents but seem to be of special importance for the class IC type.

Induction of ventricular arrhythmia of new or multiform morphologies

A more serious form of proarrhythmia is the induction of non-sustained or sustained ventricular tachycardia of one or more new morphologies.[17] Proarrhythmic effects of this type can be observed with all antiarrhythmic agents but are more often seen with class IC drugs.

Increased frequency of ventricular tachycardia

This proarrhythmic effect might be defined as an increase in frequency (number of attacks), duration (time course of each attack) or heart rate during the attack. All class I and III agents have been associated with an increased frequency of spontaneous episodes of VT. Here again

---

Table 13.3 Exacerbation or induction of ventricular arrhythmias

1. Increased frequency of baseline ventricular ectopy (premature ventricular complexes (PVCs), non-sustained ventricular tachycardia)
2. Induction of ventricular ectopy (PVCs, non-sustained ventricular tachycardia) of new or multiform morphology or morphologies
3. Increased frequency of underlying ventricular tachycardia
4. Induction of incessant ventricular tachycardia
5. Torsade de pointes (QT interval prolongation) with polymorphic ventricular tachycardia

---

Table 13.4 Predisposing risk factors for developing drug-induced ventricular tachyarrhythmias

–age	–use of diuretics
–female gender	–use of digitalis
–depressed left ventricular ejection fraction (< 35%)	–malignant ventricular arrhythmia at presentation
–congestive heart failure	–prolonged QTc interval
–concomitant myocardial infarction	–previous history of proarrhythmia
–history of myocardial infarction	–coexistent liver or renal failure
–electrolyte imbalance	–high plasma concentration

---

class IC agents seem to produce more often those proarrhythmic effects compared to class IA and III agents.

Induction of incessant ventricular tachycardia

A dangerous and potentially life-threatening complication of antiarrhythmic drug treatment is the development of incessant ventricular tachycardia. Incessant ventricular tachycardia can be defined as a continuous ventricular tachycardia which is not terminated by DC cardioversion or overdrive pacing or VT recurs immediately after termination.

In rare cases this drug-induced ventricular tachycardia can have the same morphology as spontaneously-occurring tachycardia. In the majority of cases however, this type of tachycardia shows a broad QRS complex or in some cases a sinusoidal form with a relatively slow ventricular rate (100–160/min).

Incessant VT occurs specifically under the following conditions:

- initiation of antiarrhythmic drug therapy;
- increase of antiarrhythmic agent dose;
- depressed left ventricular function;
- history of sustained ventricular tachycardia,
- use of class IC agents.

This proarrhythmia is associated with a significant morbidity and mortality.

Patients often develop hemodynamic problems, which sometimes progress into cardiogenic shock.

Treatment of this arrhythmia includes discontinuation of the antiarrhythmic agents, emergent i.v. antiarrhythmic treatment with amiodarone in class IC-induced proarrhythmia, and in rare cases intra-aortic ballon counterpulsation for the treatment of cardiogenic shock.

Induction of Torsade de Pointes tachycardia

Definition: TdP tachycardia is a polymorphic ventricular arrhythmia that is associated with a prolonged QT interval (first described by Desertenne in 1966[18]). The ventricular rate of this tachycardia is usually in the range of 200–300 beats per min (bpm). The tachycardia is self-limiting and lasts for only a few seconds. The morphology shows a characteristic pattern with rapid changes in the QRS morphology winding around an isoelectric baseline resembling 'twisting of the points' (Fig. 13.1). Tachycardia episodes usually occur as clusters with repetitive periods. Under these conditions episodes are highly symptomatic (presyncope, syncope), whereas singular episodes can occur without any symptoms. Episodes may reoccur several times and may degenerate into ventricular fibrillation resulting in sudden cardiac death.

Torsade de pointes

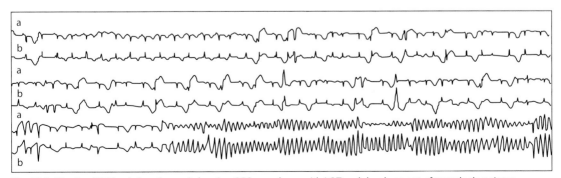

Fig. 13.1 Monitor ECG leads (continuous) showing QRS complexes with LQT and development of torsade de pointes.

By definition the term TdP should be reserved for those tachycardias that share the typical morphology *and* are accompanied by a clearly prolonged QT, QTc or QU interval. If the QT interval is normal the term polymorphic VT should be used. The typical corrected QT or QTc interval is frequently greater than 600 ms.

Key points

Torsade de Pointes (TdP)

- TdP is a polymorphic ventricular tachycardia with the QRS complexes rotating around the isoelectrical line in the ECG (see figure)
- It is usually of short duration and self-limiting, and symptoms may vary from dizziness to syncope and, if it degenerates, to ventricular fibrillation and sudden death
- TdP may occur in the acute setting but also later in the course of the antiarrhythmic treatment.

Pathophysiology: Electrophysiologically, a prolonged QT interval represents a dispersion of refractoriness within the ventricles. This electrophysiological milieu predisposes to the development of early afterdepolarizations (EADs). These EADs are oscillations of transmembrane potential that occur during repolarization of the action potential. In humans EADs have been documented in Purkinje fibers and in cardiac M cells, which are found in the deep subepicardial to mid-myocardial regions.[19]

If these EADs are sufficiently large to depolarize the cell membrane to its threshold they may induce spontaneous action potentials referred as to triggered responses. These triggered responses can be regarded as an origin of TdP tachycardias.

1. Because EADs are most prominent at reduced heart rates it is not surprising that TdP tachycardias are triggered by such a condition. With this in line, TdP tachycardia is typically initiated by an electrocardiographic pattern in which a pause (long RR interval) is followed by a premature ventricular contraction (PVC) (i.e. a long-short sequence). This PVC has a markedly prolonged repolarization phase and thus creates the milieu of EADs and triggered activity.

2. Another electrocardiographic 'condition' for TdP tachycardias is the '*TU or U wave alternans*'. This alternans is characterized by a significant beat to beat change in the TU axis. It is more often seen at higher heart rates and is less common in drug-induced TdP tachycardias than the long-short sequence.

3. A third electrocardiographic marker for TdP tachycardias is the dispersion of the QT interval. QT dispersion can be defined as the difference between the maximum and the minimum measured QT interval on the same 12-lead ECG. QT dispersion normally averages 50±15 ms. In patients with TdP tachycardias, QT dispersion is often even more than 100±40 ms.[20] It is important to note that QT dispersion is independent of total QT or QTU interval prolongation. Thus it may be another – independent of QT prolongation – risk predictor for the development of TdP tachycardias. From this perspective it is interesting that amiodarone produces less QT dispersion compared with class IA agents or sotalol, even though the absolute QT or QTU interval prolongation is similar.[21]

Could it be that this failure of amiodarone to produce a marked QT dispersion – in contrast to class IA agents and to sotalol – can explain the limited proarrhythmic potential of this drug?

Incidence: TdP tachycardias induced by antiarrhythmic agents are seen most under drug treatment with class IA agents and sotalol. The majority of cases occur with higher doses of these drugs and/or when predisposing conditions (see Table 13.4) are present.

Class I antiarrhythmic agents: When Selzer and Wray[1] published their observations in patients treated with quinidine for atrial fibrillation, they assumed that this effect represented a 'specific toxic effect of quinidine' and introduced the term 'quinidine syncope'. They described the typical features of this adverse effect: they occurred early during therapy, quinidine blood levels were low in most of their patients and signs of conventional quinidine toxicity were absent. They hypothesized 'that quinidine produces in certain individuals a specific sensitization of the myocardium by reducing the fibrillation threshold' and recommended 'the complete omission of quinidine as a therapeutic agent in such a patient'. These observations by Selzer and Wray have been confirmed by several other investigators. More than 25 years later Coplen et al[4] performed a meta-analysis of randomized trials evaluating the role of quinidine in maintenance of sinus rhythm after cardioversion from chronic atrial fibrillation. Quinidine treatment was associated with a significant increase in total mortality (2.9% in the quinidine group versus 0.8% in the control group) which may be due to quinidine-induced proarrhythmia.

TdP tachycardias also occurred during therapy with disopyramide and procainamide. TdP tachycardia has also been reported with class IB agents like lidocaine (lignocaine) or mexilitine. However this association was not conclusive. Similarly, class IC agents usually do not provoke TdP tachycardia. The same applies to propafenone although individual cases of such an arrhythmia secondary to propafenone and ajmaline were reported.[22,23]

Class III antiarrhythmic agents: In case of sotalol, TdP tachycardia is the most significant adverse reaction which occurs relatively frequently.[24]

For example, the incidence of TdP tachycardias with sotalol is dose related.[25] In patients presenting with a history of sustained ventricular tachycardia, the incidence of TdP tachycardia was 4%, while in patients with less serious ventricular arrhythmias or supraventricular arrhythmias the incidence was 1 and 1.4%, respectively. Risk factors were female

gender, excessive prolongation of the QT_C on sotalol and a history of heart failure. Haverkamp and co-workers[26] reported that TdP tachycardias occurred within 5 days of initiation of the therapy in the majority of the patients. Their patients could be divided into two groups: those who developed TdP tachycardias while taking a low sotalol dose (< 240 mg/day) usually had normal potassium level and no bradycardia. Most patients developing TdP tachycardia at high sotalol doses (> 320 mg/day) had additional provocative factors such as hypokalemia, hypomagnesemia and bradycardia.

TdP tachycardias were also seen with new agents who were called pure 'class III agents' like dofetilide, sematilide or almokalant.[26] Several case reports with TdP tachycardias due to treatment with amiodarone have also been published.[25] However, despite QT interval prolongation, the development of TdP tachycardia with amiodarone seems to be relatively rare with an estimated incidence of < 1% of amiodarone treatments.

There are case reports of patients who initially developed TdP tachycardias during therapy with a class IA antiarrhythmic agent and then these patients developed arrhythmias also on a second or third class antiarrhythmic agent ('cross-reactivity'). Individual cases of cross-reactivity have also been reported for class IA drugs and amiodarone. In other cases such cross-reactivity was not observed between sotalol and amiodarone.[27]

Predisposing factors
- Acquired QT prolongation associated with TdP tachycardia has been observed in patients with various types of cardiac diseases as well as in those without any detectable heart disease. Thus, it seems that structural myocardial changes are not a prerequisite for this particular form of proarrhythmia.
- Female preponderance has been reported. The reason for this finding is not known.

- Underlying heart disease constitutes a contributing risk factor for the occurrence of drug induced QT prolongation and TdP.[27]
- Myocardial hypertrophy, use of diuretics and congestive heart failure also play an important role as predisposing factors for developing such arrhythmias.

Thus every drug that prolongs the cardiac repolarization produces a risk of malignant ventricular arrhythmias that may lead to sudden death - early or late in the course of drug treatment. The sequence of events leading to adverse proarrhythmia may be described as follows:

Risk factor(s) → QT prolongation → TdP → VT/VF → sudden cardiac death

Heart rate corrected QT interval (QTc):

Normal range (HR 45–115)	300 – 460 ms
Borderline prolongation	450 –460 ms (in certain heart diseases)
Definite prolongation	> 550 ms
Excessive prolongation	> 600 ms

ECG diagnosis and QTc measurement: The QT interval has to be measured in the longest QT in any standard lead and U-waves have to be taken into consideration. Mistaking a T-wave component for a U wave may lead to an underestimation of the drug effect to prolong the QTc and thus the drug's proarrhythmic potential.

Treatment: Treatment includes a spectrum of therapeutic interventions:

- discontinuation of the causative agent;
- correction of any electrolyte imbalance;
- high doses intravenous magnesium sulfate (4–8 g over 1–2 h, continued by 1–2 g/h) up to the disappearance of tachycardias;
- atrial or ventricular pacing at a rate exceeding the underlying rhythm. If pacing is not available: intravenous isoproterenol.

Induction of ventricular fibrillation or sudden cardiac death

Ventricular fibrillation can be the first and last manifestation of proarrhythmia without preceding warning signs. This has been documented during Holter monitoring. In the majority of cases ventricular fibrillation is secondary to the degeneration of monomorphic or polymorphic ventricular tachycardia into this arrhythmia. In a number of these cases there were warning signs (like a increased number and duration of ventricular tachycardia episodes, new morphologies, hemodynamic deterioration) but these were often overlooked. Furthermore specifically in these patients, concomitant risk factors are nearly always present: reduced left ventricular function, clinical signs of heart failure, myocardial ischemia, malignant ventricular arrhythmias as a cause of antiarrhythmic treatment.

Prevalence of drug-induced ventricular tachyarrhythmias

The incidence of life-threatening proarrhythmia or proarrhythmia-induced ventricular fibrillation can only be estimated. In the Cardiac Arrhythmia Suppression Trial (CAST) study[5] an incidence of 4.5% arrhythmia caused death and non-fatal cardiac arrests were documented in patients treated with flecainide or encainide compared to 1.2% on placebo. The relative risk of arrhythmic death for patients receiving antiarrhythmics was a 3.6-fold increase. The patient population included in the CAST study consisted of asymptomatic or mildly symptomatic patients with ventricular ectopy following myocardial infarction.

In patients with sustained ventricular tachyarrhythmias and severely depressed left ventricular function and/or in the presence of ischemia the incidence of life-threatening proarrhythmia seems to be much higher and was reported to be in the range of up to 12%. This was reported for class IA and C agents as well as for sotalol.

Therefore these agents should not be used in such patient populations anymore.

In addition, these agents should also not be given to patients with these characteristics for the treatment of supraventricular tachyarrhythmias. The only antiarrhythmic agent for this patient population is amiodarone. Compared to all other antiarrhythmic agents except beta adrenergic blockers, it produces proarrhythmic effects far less often.

In patients with no or minimal structural heart disease (e.g. LVH) the incidence of life-threatening proarrhythmia is by far less compared to that of the CAST population. This is true for treatment indication such as symptomatic ventricular tachycardia (e.g. from the right ventricular outflow tract) or for supraventricular arrhythmias. The incidence of life-threatening proarrhythmia of class I agents and for sotalol in this patient population can be estimated to be in the range of 0.5–3%. Here again beta-blocking agents and amiodarone share by far the lowest proarrhythmic potential (less than 0.5%).

HOW TO AVOID PROARRHYTHMIA

- Avoid inappropriate drug dosing – Do not extrapolate therapeutic drug dosing from normal healthy volunteers to ill patients with arrhythmias.
- Consider carefully changes in renal and hepatic drug clearance as well as drug interactions.
- Monitor patients closely who are receiving antiarrhythmic drug therapy – Be aware of factors predisposing to proarrhythmia and of the clinical and electrocardiographic warning signs.
- Start antiarrhythmic therapy during telemetric monitoring. This strategy is obligatory for the initiation of antiarrhythmic therapy in patients with potential risk factors or malignant ventricular arrhythmias.
- Be sure of the indications for your antiarrhythmic drug therapy.

Practical preventive measures to avoid LQT:

- Always measure baseline QT in the ECG
- Select patients without congestive heart failure and left ventricular hypertrophy
- Check electrolyte status and renal function frequently
- Avoid hypo-kalaemia
- Do not use quinidine, and use sotalol, ibutilide, dofetilide only in certain indications
- Initiate antiarrhythmic therapy in hospital during ECG monitoring

References

1. Selzer A, Wray HW. Quinidine syncope; paroxysmal ventricular fibrillation occurring during treatment of chronic atrial arrhythmias. Circulation 1964; 30:17–26.
2. Darpö B. Spectrum of drugs prolonging QT interval and the incidence of torsades de pointes. Eur Heart J Supplements 2001; 3(suppl K):K 70–K 80.
3. Wyse DG, Waldo AL, DiMarco JP, et al. A comparison of rate control and rhythm control in patients with atrial fibrillation. N Engl J Med 2002; 347 (23):1825-1833.
4. Coplen SE, Antman EM, Berlin JA, et al. Efficacy and safety of quinidine therapy for maintenance of sinus rhythm after cardioversion. A metaanalysis of randomized control trials. Circulation 1990, 82:1106–1116.
5. The Cardiac Arrhythmia Suppression Trial (CAST) Investigators. Increased mortality due to encainide or flecainide in a randomized trial of arrhythmia suppression afte myocardial infarction. N Engl J Med 1989; 321:406–412.
6. Talley JD, Wathen MS, Jurst JW. Hyperthyroid-induced atrial flutter-fibrillation with profound sinoatrial nodal pauses due to small doses of digoxin, verapamil, and propanolol. Clin Cardiol 1989; 12:45–47.
7. Labarre A, Strauss JC, Scheinmann MM, et al. Electrophysiologic effects of disopyramide phosphate on sinus node function in patients with sinus node dysfunction. Circulation 1979; 59:226.
8. Touboul P, Atallah G, Gressard A, et al. Effects of amiodarone on sinus node function in man. Br Heart J 1979; 42:573–578.
9. Falk RH. Proarrhythmia in patients treated for atrial fibrillation or flutter. Ann Intern Med 1992; 117:141–150.
10. Rawles JM, Metcalfe MJ, Jennings K. Time of occurrence, duration, and ventricular rate for paroxysmal atrial fibrillation: the effect of digoxin. Br Heart J 1990; 63: 225–227.
11. Shenasa M, Kus T, Fromer M, et al. Effect of

intravenous and oral calcium antagonists (diltiazem and verapamil) on sustenance of atrial fibrillation. Am J Cardiol 1988; 62:403–407.

12. Kasanuki H, Ohnishi S. Verapamil increasing inducibility and persistence of atrial fibrillation. Circulation 1986; 74: II. Abstract.

13. Feld GK, Chen PS, Nicod P, et al. Possible atrial proarrhythmic effects of class IC antiarrhythmic agents. Am J Cardiol 1990; 66:378.

14. Reithmann C, Hoffman E, Spitzlberger G, et al. Catheter ablation of atrial flutter due to amiodarone therapy for paroxysmal atrial fibrillation. Eur Heart J 2000; 21:565–572.

15. Geelen P, Brugada P. Hybrid therapy for atrial fibrillation. Eur Heart J 2000; 21:509–510.

16. Robertson CE, Miller HC. Extreme tachycardia complicating the use of disopyramide in atrial flutter. Br Heart J 1980; 44:602–603.

17. Velebit V, Podrid P, Lown B, et al. Aggravation and provocation of ventricular arrhythmias by antiarrhythmic drugs. Circulation 1982; 65:886–894.

18. Desertenne F. La tachycardie ventriculaire a deux foyers opposes veriables. Arch Mal Coeur 1966; 59:263–272.

19. Antzelevitch C, Sicouri S. Clinical relevance of cardiac arrhythmias generated by afterdepolarizations: role of M cells in the generation of U waves, triggered activity and torsade de pointes. J Am Cardiol 1994; 23:259–277.

20. Hii JT, Wyse DG, Gillis AM, et al. Precordial QT interval dispersion as a marker of torsade de pointes. Disparate effects of class IA antiarrhythmic drugs and amiodarone. Circulation 1992; 86:1376–1382.

21. Van de Loo A, Klingenheben T, Hohnloser SH. Amiodarontherapie nach Sotalol-induzierter Torsade de pointes : QT-Verlängerung und QT-Dispersion zur Differenzierung proarrhythmischer Effekte. Z Kardiol 1994 ; 83 :887–890

22. Hii JT, Wyse DG, Gillis AM, et al. Propafenon-induced torsade de pointes: cross reactivity with quinidine. PACE 1991; 14:1568–1570.

23. Kaul U, Mohan JC, Marula J, et al. Ajmaline-induced torsade de pointes. Cardiology 1985; 72:140–143.

24. Kehoe R, Zheutlin TA, Dunnington CS, et al. Safety and efficacy of sotalol in patients with drug refractory sustained ventricular tachyarrhythmias. Am J Cardiol 1990; 65:58A–64A.

25. Mattioni TA, Zheutlin TA, Sarmiento JJ, et al. Amiodarone in patients with previous drug-mediated torsade de pointes. Ann Int Med 1989; 111:574–580.

26. Haverkamp W, Hördt M, Hindricks G, et al. Torsade de pointes induced by d,l-sotalol. Circulation 1993; 88 (suppl):1872.

27. Haverkamp W, Shenasa M, Borggrefe M, et al. Torsade de pointes. In: Zipes DP, Jalife J, eds. Cardiac electrophysiology. From cell to bedside. 2nd edn, Philadelphia: Saunders; 1995:885–889.

References to recent reviews

Haverkamp W, Eckhardt L, Mönnig G, et al. Clinical aspects of ventricular arrhythmias associated with QT prolongation. Eur Heart J Supplements 2001; B(suppl K): K81–K88.

Napolitano C, Priori SG. Genetics of ventricular tachycardia. Curr Opin Cardiol 2002; 17:222–228.

MANAGEMENT

CHAPTER 14

Paroxysmal, persistent and permanent AF

John Godtfredsen MD FESC

Herlev University Hospital, Herlev, Denmark

> Guidelines are to be interpreted and matched to cases not the other way around

Introduction

The heterogeneity of the clinical presentations of atrial fibrillation (AF) implies that there are no such things as a standardized general management, a streamlined specific medical therapy or a cook-book approach to any given patient.

On the other hand in the excellent international guidelines[1] the best available evidence from the literature has been interpreted and evaluated by acknowledged experts. These current guidelines procure carefully weighted recommendations for treatment of paroxysmal, persistent and permanent AF ranked in such a way that the responsible physician is enabled to deliver up-to-date evidence-based therapy to his patients. Even then he may sometimes need to interpret the guidelines in order to achieve efficient results in particular patients.

The current international guidelines are based not only on the best available evidence but also on a rather new classification of AF which constitutes the framework for good clinical practice.

All this said, modern AF treatment is complex and in some areas, e.g. maintenance of sinus rhythm after cardioversion, outright unsatisfactory with a rather poor outcome.

The proper management of AF therefore requires expertise, good clinical judgment and a carefully tailored approach to each patient, and as stressed in the guidelines any therapeutical choice should be based on the total arrhythmia burden, the type of underlying heart disease, the severity of symptoms, the risk of side-effects and the patients' preferences.

Since AF is generally a benign condition, safety in the selection of pharmacological treatment always must have priority over drug efficacy. This important viewpoint is very much in keeping with the upcoming solution to the old problem of whether rhythm control or heart rate control is preferable in the long-term management of AF. There is now very good evidence from the recent

Pharmacologic Intervention in Atrial Fibrillation (PIAF)[2], Strategies of Treatment of Atrial Fibrillation (STAF), Atrial Fibrillation Follow-up Investigation of Rhythm Management (AFFIRM)[3] and Rate Control versus Electrocardioversion for persistent atrial fibrillation (RACE) that heart rate control is just as good or even better than rhythm control in this respect.[4]

TAXONOMY OF AF

A precise, succinct and logical classification of AF has been difficult to provide. The reason is that so many sets of criteria for classification may be used, e.g. underlying etiology, course over time (temporal course), cardiac mechanics, i.e. hemodynamic status, the electrocardiogram (ECG), the electrophysiological background, autonomic status, size of f waves, and even the age of the patient may pertain.

Classification is necessary especially in heterogeneous disease states (as AF) with the purpose of facilitating comparisons in the literature and trials, constituting a framework for management principles and being both sufficiently simple and exhausting to be of any use in daily clinical work.

An episode of AF needs a classification but the circumstances are not always sufficient for an exhausting definition since so many options are available, and because the temporal course plays an important role, a useful classification may only be operational after some time has elapsed.

There is now international consensus on the classification, as shown in Figure 14.1.

It takes into account the earlier (rather inconsistent) nomenclature and synonyms, and recent developments regarding specific treatment according to types of AF thus aligning classification and management in a meaningful way. These criteria for classification do not include ECG variables or symptoms and the term 'chronic AF' is out of (official) use.

Also several AF types are discernible on intracardiac electrograms according to the

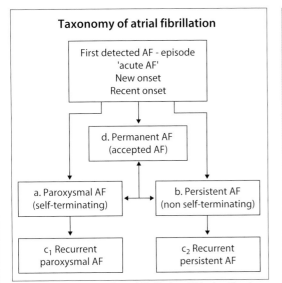

Taxonomy of atrial fibrillation

First detected AF - episode
'acute AF'
New onset
Recent onset

d. Permanent AF
(accepted AF)

a. Paroxysmal AF
(self-terminating)

b. Persistent AF
(non self-terminating)

c₁ Recurrent
paroxysmal AF

c₂ Recurrent
persistent AF

Fig. 14.1 Taxonomy of atrial fibrillation. This classification is the basis for current principles of treatment of the various types of atrial fibrillation. a: Episodes last ≤ 7 days, mostly < 24 h; b: Episodes last usually > 7 days; c: Considered recurrent with ≥ two episodes; d: Failed or not attempted cardioversion.

atrial deflection morphology. Such niceties as for example focal AF has claimed classificational merit, but by and large electrophysiological classification is of little or no clinical use.

But even this new classification is not perfect, so some comments are necessary:

- new onset AF is not equal to the first episode;
- persistent AF may include various forms of paroxysmal AF;
- permanent AF is not equal to 'never sinus rhythm again';
- acute AF still seems a relevant operational term at least regarding clinical presentation

Some special types or presentations of AF are not clearly contained in the classification above, mainly because they are complications of, and specifically linked to, precipitating causes, the treatment of which usually abolishes the episode of AF which may then never recur. Such examples are postsurgical AF, and AF in the course of acute myocardial infarction, pericarditis, hyperthyroidism and pulmonary diseases.

Other rather rare or special forms of AF include the following:

- vagal AF (Coumel) occurring after meals, late after stress/exercise, during sleep and never between breakfast and lunch, may be categorized as paroxysmal AF.
- so-called 'lone AF'; this term applies to young patients < 60 years without any discernible underlying heart disease and a good prognosis;
- valvular AF is usually designed as being a complication to (rheumatic) mitral diseases or AF in patients with a prosthetic heart valve.

MANAGEMENT OF AF

The treatment objectives in AF are precise and simple (Table 14.1) and the means for achieving the goals listed in Table 14.1 are many – both general and more specific. For example heart failure accompanies AF in about one-third of all cases and should be addressed accordingly.

Risk stratification regarding thromboembolic prevention is also mandatory and is dealt with in Chapters 7 and 18.

The more specific treatment modalities comprise:

1. cardioversion to sinus rhythm either by antiarrhythmic drugs (AAD) or by electrical direct current (DC) shock [electrocardioversion (ECV)];
2. maintaining sinus rhythm after cardioversion either by AAD or by (some curative) non-pharmacological method; and
3. rate control either by rate controlling drugs (RCD) or by electrophysiological methods (His bundle ablation and pacemaker).

Table 14.1 Treatment objectives in AF

Symptom relief
Reduction in thromboembolic events
Avoid or treat concomitant heart failure

The electrophysiologically guided non-pharmacological interventions are dealt with in Chapters 3 and 19.

The main treatment principles and modalities are shown in Tables 14.2 and 14.3, which form the basis for the structure

of this chapter. The treatment of acute AF is dealt with in more detail in Chapter 15.

SUBTYPES OF AF AND DRUG MANAGEMENT

First detected episode

Paroxysmal AF

Paroxysmal AF when first detected needs usually no treatment. AAD drugs may be used to speed up cardioversion, and rate control and CHF treatment (even acute ECV) may be necessary to combat accompanying severe heart failure, angina pectoris or hypotension.

AADs with proven efficacy are: (class I recommendation) ibutilide i.v.; flecainide or propafenone orally or i.v.; (class IIa) amiodarone i.v. if heart rate control is essential in the presence of CHF. Procainamide i.v. and quinidine orally are rarely used nowadays. Digoxin and sotalol are not recommended (class III).

Persistent AF

Persistent AF when first detected can only be so labeled if the patient's history points

---

Table 14.2 AF treatment: principles, options and modalities

Treatment
AAD
for cardioversion
for maintenance of sinus rhythm
ECV
RCD
Non-pharmacological correction of AF
EP guided treatment
ATT
vitamin K antagonists (warfarin)
ASA, low molecular weight heparin
Treatment of CHF

AAD, antiarrhythmic drugs; ASA, acetyl salicylic acid; ATT, antithrombotic therapy; CHF, concomitant heart failure; ECV, electrical cardioversion; EP, electrophysiology; RCD, rate controlling drugs.

Table 14.3 AF treatment according to classification

Type of AF (Fig.14. 1)	Treatment option: Items in parenthesis only on certain indications
A. Paroxysmal AF	No therapy; AAD to speed up cardioversion; (RCD); (ECV); (CHF-Rx); ATT (LMWH)
B. Persistent AF	RCD; ATT warfarin; AAD cardioversion; ECV
C_1. Recurrent paroxysmal AF	– Symptoms: RCD; ATT + Symptoms: RCD; ATT; AAD maintenance; EP
C_2. Recurrent persistent AF	– Symptoms: RCD; ATT + Symptoms: RCD; ATT; ECV; AAD maintenance; EP
C. +/- Heart disease	See correlative essays below
D. Permanent AF	RCD; ATT long-term; EP

AAD, antiarrhythmic drugs; ATT, antithrombotic therapy; CHF-Rx, concomitant heart failure; ECV, electrical cardioversion; EP, electrophysiology; LMWH, low molecular weight heparin; RCD, rate controlling drugs.

---

to a duration of > 7 days. In many cases especially in elderly patients with mild symptoms and perhaps a faint memory this presentation may just as well be permanent AF (see below).

The aim of treatment is to electively obtain sinus rhythm and maintain it when AF is considered undesirable or hemodynamically threatening in a given patient.

Rate control and anticoagulation [with international normalized ratio (INR) at target for 3–4 weeks] are both first line treatments to be followed by elective cardioversion either electrically or with (DC shock preceding) antiarrhythmic drugs depending on the urgency for obtaining sinus rhythm and the duration of the AF episode. An AAD for cardioversion is much more effective if applied as early as possible within 7 days after AF onset/ detection.

Unless there is good clinical and echocardiographic evidence that the index AF episode in fact has lasted for very long and the prognosis for maintaining sinus rhythm therefore is very poor most cardiologists would favor at least one attempt at cardioversion. Two recent randomized studies suggest that if a second attempt at restoring sinus rhythm fails there is little to be gained from a third cardioversion[5] (see the section on treatment of recurrent persistent AF below).

AADs proven to be effective are: (class I) dofetilide orally; (class IIa) amiodarone orally or i.v.; ibutilide i.v.; (class IIb) flecainide orally or propafenone orally or i.v.

Digoxin may be used but only if concomitant CHF is present, and sotalol (if angina pectoris is present) should be replaced with another beta-blocker without sotalol's propensity to proarrhythmia (class III).

When (pre-)treated with an AAD about 7–10% of the patients may convert to sinus rhythm in the interval before the planned DC shock 3–4 weeks ahead, and if sinus rhythm is achieved, long-term AAD treatment is not considered necessary.

Recurrent episodes

Recurrent paroxysmal AF

In recurrent paroxysmal AF the choice of treatment depends on the patient's symptoms. If symptoms are absent or minor and/or the episodes of AF are very infrequent there is no indication for AADs. Only rate control as short-term palliation and anticoagulation if thromboembolic risk factors are present is required.

In case of disabling symptoms, rate control and AADs for maintenance of sinus rhythm as well as anticoagulation are required. AADs of proven efficacy and safety when no underlying heart disease [coronary artery disease (CAD), CHF or left ventricular hypertrophy (LVH)] is present are: flecainide, propafenone or sotalol (or an other beta-blocker) as first line drugs vs. amiodarone and dofetilide. Flecainide and propafenone has the advantage that home treatment ('pill-in-the pocket' approach) is possible after a trial in hospital has demonstrated their safety including pretreatment with verapamil or a beta-blocker to avoid 1:1 AV conduction should atrial flutter develop; the beta-blockers' advantage is their effect in adrenergic mediated AF and the rate controlling effect.

In patients with underlying heart disease (especially heart failure) amiodarone or dofetilide are first choice drugs. In cases with very frequent episodes of AF and/or with very rapid heart rates during an episode non-pharmacological treatment should be considered.

Combination of AADs may be useful if single drug treatment fails. Beta-blockers, amiodarone and flecainide/propafenone may all be combined, but beware of proarrhythmia and monitor the QT interval in such cases, and remember that left ventricular function is depressed by most AADs.

Recurrent persistent AF

Recurrent persistent AF represents a difficult type of AF to treat, particularly cumbersome is the need for repeated DC conversion whenever sinus rhythm relapses into AF and the long-term outlook is poor regarding complications despite aggressive treatment with serial cardioversions and use of AAD combinations.

Most of these patients have recognized risk factors for AF recurrence: 80% have some underlying heart disease, they are elderly or have been in (and out of) AF for many months or years. Given the disappointingly low proportion of these patients that stay in sinus rhythm after say 4 years, it is no wonder that other treatment options (i.e. electrophysiological methods and the recent quest for permanency instead of persistent AF) have been developed.

Still some few patients may have such troublesome symptoms and perhaps threatening tachycardia-induced cardiomyopathy during AF that aggressive antiarrhythmic therapy is warranted in these cases.

The AADs available in persistent AF are generally the same as in section C_1 above and with the same reservations and limitations regarding presence of heart disease and the risk of proarrhythmia.

After the publication of the PIAF[2], STAF, AFFIRM[3] and RACE trials which are all in concordance regarding the results that heart rate control is just as good as rhythm control, it is to be expected that the group of patients with recurrent persistent AF shall more or less disappear in favor of an early acceptance of AF being permanent.

Permanent state

Permanent AF

Permanent AF is the 'end stage' of AF, often by natural course or by deliberate decision jointly taken by the physician responsible and the patient after full information has been given regarding the previous AF history, the present and future treatment options and their complications.

The aim of therapy is to minimize symptoms, to prevent thromboembolism and to prevent (further) development of CHF.

The rate controlling drugs available are: (class I) digoxin especially in case of systolic heart failure with dilated ventricles; beta-blockers are very effective and can often be combined with digoxin to achieve better rate control during exercise; the calcium antagonists verapamil and diltiazem are the preferred drugs in patients with chronic obstructive lung disease, and as with beta-blockers caution must be exercised when overt left ventricular dysfunction and clinical heart failure is present, and careful dose titration is necessary in these conditions. For all these drugs the most important side-effects are excessive bradycardia, heart block (impaired AV node conduction) and hypotension particularly when drug combinations are used.

Amiodarone (class IIb) is not a first line drug for rate control, but may be used in case of more severe heart failure.

Non-pharmacological regulation of AV nodal conduction and various pacing modalities are therapeutical options when rate control with drugs fail.

CHOICE OF DRUGS BASED ON UNDERLYING HEART DISEASE

Since an episode of AF is only rarely a solitary event it is necessary in the clinical situation to be aware of the underlying etiology and to analyze for possible cardiac precipitating causes before jumping to decisions on antiarrhythmic therapy. In as many as one-third of all cases of newly detected clinical AF a more or less obvious cardiac precipitating cause may be present (see Ch. 5). Most frequent among these are heart failure, CAD (symptomatic or asymptomatic), hypertensive heart disease and more seldom the pre-excitation syndromes.

Heart failure (CHF)

CHF leads to AF when the atrial wall is stretched and AF leads to CHF when the heart rate is exhaustingly rapid for a certain time (so-called tachycardia-induced cardiomyopathy). In case of overt CHF, therapy with digoxin is often a judicious choice and for further rate control or maintenance of sinus rhythm both amiodarone or dofetilide are safe drugs. Since CHF predisposes to proarrhythmia most other AADs are contraindicated.

Coronary artery disease (CAD)

CAD is a common underlying disease in AF the frequency ranging from 17 to 42% (see Table 5.3 in Ch. 5). In patients with stable CAD, i.e. angina pectoris, beta-blockers for rate control (and sotalol for sinus rhythm maintenance) are first-line drugs, whereas flecainide and propafenone are contraindicated. Amiodarone and dofetilide are second-line drugs especially with concomitant CHF.

Hypertensive heart disease (HHD)

In patients with LVH diagnosed by echocardiography there is an increased risk of proarrhythmia (torsade de pointes). AADs that prolong the QT interval are therefore contraindicated. In the absence of CAD and severe LVH (LV wall thickness ≥ 14 mm) propafenone and flecainide can be used with amiodarone as second-line drug. When severe LVH is present amiodarone becomes a first-line drug preferably after a trial during ECG monitoring and check of the QT interval.

Wolff-Parkinson-White syndrome

In acute AF with Wolff-Parkinson-White (WPW) syndrome (see Fig. 15.1) prompt DC cardioversion is indicated and it is critically important to avoid all AADs that influence the AV node conduction, i.e. digoxin, verapamil, diltiazem or beta-

blockers. If the patient is clinically stable and ECV not immediately available, i.v. procainamide may be used to cardiovert AF to sinus rhythm. Elective radio frequency ablation of the accessory pathway is the preferred ultimate treatment in symptomatic patients.

SUMMARY OF THE MOST IMPORTANT EVIDENCE-BASED RECOMMENDATIONS RANKED BY CLASS

Definitions

Class I : The treatment is useful and effective.
Class II: Conflicting evidence and/or divergence of opinion about the usefulness/efficacy of a treatment.
Class IIa: The weight of evidence or opinion is in favor of the treatment.
Class IIb: Usefulness/efficacy is less well established by evidence or opinion.
Class III: Evidence and/or general agreement that the treatment is not useful/effective and in some cases even may be harmful.

Recommendations for cardioversion of AF

Class I

- Acute DC cardioversion in paroxysmal AF with severe CHF, angina pectoris or hypotension not responding promptly to pharmacological rate control.
- DC cardioversion in patients with unacceptable symptoms.

Class IIa

- DC or pharmacological cardioversion in paroxysmal AF to speed up

(spontaneous) conversion to sinus rhythm.
- DC cardioversion in persistent AF when early recurrence is unlikely.
- Repeat cardioversion followed by AAD for maintenance of sinus rhythm after first relapse without AADs.

Class IIb

- AAD for cardioversion in persistent AF.
- Out-of-hospital administration of AADs in first detected paroxysmal or persistent AF without heart disease when safety is not established in the particular patient.

Class III

- Cardioversion in patients with spontaneous alteration between AF and sinus rhythm over short time periods (this is NOT recommended)

Recommendations for AAD in maintenance of sinus rhythm

Class I

- Select AADs for maintenance based on safety.
- Treat precipitating causes of AF before using AADs.

Class IIa

- Use AAD (or rate control drug) to prevent tachycardia-induced cardiomyopathy.
- Rare and symptom-free AF recurrences may be a successfull outcome of AAD use.

Class IIb

- Use AAD combinations when single drug therapy fails.

Class III

- Do not use AADs in patients with a high-risk profile for proarrhythmia.
- Do not use AADs in patients with sick sinus syndrome or AV block unless a pacemaker is implanted.

Recommendations for heart rate control

Class I

- The physiological range of heart rate in AF [60–80 beats per min (bpm) at rest and 90–115 bpm during moderate exercise] should be pursued with beta-blockers or calcium antagonists.
- In acute AF intravenous beta-blockers and calcium antagonists (verapamil, diltiazem) should be used to slow heart rate in the absence of an accessory pathway and overt CHF or hypotension.

Class IIa

- Combination of digoxin and beta-blockers/calcium antagonists can be used on an individual basis but bradycardia must be avoided.
- Non-pharmacological therapy can be used when drugs fail.

Class IIb

- Digoxin may be used as the sole drug for heart rate control in persistent AF.
- Acute cardioversion is required in patients with very rapid tachycardia or hemodynamic instability in AF involving conduction over an accessory pathway (WPW).

Class III

- Digoxin as the sole drug to control a rapid heart rate in paroxysmal AF (is NOT recommended).
- Catheter ablation without prior drug therapy to control AF (is NOT recommended).

Table 14.4 Electrical therapies in AF (Adapted from Camm[6])

	Pacemaker (atrial or dual chamber)	IAD	Ablation Procedure
Ideal candidate	Recurrent AF with a background of spontaneous or iatrogenic sinus bradycardia (Sick sinus node).	Rare occurrences of highly symptomatic and persistent AF refractory to drugs	Paroxysmal AF in younger patients with frequent atrial ectopy between attacks
Advantages	No compliance problems Easily achieved May be combined with IAD or ICD	Acute or early AF termination. Reduced emergency room visits May be combined with ICD and pacemaker	No compliance problems Potential 'cure' Anticoagulant therapy may not be needed long term
Disadvantages	Expensive. Efficacy uncertain Special device may be needed Electrode placement may be difficult	Very expensive Painful intracardiac shocks Compliance uncertain Potential pro-arrhythmia	Very expensive Uncertain efficacy long term Time consuming procedure Adverse complications

IAD, implantable atrial defibrillator; ICD, implantable cardioverter-defibrillator

A SHORT NOTE ON NON-PHARMACO-LOGICAL TREATMENT IN AF

See Chapter 20 for more details.

Electrophysiologically guided therapy depends on:

- the patient's clinical state (hemodynamics during AF and underlying heart disease);
- symptom frequency and severity;
- the electrophysiological mechanism of the particular case.

His bundle ablation and pacemaker implantation is a treatment option in elderly patients with permanent AF and intolerably high heart rates when all drug attempts at rate control have failed.

Hybrid therapy, i.e. isthmus ablation in cases where AAD treatment in AF leads to atrial flutter, has a success rate of about 50%.

Focal ablation, pulmonary vein isolation and catheter Maze are all reserved for younger patients with a heavy arrhythmia burden and failed AAD therapy.

Success rates for the ablations are allegedly 70–90% in selected centers, and the risks are: pulmonary vein stenosis in 1–2.5% and thromboembolism in < 1%.

Pulmonary vein isolation should NOT be attempted in patients more than 70 years old, in permanent AF, when the left atrium is > 5.5 cm, and if CHF or severe hypertension is present.

A combination of (repeat) focal ablation and AAD, may be clinically useful. Therefore the approach 'wait and see' after the first (or second) ablation before any new attempt makes sense.

References

1. Task Force Report: ACC/AHA/ESC guidelines for the management of patients with atrial fibrillation. Eur Heart J 2001; 22:1852–1923.
2. Hohnloser SH, Kuck KH, Lilienthal J for the PIAF investigators. Rhythm or rate control in atrial fibrillation – pharmacological intervention in atrial fibrillation (PIAF): a randomised trial. Lancet 2000; 356: 1789–1794.
3. The Atrial Fibrillation Follow-up Investigation of Rhythm Management (AFFIRM) Investigators. A comparison of rate control and rhythm control in patients with atrial fibrillation. N Engl J Med 2002; 347:1825–1833.

4. Singh BN. Atrial fibrillation following investigation of rhythm management: AFFIRM trial outcomes. What might be their implications for arrhythmia control? J Cardiovasc Pharmacol Ther 2002; 7:131–133.

5. Fynn SP, Garratt CJ. The effectiveness of serial cardioversion therapy for recurrence of atrial fibrillation. Eur Heart J 2002; 23:1487–1489.

6. Camm AJ. Future role of electrical therapy for atrial fibrillation: reality for all? Eur Heart J Supplements 2001; 3 (suppl P): P53–P56.

CHAPTER 15

Management of acute atrial fibrillation and other supra-ventricular arrhythmias

John Godtfredsen MD FESC
Herlev University Hospital, Herlev, Denmark

> In any acute arrhythmia it is more important to treat the patient with respect to the existing hemodynamic condition than it is to treat the electrocardiogram

ATRIAL FIBRILLATION

Introduction

All over the industrialized world the incidence of hospital admissions for acute atrial fibrillation (AF) has been rising markedly over the past decade, indeed an 'epidemic of AF' is under way.[1] In many cardiology departments caring for acute emergencies in the community the number of patients with an action-diagnosis of AF is quantitatively at a par with the number of patients with acute coronary syndromes. Since 'AF begets AF'[2] this state of affairs represents a heavy burden of initial diagnostic and therapeutical efforts to any cardiological service. Prompt treatment and a carefully planned work-up for each AF patient is mandatory in order to restore sinus rhythm, if possible, and to avoid or minimize the complications of AF in case of relapse or transition to chronic, permanent AF.

Definition of acute AF

A first ever presentation of AF is termed acute AF or new-onset AF, and will often turn out to be self-limiting and spontaneously terminating, however, in practical and operational terms any case of AF – a relapse of earlier diagnosed AF or of unknown duration – presenting with or without hemodynamic compromise and in need of acute relief of symptoms, is in this context acute.

Incidence

The incidence of acute AF in its strictest definition is not precisely known, but it may be surmised that about 25–70% of all admissions for AF are of recent-onset[3,4] and thus fall into this category. Currently in Denmark the emergency admission rate of patients with AF of all types is about 2/1000 inhabitants/year.

Clinical presentations of AF

The symptoms and types of presentation in acute AF are described in Chapter 5, and some pertinent features of AF versus other supraventricular arrhythmias are seen in Table 15.1.

Treatment

Because so many treatment options are available[5,6] and because the randomized

Table 15.1 Clinical features of various supraventricular arrhythmias at presentation

Type of arrhythmia	Relative proportion (%)	Heart rate at onset	Mean age (years)
Paroxysmal AF	65	110–140	68
Chronic AF	9	–	74
AVNRT and AVNT	13	160–180	63
Atrial flutter	13	150	71
WPW	0.5–1	180–250	53

Comments: AF is clearly the most frequent arrhythmia and characterized by elderly patients. The heart rate at presentation varies according to (previous) treatment and degree of underlying heart failure. The generally lower heart rate in AF than in the other arrhythmias is less well tolerated due to the higher age.
AVNRT, atrioventricular nodal re-entrant tachycardia; AVRT, atrioventricular re-entrant tachycardia; WPW, Wolff-Parkinson-White syndrome

When confronting any AF patient, answer the four following questions:

1. Is the ECG really showing AF?
   – and not VT, PSVT with BBB, WPW?

2. Is the heart rate critically fast?
   – HR > 180 is intolerable to many elderly and > 225 may be dangerous and degenerate to VT-VF

3. Is the patient in overt heart failure?
   – any heart disease by history; known LV function by echocardiogram

4. For how long has this episode lasted?
   – about 48 h is the limit to conversion without anticoagulation

---

BBB, bundle branch block; ECG,electrocardiogram; HR, heart rate; PSVT, paroxysmal supraventricular tachycardia; VF, ventricular fibrillation; VT, ventricular tachycardia; WPW, Wolff-Parkinson-White syndrome

---

clinical trial indicating the most appropriate, effective and safe procedure is still lacking, acute AF management is very much governed by local experience and tradition.

The treatment options are also very much dependent upon the clinical and hemodynamic condition of the individual patient, making it difficult to apply a standard 'cook-book' approach, even though many such algorithms have been proposed. Therefore good clinical practice requires not only a thorough knowledge of the general principles, but also a good deal of clinical acumen, and an especially highly individualized evaluation of the patient.

The main principles are shown in the box below, but the interpretention and translation into clinical action – tailoring the treatment individually – constitutes the skill of the therapist and requires a competent judgment of the severity of the situation.

Key points

Principles of acute AF management – in order of priority

- Control of a (too) rapid heart rate
- Treatment of concomitant heart failure
- Acute conversion to sinus rhythm (by drugs or DC)
- Acute thromboembolic prevention
- Treatment of underlying precipitating cause
- Prevention of relapse

Worst case scenario

The combination of a rapid heart rate (HR) and overt heart failure needs fast action. Morphine 10–15 mg i.v.; oxygen nasally or by mask; furosemide 40 mg i.v.; prepare for acute direct current (DC) conversion; rate control with digoxin 0.25–0.5 mg i.v. followed by metoprolol (or other beta-blocker available) 5 mg i.v. bolus, repeated 2–3 times depending on the HR response. An acute bedside echocardiography is helpful to evaluate heart size and ventricular function, although with a fast ventricular response, assessment of the latter may be difficult. If the condition is not significantly relieved within 30 min to 1 h, DC conversion with a start energy level of 200 J is indicated, preceded by a subcutaneous injection of low-molecular-weight heparin (LMWH).

Metoprolol or other beta-blockers may be substituted by calcium channel blockers, for instance diltiazem or verapamil in 10–20 mg i.v. doses, but only if echocardiography shows normal systolic ventricular function. In diastolic dysfunction [often the case in a small left ventricle with (severely) hypertrophied walls] calcium blockers are well tolerated.

Senseless intravenous antiarrhythmic polypharmacy must be avoided – especially when the ventricular function is (severely) impaired (i.e. ejection fraction < 30–35%).

Fortunately most patients are not in such severe distress at admission which leaves ample time to advance step by step, and perhaps to seek qualified advice from a more experienced colleague.

In this respect it is important to get an early impression of the presence of some underlying or concomitant (and may be precipitating) heart disease, that might be disclosed by a careful history, thorough clinical examination and cardiac auscultation, and not least by echocardiography.

Aortic stenosis, mitral stenosis, hypertrophic cardiomyopathy and severe ischemic heart disease are all particularly liable to impair the condition when, and if acute AF supervenes. Thyroid heart disease may present with a very rapid ventricular rate, that is particularly responsible to beta-blocker treatment.

Heart rate control versus acute conversion to sinus rhythm?

The answer to this question depends on the duration of the presenting episode of AF:

- when the duration is < 48 h cardioversion should be attempted (Table 15.2);
- when the duration is most likely ≥ 48 h the appropriate option is rate control.

In many cases, not least in elderly patients, the duration is unknown and one has to rely on a clinical judgement, perhaps

Table 15.2 Drugs for conversion to sinus rhythm* (Adapted from Falk[6] and Task Force Report[8])

Drug	Dose for conversion	Dose for maintenance	Comments
Flecainide	200 mg orally, repeat after 3-4 h (i.v. 2 mg /kg)	50–150 mg b.i.d.	Only for use without structural heart disease Flutter with 1:1 conduction
Propafenone	600 mg orally (i.v. 2 mg /kg)	150–300 mg b.i.d	As for flecainide
Dofetilide	0.5 mg orally b.i.d.	0.5 mg b.i.d.	Lower dose with uremia
Ibutilide	Weight ≥ 60 kg: 1 mg i.v./10 min Weight < 60 kg: 0.01 mg/kg/ 10 min Repeat x 1 if not SR within 10 min after first dose.	Not available	Not to be used in hypoK, long QT or previously known torsade de pointes
(Sotalol)	5–10 mg slowly i.v., may be repeated.	120–160 mg b.i.d.	Conversion rate rather low. Proarrhythmia risk is high
Amiodarone	6 mg/kg bolus over 30–60 min, then 1200 mg i.v. over 24 h	600 mg daily 1 week, thereafter 200 mg daily	Moderately effective, slow onset, good heart rate control. Hypotension with bolus dose
Quinidine	200 mg sulfate orally and 400 mg 1–2 h later	200–400 mg sulfate 4 times daily or 300–600 mg gluconate t.i.d.	Not much used nowadays
Procainamide	100 mg i.v. q. 5 min to max 1000 mg	1–2 g b.i.d.	Not much used nowadays
Disopyramide	200 mg orally q. 4 h to max 800 mg	100–150 mg q.i.d. or 200–300 mg slow release b.i.d.	Strong negative inotropy

* Note: Not all drugs are approved in all countries; ECG monitoring is mandatory during any drug conversion procedure in AF.

helped by the size of the left atrium by bedside echocardiography where a left atrial diameter > 40–45 mm strongly points to AF of some persistence. Medication with, for instance, digoxin or antiarrhythmic agents may also indicate that AF has been present for some time and may be recently exacerbated by some intercurrent condition, i.e. worsening congestive heart failure (CHF), pneumonia or pulmonary embolism.

Reasons for an attempt at earliest possible conversion to sinus rhythm

- To avoid the apparently immediate onset of electrical remodeling[7]
- To avoid the evolving deleterious effects of continuing the rapid heart rate (hemodynamic deterioration)
- To avoid thromboembolic complications (time-window disputed)

When the AF duration is ≥ 48 h or unknown, and the heart rate is fast and the patient is not (yet) in acute distress, heart rate control assumes priority. There are a number of drug options as shown in Table 15.3. To achieve proper rate control, a combination of drugs is often necessary, and careful titration of the dose under close ECG monitoring and frequent blood pressure readings are both mandatory since side-effects are common, notably bradycardia, AV block and hypotension.

Comments on various drug treatment options for heart rate control

Digoxin was for many years the time honored drug of choice in acute AF, but some, though not all, newer studies have failed to confirm its superiority over placebo,[9–12] and certainly the beta-blockers and calcium blockers are more effective in acutely decreasing the ventricular rate. Particularly in conditions of a high

Table 15.3 Drugs for rate control in atrial fibrillation* (Adapted from Falk[6] and Task Force Report[8])

Drug	Dose for HR-control	Dose for maintenance	Comments
Diltiazem	20 mg bolus, repeat after 25 min if necessary. Infusion 5–15 mg/h	180–300 mg daily slow release	Addition of digoxin improves rate control
Verapamil	5–10 mg i.v. over 3 min, repeat after 30 min	200 mg b.i.d., slow release	Increases digoxin level, negative inotropy
Esmolol	0.5 mg/kg i.v. bolus, then 0.05 –0.2 mg/kg/min	Not available	Hypotension: stop infusion
Metoprolol	5 mg i.v. bolus, repeated x 2 at 2 min intervals	50–200 mg b.i.d.	Useful in concomitant ischemic HD
Digoxin	0.25 mg i.v. every 2 h up to 1.5 mg	0.125–0.375 mg daily	Slow onset, but synergistic with other agents
Amiodarone	6 mg/Kg bolus over 30–60 min then 1200 mg i.v. over 24 h	600 mg daily/1 week thereafter 200 mg daily	May convert to SR, slow onset, good heart rate control. Hypotension with bolus dose
Propranolol	1–5 mg i.v. over 10 min	40–360 mg daily	Non-selective, caution with COPD

*Not all drugs are approved in all countries; ECG monitoring is mandatory during any i.v. drug injection.
COPD, chronic obstructive pulmonary disease

adrenergic drive, which often accompanies acute AF, digoxin is ineffective. In overt clinical heart failure, however, or when the left ventricular function is depressed on echocardiography, digoxin remains the favored treatment,[13] not least because of its prolonged effect, that is not matched by the acute intravenous use of beta- and calcium blockers in which the heart rate response is transient. Therefore acute combination therapy with close follow-up of the patients' condition and judicious use of all classes of drugs in proper (cautious) doses is the most succesful and wise mode of management.

In persistent AF with prolonged periods of relapse and in permanent AF digoxin may still be regarded as a useful basic drug for rate control – alone or in combination.

Beta-blockers are – but for their negative inotropic effect – generally safe for use in acute heart rate control and therefore regarded as first-line drugs. Caution and awareness is needed in heart failure and when chronic obstructive pulmonary disease (COPD) is present.

Beta-blockade combined with digoxin is also very useful in persistent and permanent AF since this combination rather effectively depresses the otherwise uncontrolled high heart rate during physical activity. One option may be the use of intravenous esmolol, which has a very short half-life, and thus rapid onset and termination of pharmacological actions.

Calcium antagonists are rather more negative inotropic than beta-blockers (and verapamil more so than diltiazem), and they are therefore contraindicated when systolic heart failure is present. These drugs are, however, useful in 'pure' diastolic heart failure (on echocardiography) and preferred in cases of concomitant COPD.

Amiodarone is particularly useful intravenously in the setting of critical illness when negative inotropy is of concern, and the other drugs are contraindicated. Heart rate control with amiodarone is usually very effective.

DC conversion

Only about 15–25% of all patients with acute AF do not respond to drug conversion, and acute DC conversion is an emergency indication only in the above mentioned worst case scenario.

Subacute DC conversion may then be necessary when in these remaining 15–25% of the patients rate control fails and they are threatened with hemodynamic instability in the near future – a situation where one has to compromise between the risk of thromboembolism and the risk of hemodynamic deteroriation, both being equally deleterious.

Some guidance is to be gained from transesophageal echocardiography, since the Assessment of Cardioversion Using Transesophageal Echocardiography (ACUTE) study showed the relative safety of early DC conversion under cover of low-molecular-heparin subcutaneously, when no thrombi were identified in the left atrium.[14]

The energy level necessary for acute transthoracic DC conversion is 200 J, gradually increased to 360 J in case of no response, and this procedure requires a short-lasting general anesthesia. Only in totally refractory AF with intolerably rapid ventricular rates when everything else has failed intracardiac DC conversion is indicated – this treatment is generally available only at tertiary centers.

Fortunately such patients are very rare in daily clinical cardiology.

Special cases of atrial fibrillation

- In WPW acute AF presents itself most commonly in younger patients with very rapid ventricular rates (often > 225) and an ECG that sometimes may mimic ventricular tachycardia (VT), (see Fig. 15.1) It is a potentially dangerous, life-threatening arrhythmia where prompt DC conversion is indicated in

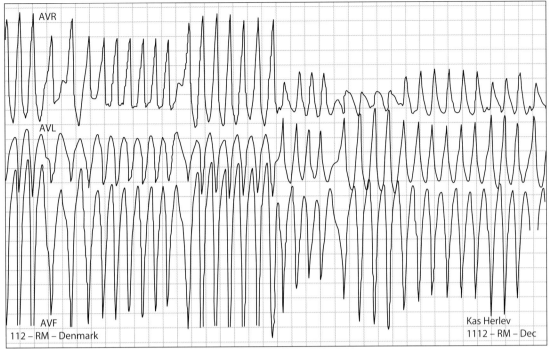

Fig. 15.1 Atrial fibrillation and Wolff-Parkinson-White syndrome (WPW), ECG paper speed 25 mm/s.

case of hemodynamic instability (low or falling blood pressure, clinical symptoms of preshock or shock). In stable patients with lower heart rates flecainide or sotalol can be used. Digoxin and verapamil are both contraindicated in WPW because of the risk of 1:1 conduction over the accessory pathway when AV conduction is blocked.

- In acute myocardial infarction AF is seen in about 15% of the patients usually when heart failure complicates the infarct. Acute beta-blocker therapy is a first line drug selection, and intravenous amiodarone second line if heart failure is prominent or if AF relapses frequently.

- Patients with very short lasting bouts of AF (minutes to half-hours) are occasionally met with in the clinic. These patients are usually younger or middle aged and have no underlying structural heart disease, and the diagnosis may (or may not) have been made by event- or Holter recording. The episodes of AF are self-terminating and more of a nuisance than an illness, and the frequency may vary from periods with many attacks to long intervals free of symptoms. Obviously neither acute drug conversion nor heart rate control is of any use because of the short duration, but sometimes a Valsalva maneuver or another vagus stimulating procedure applied very early during the attack may abolish the arrhythmia.

Thromboembolic prophylaxis

The received conventional wisdom, and a few clinical studies tell us that acute, recent onset AF with less than 48 h duration carries such a low risk of thromboembolism, that no antithrombotic prevention is justified before conversion. The reason is that thrombus formation in the left atrium takes time. But if this time is short, perhaps as little as 12 h[15] it would be safer to give all AF patients a dose of LMWH subcutaneously as soon as possible after the ECG diagnosis. This admittedly pragmatic viewpoint has been advocated with increasingly good arguments,[16] and also it satisfies another concern, namely the inappropriateness of deferring conversion to sinus rhythm in view of our certain knowledge, that the electrical remodeling which is a factor in the stability and refractoriness of established AF begins rather early.[7]

Since LMWH is almost without side effects and the chance of obtaining sustained sinus rhythm free of AF relapse is the higher the earlier conversion can be undertaken, this approach seems sensible. A prospective trial to solve this dilemma is long overdue.

The use of aspirin in acute AF has never been formally tested, and therefore its efficacy as an antithrombotic option is unknown. However, in permanent AF aspirin confers some antithrombotic protection in low-risk patients (a relative risk reduction of about 20%).[15]

Decision on eventual postconversion antiarrhythmic treatment

After termination of a first-ever bout of AF and especially if some clear extracardiac precipitating cause has been identified there is no indication for antiarrhythmic, preventive therapy. If, and when during follow-up it turns out that frequent or more long-lasting relapses do occur the time has come for deciding as to whether antiarrhythmic drugs are indicated or not (see Ch. 14).

Figure 15.2 provides an overview of management of acute atrial fibrillation.

ATRIAL FLUTTER (AFL)

Acute atrial flutter is much less common than AF (Table 15.1) and only rarely of serious clinical concern. This is because the ventricular rate seldom exceeds 150 beats per min (bpm) and often is slower due to the AV blockade varying between 2:1 and 4:1 or even more.

The ECG hallmark characteristic is – in type 1 AFL, by far the most common – the typical 'sawtooth' baseline of P waves with a frequency of 300 bpm best seen in leads II and III. With a 2:1 AV blockade this entails a rather precise and stable heart rate of close to 150 bpm which may be sustained for days or weeks without much hemodynamic disturbance unless the ventricular function has been compromised previously.

Treatment

Since patients with AFL generally present without dire distress or severely compromised ventricular function there is ample time to plan and execute the treatment strategy.

Diagnostic work-up pre- and postconversion[8]

- A careful history and physical examination to define the type and clinical course of AF, especially underlying heart disease, hyperthyroidism and alcohol abuse

- A 12-lead ECG to identify left ventricular hypertrophy, previous acute myocardial infarction, bundle branch block, pre-excitation and QT interval

- Chest X-ray in case of clinical lung disease

- Echocardiography is of invaluable significance to identify underlying heart disease and size and function of the chambers

- Blood tests of thyroid function, electrolyte status and renal funtion

- Exercise test to evaluate the adequacy of heart rate control, the (rare) occurrence of exercise-induced AF and signs of ischemic heart disease

- Event recording to evaluate rate control and occurrence of other arrhythmias (flutter)

- Transesophageal echocardiography to identify left atrial thrombus or to guide cardioversion

- Electrophysiological study when non-pharmacological treatment is contemplated

---

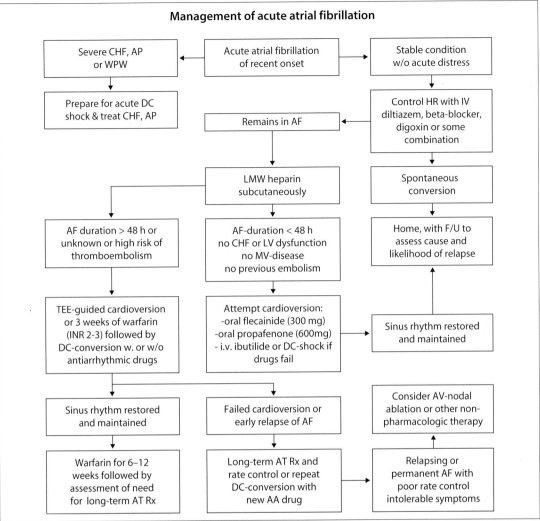

Fig. 15.2 Overview of management of acute atrial fibrillation. AA, antiarrhythmic; AF, atrial fibrillation; AT Rx, antithrombotic treatment; AP, angina pectoris; AV, atrioventricular; CHF, congestive heart failure; F/U, follow-up; HR, heart rate, LMW, low molecular weight; LV dysfct, left ventricular dysfunction; MV, mitral valve, TEE, transesophageal echocardiography; WPW, Wolff-Parkinson-White (Modified from Falk.[6])

This consists of three elements:

1. slowing the ventricular rate by increasing the AV-blockade
2. attempt at conversion to sinus rhythm
3. stratify regarding the thromboembolic risk just as in AF.

All drugs that slow the AV conduction and hence the ventricular rate may be effective: digoxin, beta- and calcium blockers are used in the same doses as in AF. If urgent ventricular slowing is necessary intravenous treatment can be used as in AF.

Flecainide and propafenone for conversion of AFL is not recommended (even though they may work) because of the risk of 1:1 AV conduction when the atrial rate is slowed.

Ibutilide when given intravenously as described in Table 15.2 has a conversion rate of about 60%, but with a small but significant risk of precipitating torsade de pointes.

In the entirely stable patient a prudent course of action is to start one or a combination of these drugs orally and then just don an expecting attitude since in 1 or

2 days time about 50% of the patients will then revert to sinus rhythm.

When this regimen fails or if the patient is initially threathened hemodynamically or it is known with certainty that the arrhythmia has already lasted for some days or weeks DC shock is the treatment of choice.[17]

AFL is very responsive to DC conversion: applied with a rather low energy level of 50–100 J more than 95% revert to sinus rhythm.[17]

In entirely refractory cases overdrive atrial pacing may be effective, but this procedure requires experienced personnel and transfer to a center with the necessary gear.

The thromboembolic prophylaxis in AFL should follow the principles outlined for AF – a pragmatic exercise – since no prospective data from randomized trials are available.

OTHER SUPRAVENTRICULAR TACHYCARDIAS (SVT)

These arrhythmias consist of several types mainly defined by their electrophysiological characteristics and properties.

Atrial tachycardias are non-AV node dependent tachycardias, AV node dependent tachycardias [AV nodal re-entrant tachycardia (AVNRT) and AV re-entrant tachycardia (AVRT)] where the AV node is involved in the mechanism of the arrhythmia.

Common features are a relatively rare prevalence compared with AF and AFL, a narrow QRS-complex on ECG and a heart rate of about 160–180 bpm, and only occasionally there is any severe hemodynamic compromise at presentation. The atrial tachycardias are sometimes precipitated by digoxin toxicity, a typical and frequent ECG feature of which is the so-called 'atrial tachycardia with block' or multifocal atrial tachycardia.

In the presence of concomitant bundle branch block or some preexcitation mechanism all these tachycardias show a broad QRS complex mimicking VT, and therefore represent a serious challenge to the diagnostic accuracy and choice of apppropriate therapy.

In the clinical, acute setting some diagnostic help is gained from two simple questions posed to the patient. [18]

An esophageal ECG may also help in the differential diagnosis between VT and an atrial tachycardia with bundle branch block.

- Have you ever had a myocardial infarction?

  and

- Have you ever had bouts of palpitations like this, subsequent to the infarction?

- If the answer is in the affirmative to both, there is a > 90% risk that the arrhythmia is ventricular

Treatment

The atrial tachycardias usually respond to the same drugs as are used in AF and AFL, with due respect towards possible concomitant heart failure. Except for digoxin which is not recommended, both calcium and beta-blockers can be used in the doses and modes of administration as outlined in Table 15.2.

Vagal maneuvers should be tried as early as possible during an attack since it may be effective in about 30% of such cases.

In case of refractory or incessant atrial tachycardias overdrive pacing, perhaps via an esophageal lead could be tried as well as DC shock if the hemodynamics become unstable. In the atrial tachycardias caused by digoxin its withdrawal is essential followed by either beta-blockade or DC shock (low energy level to start with) depending on the urgency of the situation.

In the AV node dependent tachycardias the drug of choice is *adenosine* administered as a rapid intravenous bolus of 6 or 12 mg during ECG monitoring. This gives the patient a transient feeling of heat and a flush lasting 0.5–1 min and usually terminates the arrhythmia in over 90% of the cases.

Intravenous verapamil in doses of 5–10 mg is also effective, but is not recommended if there is a broad QRS tachycardia since the mistaken intravenous treatment of VT may be deleterious.

During adenosine treatment a short lasting high grade AV block may develop, which may give a diagnostic clue on the ECG showing the atrial activity and rate.

Recalcitrant arrhythmias may be treated by esophageal overdrive pacing and if everything fails DC shock, which is rarely required.

No data are available on the need for antithrombotic prevention in these other SVT.

References

1. Chugh SS, Blackshear JL, Shen W-K, et al. Epidemiology and natural history of atrial fibrillation: clinical implications. J Am Coll Cardiol 2001; 37:371–378.
2. Wijffels MC, Kirchhof CJ, Dorland R, et al. Atrial fibrillation begets atrial fibrillation. A study in awake chronically instrumented goats. Circulation 1995; 92:1954–1968.
3. Lévy S, Maarek M, Coumel P, et al. Characterization of different subsets of atrial fibrillation in general practice in France. The ALFA Study. Circulation 1999; 99:3028–3035.
4. Davidson E, Weinberger I, Rotenberg Z, et al. Atrial fibrillation. Cause and time of onset. Arch Int Med 1989; 149:457–459.
5. Boriani G, Biffi M, Capucci A, et al. Conversion of recent-onset atrial fibrillation to sinus rhythm: effects of different drug protocols. Pacing Clin Electrophysiol 1998; 11:2470–2474.
6. Falk RH. Atrial fibrillation. N Engl J Med 2001; 344:1067–1078.
7. Goette A, Honeycutt C, Langberg JJ. Electrical remodeling in atrial fibrillation. Time course and mechanisms. Circulation 1996; 94:2968–2974.
8. Task Force Report: ACC/AHA/ESC guidelines for the management of patients with atrial fibrillation. Eur Heart J 2001; 22:1852–1923.
9. Falk RH, Knowlton AA, Bernard SA, et al. Digoxin for converting recent-onset atrial fibrillation to sinus rhythm. A randomized, double-blind study. Ann Intern Med 1987; 106:503–506.
10. Jordaens L, Trouerbach J, Calle P, et al. Conversion of atrial fibrillation to sinus rhythm and rate control by digoxin in comparison to placebo. Eur Heart J 1997; 18:643–648.
11. Hou Z-Y, Chang M-S , Chen C-Y, et al. Acute treatment of recent-onset atrial fibrillation and flutter with a tailored dosing regimen of intravenous amiodarone. A randomized, digoxin-controlled study. Eur Heart J 1995; 16:521–528.
12. The Digitalis in Acute Atrial Fibrillation (DAAF) Trial Group. Intravenous digoxin in acute atrial fibrillation. Results of a randomized, placebo-controlled multicentre trial in 239 patients. Eur Heart J 1997; 18:649–654.
13. Lévy S. Intravenous digoxin: still the drug of choice for acute termination of atrial fibrillation? Eur Heart J 1997; 18:546–547.
14. Klein AL, Grimm RA, Murray RD, et al. Use of transesophageal echocardiography to guide cardioversion in patients with atrial fibrillation. N Engl J Med 2001; 344:1411–1420.
15. Kamath S, Blann AD, Lip GYH. Platelets and atrial fibrillation. Eur Heart J 2001; 22:2233–2242.
16. Camm AJ. Atrial fibrillation: is there a role for low-molecular-weight heparin? Clin Cardiol 2001; 24 (suppl I): I15–I19.
17. Crijns HJ, Van Gelder IC, Tieleman RG, et al. Long-term outcome of electrical cardioversion in patients with chronic atrial flutter. Heart 1997; 77:56–61.
18. Tchou P, Young P, Mahmud R, et al. Useful clinical criteria for the diagnosis of ventricular tachycardia. Am J Med 1988; 84:53–56.

Further Reading

Lip GYH, Kamath S, Freestone B. Acute atrial fibrillation. Clinical Evidence 2002; 7:1–6.

CHAPTER 16

Heart rate control

Bethan Freestone MBChB MRCP

City Hospital, Birmingham, UK

Gregory Y H Lip MD FRCP DFM FACC FESC

City Hospital, Birmingham, UK

Heart rate control in atrial fibrillation is a cornerstone therapy to be implemented early

Introduction

The treatment for atrial fibrillation (AF) involves the three main facets of:

1. rate control;
2. consideration of rhythm control (involving direct current or pharmacological cardioversion); and
3. antiplatelet or anticoagulant agents for the prevention of thromboembolic complications.

In many patients who present acutely in whom conversion to sinus rhythm is delayed whilst adequate anticoagulation is awaited, or in whom cardioversion has been unsuccessful or is considered inappropriate, rate control is the primary objective of treatment. Rapid ventricular rate in association with AF can result in hemodynamic compromise with hypotension, congestive heart failure or rate related cardiac ischemia in the acute situation. In the longer term, uncontrolled AF is associated with symptoms of palpitations, dyspnea, decreased exercise tolerance and fatigue. There is also the problem of tachycardia-induced cardiomyopathy, whereby poorly controlled fast AF results in progressive ventricular dilatation and systolic dysfunction, with associated ultrastructural changes in the myocardium. Rate control in AF is therefore important and this chapter will concentrate on the pharmacological control of heart rate in AF.

Several of the antiarrhythmic drugs achieve control of ventricular response and subsequently, heart rate, better than others. This tends to be a class effect, but even within one class of antiarrhythmic there is variation in efficacy between drugs. In addition, it would appear that different therapies for rate control in AF are more beneficial in certain circumstances, for example postoperatively, on exercise, in the setting of acute myocardial infarction, and so on. This chapter will attempt to indicate where there is existing evidence for this, but will concentrate in the main on drugs for rate control, based on the Vaughan Williams classification (Table 16.1). However we should also be aware that rate control can also be achieved by non-pharmacological means, for example, by atrioventricular (AV) node ablation and pacemaker implantation.

The resting heart rate in patients with atrial fibrillation is usually in the range of 130–200 beats per min (bpm), rate control

Table 16.1 Vaughan Williams classification of antiarrhythmic drugs

Class I: Membrane stabilizing agents (fast sodium channel blockers) Ia: block Na channel and delay repolarization, increasing action potential duration	Quinidine, disopyramide, procainamide
Ib: block Na channel and accelerate repolarization, decreasing action potential duration	Lidocaine (lignocaine), mexiletine, phenytoin
Ic: pronounced Na channel blockade, little effect on repolarization	Flecanide, encainide, propafenone
Class II: Beta-blockers	Propranolol, atenolol, metoprolol, etc
Class III: Drugs which increase action potential duration	Amiodarone, bretylium, sotalol
Class IV: Calcium channel blockers	Verapamil, diltiazem

Some drugs have properties of more than one class.
Some commonly used antiarrhythmics have no place in this classification (e.g. digoxin)

in AF is generally considered to be successful in the longer term when a resting heart rate of 60–80 bpm has been achieved, although in trials this definition is variable. All drugs control heart rate in AF mainly by reduction of conduction across the AV node so that it is not the atrial activity itself that is suppressed but the ventricular response. The factors that determine the choice of drug for managing AF, as well as the management strategy are summarized in Table 16.2.

Key points

Factors that determine the choice of the drug for AF

- Nature of AF (paroxysmal or sustained)
- Treatment strategy (cardioversion or rate control)
- Co-morbid conditions (obstructive airway disease, etc)
- Ischemic and/or structural heart disease
- The rapidity with which treatment is indicated
- Patient preference

CLASS II ANTIARRHYTHMICS: BETA-BLOCKERS

Adrenergic beta-receptor blockade acts to decrease heart rate in AF predominantly by depression of conduction across the AV node, but also decreases automaticity of myocardial cells.

Beta-blockers have been shown to be effective rate control agents when compared to placebo in AF at rest, during exercise, in acute AF and postoperatively (Fig. 16.1).[1] Certain beta-blockers do appear to be more efficacious than others.

In AF, the only intravenous beta-blocker to be tested in a randomized controlled trial setting is timolol, although propranolol, metoprolol and esmolol are also available as parenteral agents and have had their efficacy demonstrated. In the trial of a timolol versus placebo in 61 patients with AF of unspecified duration with a ventricular rate of >120 bpm, at 1 h intravenous timolol had reduced the ventricular rate to <100 bpm in significantly more people than placebo (41% vs 3%, $p < 0.01$).[2]

In a systematic review of drugs used for ventricular rate control in AF, seven different beta-blockers were compared to placebo in 12 trials (including the one outlined above), and it was found that in 7 of 12 comparisons beta-blockade reduced ventricular rate at rest significantly compared with placebo.[3] All beta-blockers were efficacious during exercise.

Oral pindolol and nadolol both significantly reduced resting heart rate in AF,[4,5] whereas celiprolol and labetolol were no more efficacious than placebo at rest.[6,7] Atenolol was efficacious when tested during exercise,[8] whilst xameterol had variable results.[9,10]

All outlined evidence for beta-blockers is supportive of their rate-controlling effect in AF and this benefit, as it is assumed to be a class effect, is extended to other beta-blockers, however this evidence is limited by a lack of large randomized control trials

Table 16.2 Antiarrhythmic therapy and AF

Management strategy	Class of drug
Paroxysmal AF	Class IA, class IC, class II, class III drugs
Cardioversion of AF to sinus rhythm	Class IA, class IC and class III drugs
Rate control	Class II, class III, class IV and digoxin
Maintenance of sinus rhythm post cardioversion of AF	Class IA, class IC, class II, class III drugs

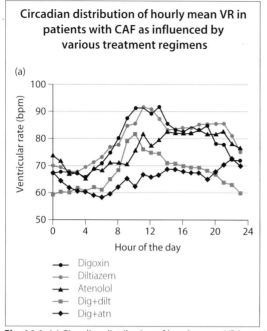

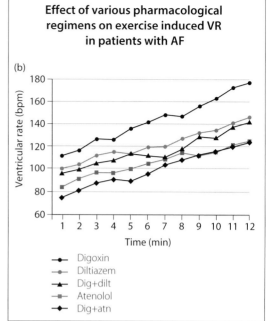

Fig. 16.1 (a) Circadian distribution of hourly mean VR in patients with CAF as influenced by various treatment regimens. (b) Effect of various pharmacological regimens on exercise induced VR in patients with AF. VR, ventricular response; CAF, chronic atrial fibrillation. Reproduced with permission from Farshi et al.[1] © 1999 The American College of Cardiology Foundation.

in this area, and indeed, for other antiarrhythmic drug use.

Although beta-blockers are effective rate control agents their use is also limited by contraindications and potential for adverse effects. For example, side-effects with beta-blockade include hypotension, or heart failure exacerbation due to a negative ionotropic effect, bradycardia or heart block, bronchospasm, impotence, peripheral vasoconstriction, fatigue, sleep disturbances, rashes and exacerbation of psoriasis.

For these reasons beta-blockade is contraindicated in those patients with a history of asthma or reversible airways disease, and in the acute situation is best avoided where there is evidence of heart failure clinically, or acutely in patients with known moderate to severe left ventricular impairment. However, for patients with left ventricular (LV) dysfunction who are stable on antifailure medications for more than a month, beta-blockers can be prognostically beneficial with gradual introduction and uptitration,[11] and could therefore

theoretically be used in chronic stable AF in association with left ventricular dysfunction for potential benefits in the treatment of both conditions.

Contraindications to beta-blockade

- in patients with a history of asthma or reversible airways disease

- in the acute situation where there is evidence of heart failure clinically

- in acute patients with known moderate to severe left ventricular impairment

CLASS IV ANTIARRHYTHMICS: CALCIUM CHANNEL BLOCKERS

The rate-limiting calcium channel blockers, namely diltiazem and verapamil, are commonly used for control of ventricular rate in atrial fibrillation (see Fig. 16.1). Again the mechanism of rate control is predominantly by slowing conduction at the AV node.

In randomized control trials, both verapamil and diltiazem are consistently superior to placebo in achieving rate control in patients with AF, both at rest and on exercise.

For diltiazem, in one trial involving 113 patients with AF or flutter of unspecified duration, with a ventricular rate of > 120 bpm, a systolic blood pressure of > 90 mmHg, and no evidence of heart failure, those receiving intravenous diltiazem (0.25mg/kg, every 2 min for 15 min) had a significant reduction in heart rate during this period in comparison to placebo (with a ventricular rate of < 100 bpm in 75% of the diltiazem group compared with 7% of placebo, $p < 0.001$).[12] The maximal reduction in heart rate with i.v. diltiazem was seen at just 4.3 min, supporting the use of this agent parenterally to achieve prompt heart rate control. Other trials of diltiazem versus placebo have allowed the use of digoxin as additional treatment in both groups.

However, in a direct comparison to digoxin, one small trial (n=30) indicated that, in patients presenting with acute AF or flutter, intravenous diltiazem had a more rapid onset of action than intravenous digoxin (with a significant reduction in mean heart rate seen by 5 min in the diltiazem group, 111 bpm with diltiazem vs 144 bpm with digoxin, $p=0.0006$).[13] A significant reduction in heart rate was not reached until 180 min with the use of intravenous digoxin.

Interestingly, another small trial using intravenous diltiazem versus placebo in a double-blind cross-over study of 37 patients presenting with rapid AF or flutter and moderate to severe congestive heart failure, suggested that diltiazem may be safely used for heart rate control in heart failure despite concerns over its negative ionotropic effect, with 36 of the 37 patients achieving a therapeutic response (> 20% reduction in heart rate), and no exacerbations of congestive failure experienced.[14] However hypotension occurred in four patients and

should be watched for, and the short follow-up period of only 4 h should be borne in mind as it does not support long-term use of calcium antagonists in patients with heart failure and AF.

Verapamil, again in trials versus placebo, significantly reduces ventricular rate within 10 min when administered intravenously,[15,16] supporting its use in AF for rapid ventricular rate control. Numerous additional small trials have shown oral verapamil to be an effective rate control agent in AF. Versus placebo, in one very small trial (n=6) verapamil produced a significant reduction in both the resting heart rate (absolute reduction of 22 bpm, $p < 0.01$) and heart rate on exercise (absolute reduction of 21, $p < 0.05$).[17] In four trials of verapamil versus placebo, in which digoxin was permitted as an additional therapy, verapamil still consistently reduced heart rate.[9,17–19]

In comparative trials of verapamil versus diltiazem there were no significant differences in rate control or measures of systolic function between the two agents, although hypotension was noted in more patients given verapamil.[17,20] On exercise, in patients with AF, both diltiazem and verapamil have been shown to reduce mean heart rate and improve exercise tolerance, particularly in comparison to digoxin.[8,19]

Side-effects with the calcium antagonists include hypotension because of a reduction in cardiac output seen with calcium antagonists, due partly to a negative ionotropic effect, but also the vasodilatation these agents produce due to smooth muscle relaxation. As with beta-blockers, calcium blockers can also precipitate worsening cardiac failure in patients with LV impairment. Although the small study with diltiazem outlined above indicated that LV impairment should not be an absolute contraindication for its use as a rate control agent in heart failure, calcium channel blockers should still be used with caution for rate control in AF in such patients, and other rate control measures (such as direct current cardioversion, or the use of amiodarone or digoxin in the less compromised) should be implemented in patients with signs of congestive cardiac failure or hemodynamic compromise. Furthermore, both verapamil and diltiazem can cause bradycardia or AV block. Verapamil through smooth muscle relaxation is also associated with constipation as a relatively common side-effect, especially in the elderly. Other side-effects associated with both diltiazem and verapamil include flushing, headache, dizziness, ankle edema, gastrointestinal upset, allergic responses, skin rashes, gingival hyperplasia, and both have also been associated with increased prolactin levels and gynecomastia as a rare side-effect.

In summary therefore, both verapamil and diltiazem are efficacious rate control agents for use in AF, have a faster onset of action than digoxin when given parenterally in randomized control trials, and diltiazem has been used safely for acute rate control in the setting of heart failure in one small trial.

Contraindications to calcium antagonists

- in patients that are hypotensive
- in patients with a history of syncope, bradycardia or AV block
- in the acute situation where there is evidence of heart failure clinically
- in acute patients with known moderate to severe left ventricular impairment

DIGOXIN

Digoxin

Digoxin is not the drug of choice for rate control in AF, and should be given in preference to other agents only in patients with severe LV dysfunction, or in combination with other agents such as beta-blockers and rate limiting calcium antagonists

Other drugs are slowly replacing digoxin, once considered the mainstay of treatment for AF rate response, as primary AF treatment, due to the limitations of digoxin in terms of its efficacy and side-effects.

As digoxin mainly acts to enhance parasympathetic activity, its effect on rate control is reduced during times of sympathetic activation, as occurs for example in acute cardiac failure, sepsis, myocardial infarction and so on. It therefore has reduced efficacy for rate control in such instances.

In trials versus placebo, results with digoxin are inconsistent, with digoxin showing only equivalence in terms of rate control in AF in two studies, but in three studies a reduction in resting heart rate was demonstrated. One larger randomized control trial involving 239 patients compared intravenous digoxin with placebo, but verapamil was allowed as an additional therapy for rate control in both groups, so the difference in rate control between the two groups cannot be attributed to digoxin alone, although it was significant ($p < 0.0001$).[21]

Studies also evaluating digoxin for heart rate control on exercise, have confirmed its lack of efficacy, with two trials reporting no significant difference between digoxin and placebo, although measurements of exercise tolerance did seem to be improved in the digoxin groups with improved cardiac output for patients on digoxin in one of the trials[17] and a longer time spent on the treadmill in the digoxin group in another.[10]

In chronic AF, control of ventricular rate during exercise is poor for patients on digoxin unless a calcium channel blocker or beta-blocker are used in combination. In trials of digoxin versus calcium channel blockers, there is a definite trend towards better heart rate control at rest and on exercise with calcium channel blockers. Verapamil certainly allowed patients to exercise longer on the treadmill overall than the group on digoxin in one trial.[18] Comparative trials of digoxin versus beta-blockers in AF appear to show little difference for rate control at rest, but improved rate control with beta-blockers on exercise.[4,10]

Another of the drawbacks of digoxin is its slow onset of action, the peak action of digoxin is typically delayed, taking 6–12 h to reduce ventricular rate to < 100 bpm.

Digoxin has a narrow therapeutic index, and side-effects are more common at increased plasma levels. Indeed, digoxin has many potential unwanted side-effects including gastrointestinal upset, lethargy, dizziness and confusion. Cardiac side-effects include complete heart block, the promotion of ventricular extrasystoles and possible ventricular tachycardia or ventricular fibrillation. Hypokalemia can also precipitate cardiac side-effects. Glycoside toxicity is often indicated by the onset of nausea, vomiting, dizziness and confusion in a patient taking digoxin and this patient is in danger of life-threatening cardiac arrhythmias.

Digoxin toxicity is often seen in association with renal impairment, as digoxin is eliminated via the kidneys, and due to its long half-life and narrow therapeutic range can accumulate to toxic levels reasonably quickly.

The limitations of digoxin in terms of its only modest rate control, side-effects and potential for toxicity, dependence on renal excretion, slow onset of action and need for stepwise loading all reduce the favorability for the use of this drug as a primary rate control agent in AF. In addition, digoxin is no better than placebo for reversion of AF to sinus rhythm[21,22] and in the setting of paroxysmal AF digoxin can paradoxically increase the frequency and prolong the duration of episodes of AF.[23,24]

For these reasons, digoxin should not be the drug of choice when deciding on treatment for rate control in AF, and should be given in preference to other agents perhaps only in patients with severe LV dysfunction, or in combination with other agents such as beta-blockers and rate limiting calcium antagonists.

CLASS III ANTIARRHYTHMICS: AMIODARONE AND SOTALOL

Class III antiarrhythmics act to increase the action potential and the refractoriness of myocardial tissue without slowing conduction and should therefore be ideal agents for the treatment of re-entrant arrhythmias such as AF to restore sinus rhythm. However, both amiodarone and sotalol have additional rate control advantages.

Amiodarone

Amiodarone is generally regarded as a rhythm control agent rather than a rate control agent in AF.

However, intravenous amiodarone has been used to control heart rate in recent onset AF but probably does this, not by pure class III antiarrhythmic actions, but by beta adrenoreceptor and calcium channel receptor blockade properties.[25] Data for amiodarone as a rate control agent comes, in the main, from trials in which the primary objective was assessment of amiodarone as a treatment for pharmacological cardioversion in acute AF.

In one such trial of amiodarone versus placebo (in which digoxin was permitted as adjuvant therapy in both groups), at 24 h, in those patients who had not returned to sinus rhythm, treatment with amiodarone was associated with a slower ventricular rate (82 ± 15 bpm in amiodarone group versus 91 ± 23 bpm in controls, $p=0.022$).[26]

In a randomized digoxin-controlled study, intravenous amiodarone significantly reduces heart rate by 6 h (from a mean heart rate of 157 ± 20 to 96 ± 25), also supporting its use for relatively prompt rate control.[27] When compared to flecainide, intravenous amiodarone also was shown to promptly reduce heart rate in recent onset AF, whereas flecainide was no more effective than placebo.[28]

In a small trial involving 60 critically ill patients on intensive care with supraventricular arrhythmias, intravenous amiodarone showed at least equivalence to intravenous diltiazem for ventricular rate control, with an over 30% reduction in heart rate achieved in 70% of patients on diltiazem, 55% of patients given an amiodarone bolus, and 75% of patients given amiodarone as a bolus followed by infusion.[29]

Evaluation of amiodarone in heart failure was addressed in one trial involving 667 patients with congestive cardiac failure, 103 of whom had AF. Ventricular rate control, assessed over 24 h using Holter monitoring, when assessed at 2 weeks, 6 months and 12 months was significantly reduced in the amiodarone group, supporting its use as a rate control agent in patients with AF and heart failure.[30]

Unfortunately, the side-effects of amiodarone are numerous and include photosensitivity, skin discoloration, alopecia, rashes, thyroid dysfunction (either hyper- or hypothyroidism), hepatitis, peripheral neuropathy or myopathy, corneal microdeposits, and rarely optic neuritis or pulmonary toxicity. Like all other antiarrhythmics, amiodarone can also be associated with cardiac side-effects including bradycardia and heart block, but is also associated with an increased frequency of *torsade de pointes* as well as monomorphic ventricular tachycardia and ventricular fibrillation.

The many drug interactions possible with amiodarone, particularly that with warfarin, are another drawback to its widespread use in AF. Thus, the potential for adverse effects with amiodarone limits the use of this drug for rate control in AF, and because of this it tends to be used only when other drugs have failed or are contraindicated. However, as amiodarone has no significant negatively ionotropic or vasodilatory actions, it is often the drug of

---

Amiodarone

- The potential for adverse effects limits the use for rate control in AF, and because of this it should be used only when other drugs have failed or are contraindicated
- Amiodarone has no significant negatively inotropic or vasodilatory actions, and is often the drug of choice in patients with heart failure or hypotension despite its unfavourable side-effect profile.

---

choice in patients with heart failure or hypotension despite its unfavourable side-effect profile.

Alternative class III antiarrhythmics with an improved side-effect profile are currently in development and ibutilide and dofetilide are other such agents already being used in the USA, but for cardioversion rather than rate control.[31,32]

Sotalol

As an antiarrhythmic with both class II and class III effects sotalol has long been used preferentially for rate and potential rhythm control benefits in AF. However, as a rhythm control agent in AF in actual randomized control trials sotalol has been disappointing considering its promising theoretical benefit.[33] Available trials are limited by their size and relatively low doses of sotalol used, and its potential benefit for conversion (if effective at higher doses), is its additional rate control action which means there is no requirement for the introduction of extra medications for rate control.

Sotalol was inferior to quinidine, for example, in converting recent onset AF to sinus rhythm in one trial,[34] and is comparable with placebo in AF of longer duration.[35] Studies report pharmacological cardioversion rates ranging from 8 to 49% with sotalol, but overall do not support the use of this drug for efficient conversion of AF to sinus rhythm.[33]

However, in the available trials, of those patients not attaining conversion to sinus rhythm, heart rate was controlled by its beta-blockade actions, and sotalol does seem to be an effective rate control agent. In a randomized placebo controlled trial in patients with acute spontaneous or induced AF (n=83), there was no significant increase in conversion rate with intravenous sotalol when compared with placebo, but a reduction of > 20% in ventricular rate within 30 min was achieved in the sotalol group more frequently than those on placebo.[35]

Side-effects of sotalol encompass both its class II and class III actions. For example, non-cardioselective beta-blockade can cause bronchospasm, heart block and exacerbation of heart failure, but due to class III actions it has also been associated with an increased incidence of torsade de pointes and other ventricular arrhythmias. For these reasons it is regarded by some as a beta-blocker with more side-effects and few of the potential benefits of a class III agent in the lower doses at which it is commonly used.

Sotalol

- Is an effective rate control agent, but it is highly proarrhythmic
- It is regarded by some as a beta-blocker with more side-effects and few of the potential benefits of a class III agent in the lower doses at which it is commonly used

CLASS I ANTIARRHYTHMICS

As with class III antiarrhythmics, the primary use of class Ia and Ic agents for AF and flutter is for pharmacological cardioversion to return the patient to sinus rhythm or to keep the patient with paroxysmal AF in sinus rhythm, rather than as rate control agents. However in trials for class Ic agents looking at efficacy of these agents for cardioversion in AF, in those patients who do not revert to sinus rhythm, rate is better controlled on propafenone than on placebo.

In two small studies this rate control action with propafenone has been demonstrated in comparison to placebo. In a study comparing intravenous propafenone to placebo, in the 17 patients who did not cardiovert in the propafenone group, a reduction in ventricular rate was reported (from 146 at baseline to 109 bpm).[36] In the other study of intravenous propafenone versus placebo, this time in 182 patients with recent onset AF, in the nine patients who did not convert to sinus rhythm the mean ventricular rate was significantly reduced over the 24 h follow-up period (from 143 ± 16 to 101 ± 18 bpm, $p < 0.0005$).[37] This evidence does not of course advocate the use of propafenone as a rate control agent, but in patients with acute AF in whom attempted pharmacological cardioversion is the management strategy, propafenone does offer modest rate control.

Flecainide has no such evidence for a rate control effect, and in one trial in which the rate control effect of flecainide was reported, flecainide was no more effective than placebo at slowing ventricular rate in those patients not cardioverted.[28] Similarly, evidence for rate control with class Ia agents (e.g. quinidine) does not exist, and if such agents are used for pharmacological cardioversion in acute AF, then adjunctive rate control agents are used until sinus rhythm is achieved.

Class I agents are associated with proarrhythmic potential side-effects, perhaps even more so than class III drugs, and their use is reserved for prophylactic prevention in paroxysmal AF and pharmacological cardioversion or facilitation of DC cardioversion, not for rate control in AF

OTHER CONSIDERATIONS FOR PHARMACOLOGICAL RATE CONTROL

Combination therapy

Potentially, combination antiarrhythmic use for improved rate control in AF has the hazard of the side-effects of both therapies, and increased risk of heart block or symptomatic pauses associated with treatment.

For rate control in AF, digoxin has been traditionally used as initial treatment, but due to its reduced efficacy and subsequent exacerbation of symptoms at times of increased sympathetic output (e.g. exercise, chest infection, acute heart failure), other agents are often added in.

Reflective of this, the majority of trials of drug combinations for rate control in AF involve evaluation of digoxin with another agent, versus digoxin alone or placebo (as summarized in a systematic review by Segal et al[3]). Of eight trials identified, comparing the combined effects of digoxin and calcium channel blocker with digoxin, seven found a significant decrease in mean resting heart rate with the combination therapy versus digoxin. In six of the studies, effect during exercise was also evaluated, and a statistically significant difference was also found for heart rate control during exercise in favor of the calcium channel blocker–digoxin combination in comparison with digoxin alone. Similarly trials examining the use of a combination of a beta-blocker and digoxin have found a reduced resting heart rate in comparison with digoxin alone in all combinations except labetolol–digoxin, and in all studies heart rate control during exercise was improved with the combination of a beta-blocker and digoxin for AF treatment.

In a comparative study, the combination of diltiazem and digoxin reduced resting heart rate more than propranolol and digoxin combination, and all three drugs given together were, not surprisingly, even more effective.[38] However, this study also demonstrated that the beta-blocker in combination with digoxin was more effective for heart rate control during exercise than diltiazem in combination with digoxin. Thus, when given in combination with digoxin, calcium channel blockers may reduce resting heart rate most effectively, and beta-blockers may reduce heart rate more effectively on exercise. Of

Combination treatment

- When given in combination with digoxin, calcium channel blockers may reduce resting heart rate most effectively, and beta-blockers may reduce heart rate more effectively on exercise

NOTE: the drug combination of verapamil plus a beta-blocker is *contraindicated* because of the high risk of complete heart block or asystole

course, the drug combination of verapamil plus a beta-blocker is *contraindicated* because of the high risk of complete heart block or asystole. Finally, amiodarone and digoxin in combination have also been shown to reduce heart rate.[39]

Rest versus exercise

As outlined above, both beta-blockers and rate-limiting calcium channel blockers are more effective than digoxin in the control of heart rate during exercise in patients with AF. However, although studies with digoxin found no significant heart rate reduction during exercise in comparison with placebo, in one study the cardiac output was higher in patients taking digoxin, and in another, time on the treadmill longer suggesting improved exercise capacity in those patients on digoxin.[8,10]

In patients on digoxin, patients who have either a beta-blocker or calcium channel blocker given in combination also have improved heart rate control on exercise, with perhaps the combination of a beta-blocker and digoxin being the most effective combination.[1]

Postoperative AF

AF occurs after cardiac surgery in an estimated 25–35% of cases.[40] Typically the arrhythmia is short-lived, but it can cause complications in terms of hemodynamic compromise and prolonged postoperative hospitalization.[41] Onset of AF tends to occur 1–5 days after surgery and is usually self-limiting. At 6–8 weeks follow-up, 90% of patients are in sinus rhythm.

Trials have largely focused on prevention of AF postcardiac surgery, with both prophylactic antiarrhythmic and pacing therapies tested. For example, sotalol, amiodarone and beta-blockade given postoperatively all seem to have some benefit in prevention of AF after cardiac surgery in randomized trials.[41–43] However, in those patients who develop postoperative AF (with no pre-existing arrhythmia), as the AF usually has a self-limited course, rate control is the mainstay of treatment. Beta-blockade is usually first-line therapy in patients with no contraindications, as beta-blockers help counteract the inevitable sympathetic overdrive postoperatively, and many of the patients will have been on beta-blockers preoperatively for their benefits in ischemic heart disease. Data from a recent meta-analysis are summarized in Fig. 16.2a–c.[44–85] This meta-analysis also confirms the

β-blockers versus placebo or no treatment for the prevention of postoperative AF in patients undergoing heart surgery

(a)	Number of randomized patients	Weight (%)	OR (95% CI random)	OR (95% CI random)
Stephenson [44]	42	0.2	2.33 (0.2, 27.91)	
Salazar [45]	223	3.5	0.41 (0.17, 0.99)	
Oka [46]	54	2.0	0.14 (0.03, 0.70)	
Mohr [48]	103	3.6	0.22 (0.08, 0.59)	
Silverman [48]	100	2.7	0.16 (0.04, 0.61)	
Williams [49]	60	1.1	0.16 (0.02, 1.43)	
Abel [50]	91	3.1	0.38 (0.14, 0.90)	
Ivey [51]	109	1.5	0.79 (0.27, 2.31)	
Ormerod [52]	60	1.4	0.46 (0.13, 1.72)	
White [53]	41	1.2	0.31 (0.07, 1.43)	
Myhre [54]	36	1.4	0.17 (0.03, 0.98)	
Janssen [55]	89	2.7	0.32 (0.11, 0.92)	
Matangi [56]	164	3.1	0.41 (0.17, 1.02)	
Materne [57]	71	2.3	0.06 (0.01, 0.53)	
Rubin [58]	77	2.4	0.32 (0.11, 0.95)	
Daudon [59]	100	4.1	0.01 (0.00, 0.25)	
Vecht [60]	132	1.3	0.69 (0.21, 2.30)	
Khuri [61]	141	3.0	1.34 (0.68, 2.61)	
Lamb [62]	60	1.9	0.07 (0.01, 0.58)	
Martinussen [63]	75	0.8	1.17 (0.31, 4.42)	
Matangi [64]	70	1.6	0.78 (0.27, 2.14)	
Babin-Ebel [65]	64	2.0	0.15 (0.03, 0.72)	
Ali [66]	210	6.7	0.34 (0.18, 0.64)	
Paull [67]	100	2.0	0.90 (0.36, 2.22)	
Gun [68]	500	10.1	0.50 (0.31, 0.80)	
Wenke [69]	200	7.2	0.07 (0.02, 0.21)	
Cybulsky [70]	1000	27.0	0.71 (0.55, 0.92)	
Total	3840	100.0	0.39 (0.28, 0.52)	

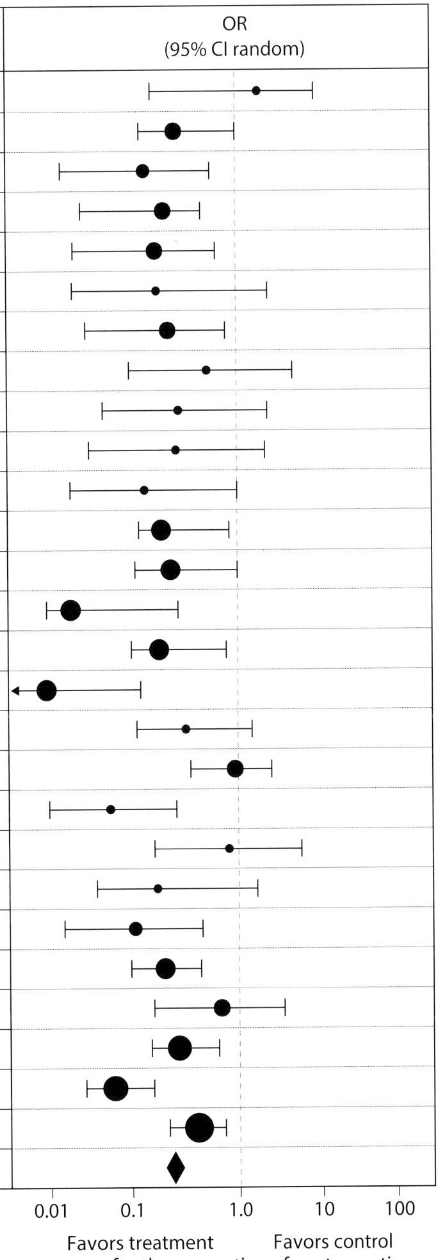

0.01　0.1　1.0　10　100
Favors treatment　　Favors control

Fig. 16.2 β-blockers (a), sotalol (b) and amiodarone (c) versus placebo or no treatment for the prevention of postoperative AF in patients undergoing heart surgery. Reproduced with permission from Crystal et al.[85]

Sotalol versus placebo or no treatment for the prevention of postoperative AF in patients undergoing heart surgery

(b)	Number of randomized patients	Weight (%)	OR (95% CI random)	OR (95% CI random)
Evrard [71]	206	18.8	0.22 (0.11, 0.42)	
Gomes [43]	85	7.3	0.24 (0.08, 0.72)	
Jacquet [72]	36	3.7	0.45 (0.09, 2.26)	
Jannsen [55]	91	2.3	0.05 (0.01, 0.38)	
Nystrom [73]	101	7.4	0.27 (0.01, 0.80)	
Pfisterer [74]	255	21.9	0.46 (0.27, 0.79)	
Suttorp [75]	300	21.0	0.44 (0.25, 0.78)	
Weber [76]	220	19.6	0.48 (0.26, 0.86)	
Total	1294	100.0	0.35 (0.26, 0.49)	

0.001 0.02 1.0 50 1000
Favors treatment   Favors control

P< 0.00001

Amiodarone versus placebo or no treatment for the prevention of postoperative AF in patients undergoing heart surgery

(c)	Number of randomized patients	Weight (%)	OR (95% CI random)	OR (95% CI random)
Butler [77]	120	4.1	0.36 (0.11, 1.21)	
Daoud [42]	124	10.5	0.29 (0.14, 0.62)	
Dorge [78]	150	11.5	0.57 (0.28, 1.18)	
Giri [79]	220	17.7	0.51 (0.21, 1.22)	
Guarnieri [80]	300	28.2	0.61 (0.39, 0.98)	
Hohnloser [81]	77	2.3	0.20 (0.04, 1.03)	
Lee [82]	150	8.5	0.27 (0.11, 0.62)	
Redle [83]	143	11.4	0.67 (0.32, 1.39)	
Treggiari-Venzi [84]	100	5.9	0.44 (0.16, 1.21)	
Total	1384	100.0	0.48 (0.37, 0.61)	

0.01 0.1 1.0 10 100
Favors treatment   Favors control

P< 0.00001

Fig. 16.2, *cont'd*.

increased length of stay associated with postoperative AF (Fig. 16.3).[85]

It should be noted that rate limiting calcium channel blockers can be used for ventricular rate control where beta-blockers are contraindicated. Intravenous digoxin is also used but there is little evidence for this.

Post myocardial infarction

AF is also a common cardiac arrhythmia seen following a myocardial infarction. It can complicate up to 20% of cases. Typically, patients developing AF post myocardial infarction do worse, compared with those who remain in sinus rhythm,

Effect of treatment on hospital length of stay

	Number of randomized patients	Difference, days (95% CI random)	
Beta-blockers	1200	2.33 (0.2, 27.91)	
Sotalol	808	0.41 (0.17, 0.99)	
Amiodarone	944	0.14 (0.03, 0.70)	
Biatrial pacing	744	0.22 (0.08, 0.59)	

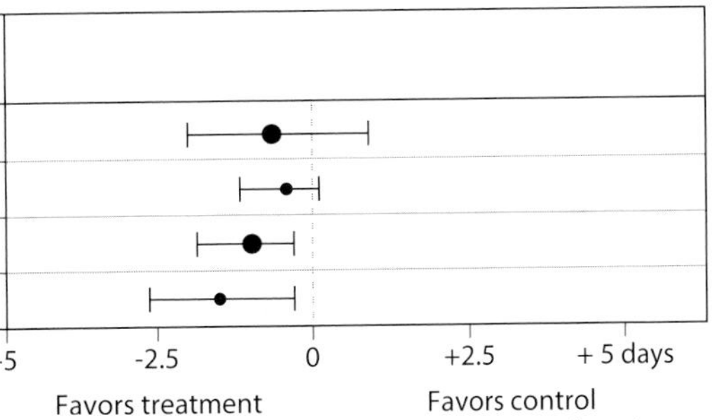

-5   -2.5   0   +2.5   + 5 days

Favors treatment   Favors control

Fig. 16.3 Effect of treatment on hospital length of stay. There was no evidence that reducing postoperative AF reduced stroke. However, data on stroke are incomplete. Reproduced with permission from Crystal et al.[85]

these patients tend to have a poorer prognosis and larger myocardial infarcts.[86–88]

Evidence from the GISSI-2 trial also showed an increased mortality in those patients who developed AF post myocardial infarction compared with those who remained in sinus rhythm even in the thrombolytic era, both in hospital and at 6 months follow-up.[89]

Whether AF itself causes increased mortality, or is just an indicator of comorbidities in the post myocardial infarction setting that are prognostically unfavorable, is unclear. In the acute setting, control is certainly important, to reduce the workload on an already ischemic, and infarcting myocardium.

Beta-blockers would be the drugs of choice in AF complicating an acute myocardial infarction in those with no contraindications due to their efficacy as rate control agents even in the setting of increased sympathetic drive, and for their prognostic benefits post myocardial infarction.[90] In those patients with reversible airways disease, a rate limiting calcium channel blocker would be a reasonable alternative, although there is less evidence from randomized control trials.

For those patients with evidence of cardiac failure or hypotension, amiodarone is often used because of its minimal negative ionotropic effect in comparison with other agents. It also has the advantage of potentially suppressing ventricular arrhythmias which are common in the post myocardial infarction setting, as well as potential rhythm control benefits. However, it should be used at increased doses intravenously for optimal rate control effects.

Digoxin administration post myocardial infarction has been associated with increased mortality, and should therefore be avoided if at all possible.[91] Class Ic agents as well as being ineffective for rate control, should also be avoided in people with ischemic heart disease and heart failure. This follows the CAST trial in which flecainide and encainide were given for arrhythmia suppression after myocardial infarction, but in which there was an excess of proarrhythmic side-effects and subsequent increased mortality in the group on antiarrhythmics.[92]

AF in myocardial infarction

- Beta-blockers are the drugs of choice in patients with no contraindications due to their efficacy as rate control agents even in the setting of increased sympathetic drive, and for their prognostic benefits post myocardial infarction

- In patients with reversible airways disease, a rate limiting calcium channel blocker is a reasonable alternative

- Amiodarone is often used because of its minimal negative inotropic effect in patients with heart failure. However, it should be used at increased doses intravenously for optimal rate control effects

In the setting of heart failure

For patients with both AF and LV dysfunction, rate control agents with minimal negative iontropic effects are often favored. This means that traditionally digoxin with its positive inotropic actions and amiodarone with its minimal negative ionotropic effects have been regarded as first-line agents.

Digoxin does have potential benefits in heart failure patients in terms of reduced morbidity and rehospitalization rates, but there has been no prognostic benefit demonstrated.[93] These potential benefits plus rate control actions still make it a good choice for the patient with AF and stable heart failure. However, in acute heart failure, the associated sympathetic overdrive often obliterates its actions as an effective rate control agent.

The use of amiodarone for effective rate control in heart failure is backed by randomized control trials, as outlined above, and it would certainly be the drug of choice for patients with AF and left ventricular dysfunction based on this evidence. However, its side-effect profile often limits prescribing.

Beta-blockers, previously contraindicated in heart failure because of their negative ionotropic effect, may be introduced slowly in stable heart failure and uptitrated as tolerated, with proven prognostic benefit.[11] In the patient with heart failure and AF, beta-blockers could be introduced for this purpose and additional rate control actions.

One small trial (n=14) of carvedilol in chronic heart failure patients already on digoxin, showed a significant reduction in the patients resting heart rate and maximal heart rates on exercise and an increased exercise time (all $p< 0.001$), as well as a symptomatic improvement in exercise intolerance and palpitations.[94]

Calcium channel blockers are also traditionally avoided for AF rate control in patients with heart failure, but evidence from one small randomized control trial reported the safe use of intravenous diltiazem in the acute setting to control rate, with only hypotension as a potential side-effect, but no exacerbations of heart failure reported.[14] This is possibly because of the hemodynamic consequences of the fast ventricular rate in uncontrolled AF being more contributory to the heart failure presentation, than the presence of pre-existing left ventricular myocardial hypokinesis in these patients. Further trials are required before these antiarrhythmics are used longer term in patients with moderate to severe LV dysfunction and AF.

Non-pharmacological methods

For AF that is refractory to pharmacological rate control, or in the patient who is very symptomatic even with perceived adequate rate control, there are alternatives.

Failure to control the ventricular rate in AF can be treated by the 'ablate and pace' approach, which involves ablation of the Bundle of His to create AV blockade and permanent ventricular pacing.[95] This method controls ventricular rate effectively, but there is no restoration of atrioventricular synchrony, or suppression of atrial activity so the patient can still be symptomatic with palpitations and dyspnea, despite a regular ventricular rate. The patient is also under the disadvantage of being made pacemaker dependent, so it is often a method reserved for the more elderly, or as a last resort in the patient completely resistant to all pharmacological methods.

Pacemakers are often required in the setting of sick sinus syndrome where there are often periods of AF interspersed with sinus rhythm, sinus bradycardia and even sinus arrest, and where adequate rate control therapy can worsen periods of bradycardia or prolong pauses. In these cases, both antiarrhythmic drugs and pacing may be necessary. The pacemaker used should be atrial or dual-chamber as ventricular pacing alone can provoke AF in periods of sinus rhythm or sinus bradycardia.[96]

Operative options are also available, including the Maze procedure or pulmonary vein isolation, but these are to 'obliterate' AF rather than for rate control. Both seem to be effective procedures but require major operative intervention and pacing is often required postoperatively.

SUMMARY

Beta-blockers, calcium antagonists and digoxin all effectively reduce heart rate in AF, both in the acute setting and long term, with proven advantages in certain settings and limitations in others (as summarized in Tables 16.3 and 16.4).

Drug choice for rate control should therefore take into consideration associated

Table 16.3 Drugs commonly used in atrial fibrillation

	Route of administration	Loading dose (if required)	Maintenance dose
Class I			
Quinidine	Oral	Nil	200–400 mg 3–4 times a day
Flecainide	Oral	Nil	50 mg twice a day Max 150 mg twice a day
Flecainide	Intravenous	2 mg/kg over 10–30 min. Max 150 mg.	1.5 mg/kg for 1 h. Then, 100–250 mcg/kg/h up to a max of 600 mg/d.
Propafenone	Oral	Nil	150 mg 3 times/d increased gradually over days to max. 300 mgs 3 times a day (if > 70 kg)
Class II			
(e.g.) Metoprolol	Oral Intravenous	Nil 5–15 mg, at rate 1–2 mg/min	25–100 mg × 2
Class III			
Sotalol	Oral	Nil	40 mg twice a day increased gradually over days to max 160 mg twice a day
Amiodarone	Oral	200 mg 3 times a day for 1 week. 200 mg twice a day for next week	200 mg/d
	Intravenous	5 mg/kg over 20–120 min	Max1.2 gm/d (including loading dose)
Class IV			
Diltiazem	Oral and (not UK) Intravenous	60–180 mg × 3	
Verapamil	Oral Intravenous	Nil 5–10 mg i.v.	40–160 mg × 3
Digoxin	Oral Intravenous	1–1.5 mg/d in divided doses 0.5–1 mg max. given in fractions over 10–20 mins up to 4 hourly	62.5–500 mcg /d nil

Table 16.4 Strategies for heart rate control in atrial fibrillation

	Clinical evidence grade	Control of resting heart rate	Control of exercise heart rate	Thrombo-embolic risk still present?	Symptomatic benefit	Haemo-dynamic benefit
Digoxin monotherapy	B	Yes	No	Yes	+	+
Digoxin + betablocker or calcium antagonist	B	Yes	Yes	Yes	++	+
Radiofrequency ablation + pacemaker	B	Yes	Yes	Yes	++	++
Radiofrequency modification	C	Yes	Yes	Yes	+++	+++

comorbidities in which the chosen antiarrhythmic may be of potential benefit (for example preferential use of a beta-blocker in a patient with coronary artery disease), or in which the antiarrhythmic may be detrimental and is therefore contraindicated (for example use of a beta-blocker in a patient with reversible airways disease causing bronchospasm) (Table 16.5).

The choice of rate control agent should also take into account the setting in which the AF is occurring, that is, acute or

Table 16.5 Drug options for AF with comorbid conditions

AF with hypertension
Beta blockers, calcium channel blockers

AF with ischemic heart disease
Beta-blockers, calcium channel blockers

AF with heart failure
Digoxin, amiodarone, beta-blocker (with caution, in patients on optimal therapy)

AF with thyrotoxicosis
Non-specific beta blocker

Lone AF in young healthy individual (paroxysmal)
Class IC, sotalol, beta-blockers

chronic, association with heart failure, and the individual patient needs in terms of exercise capacity and symptom control. It should be noted that all of these agents (with the exception of class Ic antiarrhythmics), should not be used in patients with evidence of an accessory pathway, as slowing preferentially at the AV node can result in rapid 1:1 conduction of fibrillatory waves down the accessory pathway with resultant ventricular fibrillation.

Although rate control has always been considered important in the treatment of AF, rhythm control has always been thought to be preferable and is often the primary focus of treatment. Restoration and maintenance of sinus rhythm has always been assumed to be superior to rate control in AF, both in terms of short-term benefits and long-term outcome, but there was, until recently no prospective data to compare the approach of rate control and anticoagulation with attempted cardioversion.

Several trials have attempted to address this. The Pharmacological Intervention in Atrial Fibrillation (PIAF) trial, attempted to compare pharmacological rate control (with diltiazem), with pharmacological rhythm control (with amiodarone), in terms of symptom control, in 252 patients with AF of 7 days to 360 days duration.[97] There was restoration of sinus rhythm in 23% of patients given amiodarone. Over a 1-year follow-up period there was no significant difference in symptomatic improvement or quality of life scores between the two groups, but exercise tolerance (quantified by distance walked on a 6 min walk test) was better in the rhythm control group. However, the rate of hospitalization in this group was significantly higher than the rate control group [87 of 127 (69%) patients on amiodarone vs 30 of 125 (24%) patients on diltiazem, p=0.001] and the adverse event rate on amiodarone was also higher.

The Atrial Fibrillation Follow-up Investigation of Rhythm Management (AFFIRM) Study randomized patients with AF to ventricular rate control and anticoagulation or rhythm control and anticoagulation therapeutic strategies.[98] Preliminary data suggests that there was no difference between groups in terms of mortality (Fig. 16.4).

This suggests that if patients with AF are adequately rate controlled and anticoagulated their long-term outlook is the same as those treated with a more aggressive rhythm control strategy. Therefore in view of the potential hazards of pursuing sinus rhythm with possible class I and III antiarrhythmic side-effects, and with adverse events associated with direct current (DC) cardioversion, attempts at restoration of sinus rhythm should perhaps be considered only in those patients with symptomatic AF of short duration.

With this evidence from PIAF and AFFIRM trials, rate control and anticoagulation could well become the mainstay of treatment for AF in the future.

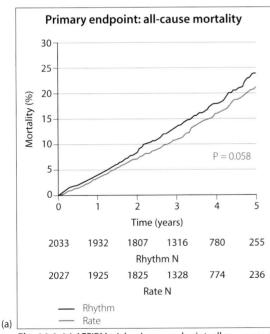

(a)

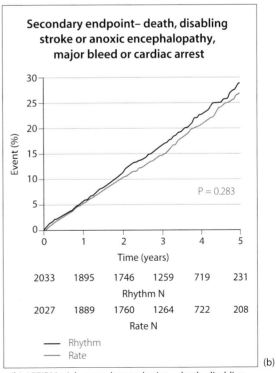

(b)

Fig. 16.4 (a) AFFIRM trial: primary endpoint: all-cause mortality. (b) AFFIRM trial: secondary endpoint – death, disabling stroke or anoxic encephalopathy, major bleed or cardiac arrest.

References

1. Farshi R, Kistner D, Sarma JS, et al. Ventricular rate control in chronic atrial fibrillation during daily activity and programmed exercise: a crossover open label study of five drug regimens. J Am Coll Cardiol 1999; 33: 304–310.

2. Sweany AE, Moncloa F, Vickers FF, et al. Antiarrhythmic effects of intravenous timolol in supraventricular arrhythmias. Clin Pharmacol Ther 1985; 37:124–127.

3. Segal JB, Macnamara RL, Miller MR, et al. The evidence regarding the drugs used for ventricular rate control. J Fam Pract 2000; 49:47–58.

4. Wong CK, Lau CP, Leung WH, et al. Usefulness of labetolol in chronic atrial fibrillation. Am J Cardiol 1990; 66:1212–1215.

5. Myers J, Atwood JE, Sullivan M, et al. Perceived exertion and gas exchange after calcium and beta-blockade in atrial fibrillation after calcium and beta-blockade in atrial fibrillation. J Appl Physiol 1987; 63:97–104.

6. Lin SK, Morganroth J, Heng M, et al. Effect of orally administered celiprolol in patients with chronic atrial fibrillation. J Cardiol Pharm 1986; 8(Suppl 4):S112–115.

7. Koh KK, Song JH, Kwon KS, et al. Comparative study of efficacy and safety of low dose diltiazem or betaxolol in combination with digoxin to control ventricular rate in chronic atrial fibrillation: randomised crossover study. Int J Cardiol 1995; 52:167–174.

8. Lewis RV, McMurray J, McDevitt DG. Effects of atenolol, verapamil and xamoterol on heart rate and exercise tolerance in digitalised patients with chronic atrial fibrillation. J Cardiovasc Pharmacol 1989; 13:1–6.

9. Lundstrom T, Moor E, Ryden L. Differential effects of xamoterol and verapamil on ventricular rate regulation in patients with chronic atrial fibrillation. Am Heart J 1992; 124:917–923.

10. Ang EL, Chan WL, Cleland JG, et al. Placebo-controlled trial of xameterol versus digoxin in chronic atrial fibrillation. Br Heart J 1990; 64:256–260.

11. CIBIS-II Investigators. The Cardiac Insufficiency Study II (CIBIS-II): a randomised trial. Lancet 1999; 353:9–13.

12. Salerno DM, Dias VC, Kleiger RE, et al. Efficacy and safety of intravenous diltiazem for the treatment of atrial fibrillation and flutter: the Diltiazem-Atrial Fibrillation/Flutter Study Group. Am J Cardiol 1989; 63:1046–1051.

13. Schreck DM, Rivera AR, Tricarico VJ. Emergency management of atrial fibrillation and flutter: intravenous diltiazem versus intravenous digoxin. Ann Emerg Med 1997; 29:135–140.

14. Goldenberg IF, Lewis WR, Dias VC, et al. Intravenous diltiazem for the treatment of patients with atrial fibrillation or flutter and moderate to severe congestive heart failure. Am J Cardiol 1994; 74:884–889.

15. Aronow WS, Ferlinz J. Verapamil versus placebo in atrial fibrillation and atrial flutter. Clin Invest Med 1980; 3:35–39.

16. Waxman HL, Myerberg RJ, Appel R, et al. Verapamil for control of ventricular rate in paroxysmal supraventricular tachycardia and atrial fibrillation or flutter: a double blind randomised cross-over study. Ann Int Med 1981; 94:1–6.

17. Lewis RV, Irvine N, McDevitt DG. Relationships between heart rate, exercise tolerance and cardiac output in atrial fibrillation: the effects of treatment with digoxin, verapamil and diltiazem. Eur Heart J 1988; 9:777–781.

18. Panidis IP, Morganroth J, Baessler C. Effectiveness and safety of oral verapamil to control exercise-induced tachycardia in patients with atrial fibrillation receiving digitalis. Am J Cardiol 1983; 52:1197–1201.

19. Lundstrom T, Ryden L. Ventricular rate control and exercise performance in chronic atrial fibrillation: effects of diltiazem and verapamil. J Am Coll Cardiol 1990; 16:86–90.

20. Phillips BG, Gandhi AJ, Sanoski CA, et al. Comparison of intravenous diltiazem and verapamil for the acute treatment of atrial fibrillation and flutter. Pharmacotherapy 1997; 17:1238–1245.

21. DAAF Trial group. Intravenous digoxin in acute atrial fibrillation. Results of a randomised placebo-controlled multicentre trial in 239 patients. The Digitalis in Acute Atrial Fibrillation Trial Group. Eur Heart J 1997; 18:649–654.

22. Jordeans L, Trouerbach J, Calle P, et al. Conversion of atrial fibrillation to sinus rhythm and rate control by digoxin in comparison to placebo. Eur Heart J 1997; 18:643–648.

23. Rawles JM, Metcalf MJ, Jennings K. Time of occurrence, duration and ventricular rate of paroxysmal atrial fibrillation: the effect of digoxin. Br Heart J 1990; 63:225–227.

24. Lip GYH, Li Saw Hee FL. Paroxysmal atrial fibrillation. QJM 2000; 94:665–678.

25. Wellens HJJ, Brugada P, Abdollah H, et al. A comparison of the electrophysiological effects of intravenous and oral amiodarone in the same patient. Circulation 1984; 69:120–124.

26. Galve E, Rius T, Ballester R, et al. Intravenous amiodarone in treatment of recent onset atrial fibrillation: results of a randomised control study. J Am Coll Cardiol 1996; 27: 1079–1082.

27. Hou ZY, Chang MS, Chen CY, et al. Acute treatment of recent onset atrial fibrillation and flutter with a tailored dosing regimen of intravenous amiodarone. A randomised digoxin-controlled study. Eur Heart J 1995; 16:521–528.

28. Donovan KD, Power BM, Hockings BE, et al. Intravenous flecainide versus amiodarone for recent onset atrial fibrillation. Am J Cardiol 1995; 75:693–697.

29. Delle KG, Geppert A, Neubteufl T, et al. Amiodarone versus diltiazem for rate control in

critically ill patients. Crit Care Med 2001; 29:1149–1153.

30. Deedwania PC, Singh BN, et al. Spontaneous conversion and maintenance of sinus rhythm by amiodarone in patients with heart failure and atrial fibrillation: Observations from the Veterans Affairs Congestive Heart Failure Survival Trial. Circulation 1998; 98:2574–2579.

31. Foster RH, Wilde MI, Markham A. Ibutilide. A review of its pharmacological properties and clinical potential in the acute management of atrial flutter and atrial fibrillation. Drugs 1997; 54:312–330.

32. Vos MA, Golitsyn SR, Stangl K, Ruda MY, et al. Superiority of ibutilide (a new class III agent) over DL-sotalol in converting atrial flutter and atrial fibrillation. The Ibutilide/Sotalol Comparator Study Group. Heart 1998; 79:568–575.

33. Ferreira E, Sunderji R, Gin K. Is oral sotalol effective in converting atrial fibrillation to sinus rhythm? Pharmacotherapy 1997; 17:1233–1237.

34. Halinen MO, Huttunen M, Paakinen S, et al. Comparison of sotalol with digoxin-quinidine for conversion of acute atrial fibrillation to sinus rhythm. Am J Cardiol 1995; 76:495–498.

35. Sung RJ, Tan HL, Karagounis L, et al. Intravenous sotalol for the termination of supraventricular tachycardia and atrial fibrillation/flutter: a multicentre randomised double-blind placebo-controlled study. Am Heart J 1995; 129:739–748.

36. Fresco P, Proclemer A, Pavan A, et al. Intravenous propafenone in paroxysmal atrial fibrillation: a randomised, placebo controlled, multicentre clinical trial. Paroxysmal Atrial Fibrillation Italian Trial (PAFIT)-2 Investigators. Clin Cardiol 1996; 19:409–412.

37. Bellandi F, Cantini F, Pedone T, et al. Effectiveness of intravenous propafenone for conversion of recent onset atrial fibrillation: A placebo controlled study. Clin Cardiol 1995; 18:631–634.

38. Dahlstrom CG, Edvardson N, Nasheng C, et al. Effects of diltiazem, propranolol, and their combination in the control of atrial fibrillation. Clin Cardiol 1992; 15:280–284.

39. Zehender M, Hohnloser S, Muller B, et al. Effects of amiodarone versus quinidine and verapamil in patients with chronic atrial fibrillation: results of a comparative study and a 2-year follow-up. J Am Coll Cardiol 1992; 19:1054–1059

40. Bharucha DB, Kowey PR. Management and prevention of atrial fibrillation after cardiovascular surgery. Am J Cardiol 2000; 85:20D–24D.

41. Kowey PR, Taylor JE, Rials SJ, et al. Meta-analysis of the effectiveness of prophylactic drug therapy in preventing supraventricular arrhythmias early after coronary artery bypass grafting. Am J Cardiol 1992; 69:963–965.

42. Daoud EG, Strickberger S-A, Man KC, et al. Preoperative amiodarone as prophylaxis against atrial fibrillation after heart surgery. N Engl J Med 1997; 337:1785–1791.

43. Gomes JA, Ip J, Santoni-Rugui F, et al. Oral D,1 sotalol reduces the incidence of post operative atrial fibrillation in coronary artery bypass surgery patients: a randomised double-blind, placebo-controlled study. J Am Coll Cardiol 1999; 34:334–339.

44. Stephenson LW, MacVaugh H 3rd, Tomasello DN, et al. Propranolol for prevention of postoperative cardiac arrhythmias: a randomized study. Ann Thorac Surg 1980; 29:113–116.

45. Salazar C, Frishman W, Friedman S, et al. β-blockade therapy for supraventricular tachyarrhythmias after coronary surgery: a propranolol withdrawal syndrome? Angiology 1979; 30:816–819.

46. Oka Y, Frishman W, Becker RM, et al. Clinical pharmacology of the new beta-adrenergic blocking drugs, part 10: β-adrenoceptor blockade and coronary artery surgery. Am Heart J 1980; 99:255–269.

47. Mohr R, Smolinsky A, Goor DA. Prevention of supraventricular tachyarrhythmia with low-dose propranolol after coronary bypass. J Thorac Cardiovasc Surg 1981; 81:840–845.

48. Silverman NA, Wright R, Levitsky S. Efficacy of low-dose propranolol in preventing postoperative supraventricular tachyarrhythmias: a prospective, randomized study. Ann Surg 1982; 196:194–197.

49. Williams JB, Stephenson LW, Holford FD, et al. Arrhythmia prophylaxis using propranolol after coronary artery surgery. Ann Thorac Surg. 1982; 34:435–438.

50. Abel RM, van Gelder HM, Pores IH, et al. Continued propranolol administration following coronary bypass surgery: antiarrhythmic effects. Arch Surg 1983; 118:727–731.

51. Ivey MF, Ivey TD, Bailey WW, et al. Influence of propranolol on supraventricular tachycardia early after coronary artery revascularization: a randomized trial. J Thorac Cardiovasc Surg 1983; 85:214–218.

52. Ormerod OJ, McGregor CG, Stone DL, et al. Arrhythmias after coronary bypass surgery. Br Heart J 1984; 51:618–621.

53. White HD, Antman EM, Glynn MA, et al. Efficacy and safety of timolol for prevention of supraventricular tachyarrhythmias after coronary artery bypass surgery. Circulation 1984; 70:479–484.

54. Myhre ES, Sorlie D, Aarbakke J, et al. Effects of low dose propranolol after coronary bypass surgery. J Cardiovasc Surg (Torino) 1984; 25:348–352.

55. Janssen J, Loomans L, Harink J, et al. Prevention and treatment of supraventricular tachycardia shortly after coronary artery bypass grafting: a randomized open trial. Angiology 1986; 37:601–609.

56. Matangi MF, Neutze JM, Graham KJ, et al. Arrhythmia prophylaxis after aorta-coronary bypass: the effect of minidose propranolol. J Thorac Cardiovasc Surg 1985; 89:439–443.

57. Materne P, Larbuisson R, Collignon P, et al. Prevention by acebutolol of rhythm disorders

following coronary bypass surgery. Int J Cardiol 1985; 8:275–286.

58. Rubin DA, Nieminski KE, Reed GE, et al. Predictors, prevention, and long-term prognosis of atrial fibrillation after coronary artery bypass graft operations. J Thorac Cardiovasc Surg 1987; 94:331–335.

59. Daudon P, Corcos T, Gandjbakhch I, et al. Prevention of atrial fibrillation or flutter by acebutolol after coronary bypass grafting. Am J Cardiol 1986; 58:933–966.

60. Vecht RJ, Nicolaides EP, Ikweuke JK, et al. Incidence and prevention of supraventricular tachyarrhythmias after coronary bypass surgery. Int J Cardiol 1986; 13:125–134.

61. Khuri SF, Okike ON, Josa M, et al. Efficacy of nadolol in preventing supraventricular tachycardia after coronary artery bypass grafting. Am J Cardiol 1987; 60:51D–58D.

62. Lamb RK, Prabhakar G, Thorpe JA, et al. The use of atenolol in the prevention of supraventricular arrhythmias following coronary artery surgery. Eur Heart J 1988; 9:32–36.

63. Martinussen HJ, Lolk A, Szczepanski C, et al. Supraventricular tachyarrhythmias after coronary bypass surgery: a double blind randomized trial of prophylactic low dose propranolol. Thorac Cardiovasc Surg. 1988; 36:206–207.

64. Matangi MF, Strickland J, Garbe GJ, et al. Atenolol for the prevention of arrhythmias following coronary artery bypass grafting. Can J Cardiol 1989; 5:229–234.

65. Babin-Ebell J, Keith PR, Elert O. Efficacy and safety of low-dose propranolol versus diltiazem in the prophylaxis of supraventricular tachyarrhythmia after coronary artery bypass grafting. Eur J Cardiothorac Surg 1996; 10:412-416.

66. Ali IM, Sanalla AA, Clark V. β-blocker effects on postoperative atrial fibrillation. Eur J Cardiothorac Surg 1997; 11:1154–1157.

67. Paull DL, Tidwell SL, Guyton SW, et al. β blockade to prevent atrial dysrhythmias following coronary bypass surgery. Am J Surg 1997; 173:419–421.

68. Gun C, Bianco ACM, Freire RB, et al. β-blocker effects on postoperative atrial fibrillation after coronary artery by-pass surgery. J Am Coll Card. CD-ROM of Abstracts from World Cardiology Congress 3801; 1998.

69. Wenke K, Parsa MH, Imhof M, et al. Efficacy of metoprolol in prevention of supraventricular arrhythmias after coronary artery bypass grafting [in German]. Z Kardiol 1999; 88:647–652.

70. Cybulsky I, Connolly S, Gent M, et al. β blocker length of stay study (BLOSS): a randomized trial of metoprolol for reduction of postoperative length of stay. Can J Cardiol 2000; 16:238F. Abstract.

71. Evrard P, Gonzalez M, Jamart J, et al. Prophylaxis of supraventricular and ventricular arrhythmias after coronary artery bypass grafting with low-dose sotalol. Ann Thorac Surg 2000; 70:151–156.

72. Jacquet L, Evenepoel M, Marenne F, et al.

73. Nystrom U, Edvardsson N, Berggren H, et al. Oral sotalol reduces the incidence of atrial fibrillation after coronary artery bypass surgery. Thorac Cardiovasc Surg 1993; 41:34–37.

74. Pfisterer ME, Kloter-Weber UC, Huber M, et al. Prevention of supraventricular tachyarrhythmias after open heart operation by low-dose sotalol: a prospective, double-blind, randomized, placebo-controlled study. Ann Thorac Surg 1997; 64:1113–1119.

75. Suttorp MJ, Kingma JH, Peels HO, et al. Effectiveness of sotalol in preventing supraventricular tachyarrhythmias shortly after coronary artery bypass grafting. Am J Cardiol 1991; 68:1163–1169.

76. Weber UK, Osswald S, Buser P, et al. Significance of supraventricular tachyarrhythmias after coronary artery bypass graft surgery and their prevention by low-dose sotalol: a prospective double-blind randomized placebo-controlled study. J Cardiovasc Pharmacol Ther 1998; 3:209–216.

77. Butler J, Harriss DR, Sinclair M, et al. Amiodarone prophylaxis for tachycardias after coronary artery surgery: a randomised, double blind, placebo controlled trial. Br Heart J 1993; 70:56–60.

78. Dorge H, Schoendube FA, Schoberer M, et al. Intraoperative amiodarone as prophylaxis against atrial fibrillation after coronary operations. Ann Thorac Surg 2000; 69:1358–1362.

79. Giri S, White CM, Dunn AB, et al. Oral amiodarone for prevention of atrial fibrillation after open heart surgery, the Atrial Fibrillation Suppression Trial (AFIST): a randomised placebo-controlled trial. Lancet 2001; 357:830–836.

80. Guarnieri T, Nolan S, Gottlieb SO, et al. Intravenous amiodarone for the prevention of atrial fibrillation after open heart surgery: the Amiodarone Reduction in Coronary Heart (ARCH) trial. J Am Coll Cardiol 1999; 34:343–347.

81. Hohnloser SH, Meinertz T, Dammbacher T, et al. Electrocardiographic and antiarrhythmic effects of intravenous amiodarone: results of a prospective, placebo-controlled study. Am Heart J 1991; 121:89–95.

82. Lee SH, Chang CM, Lu MJ, et al. Intravenous amiodarone for prevention of atrial fibrillation after coronary artery bypass grafting. Ann Thorac Surg 2000; 70:157–161.

83. Redle JD, Khurana S, Marzan R, et al. Prophylactic oral amiodarone compared with placebo for prevention of atrial fibrillation after coronary artery bypass surgery. Am Heart J 1999; 138:144–150.

84. Treggiari-Venzi MM, Waeber JL, Perneger TV, et al. Intravenous amiodarone or magnesium sulphate is not cost-beneficial prophylaxis for atrial fibrillation after coronary artery bypass surgery. Br J Anaesth 2000; 85:690–695.

85. Crystal E, Connolly SJ, Sleik K, et al. Interventions on prevention of postoperative atrial fibrillation in patients undergoing heart surgery: a meta-analysis. Circulation 2002; 106:75–80.

86. Suguira T, Iwasaka T, Ogawa A, et al. Atrial fibrillation in acute myocardial infarction. Am J Cardiol 1985; 56:27.

87. Goldberg RJ, Seeley D, Becker RC et al. Impact of atrial fibrillation on the in-hospital and longterm survival of patients with acute myocardial infarction: a community wide perspective. Am Heart J 1990; 119: 991

88. Sakata K, Kurihara H, Iwamori K, et al. Clinical and prognostic significance of atrial fibrillation in acute myocardial infarction. Am J Cardiol 1997; 80:1522–1527.

89. Ledda A, Maggioni AP, Franzosi MG, et al. Incidence and prognostic value of paroxysmal atrial fibrillation in 111,493 patients with confirmed acute myocardial infarction treated with thrombolytic agents. J Am Coll Cardiol 1994; 23:313A.

90. First International Study of Infarct Survival (ISIS-1) Collaborative Group. Randomised trial of intravenous atenolol amongst 16027 cases of suspected acute myocardial infarction. Lancet 1986; 2:57–66.

91. Bigger JT, Fleiss JL, Rolnitzky LM, et al. Effect of digitalis on survival after acute myocardial infarction. Am J Cardiol 1985; 55:623–630.

92. The Cardiac Arrhythmia Suppression Trial Investigators. Preliminary report: effect of ecainide and flecainide on mortality in a randomised trial of arrhythmia suppression after myocardial infarction. NEJM 1989; 321:406–412.

93. The Digitalis Investigation Group. The effect of digoxin on mortality and morbidity in patients with heart failure. N Engl J Med 1997; 336:525–533.

94. Agarwal AK, Venugopalan P. Beneficial effect of carvedilol on heart rate respose to exercise in digitalised patients with heart failure in atrial fibrillation due to idiopathic dilated cardiomyopathy. Eur J Heart Fail 2001; 3:437–440.

95. Kay GN, Ellenborg KA, Guidici M, et al.The Ablate and Pace Trial: a prospective study of catheter ablation of the AV conduction system and permanent pacemaker implantation for treatment of atrial fibrillation. APT investigators. J Interv Card Electrophysiol 1998; 2:121–135.

96. Rosenqvist M, Brandt J, Schuller H. Long term pacing in sinus node disease: effects of stimulation mode on cardiovascular morbidity and mortality. Am Heart J 1988; 116:16–22.

97. Hohnloser SH, Kuck K, Lilienthal J. Rhythm or rate control in atrial fibrillation – Pharmacological Intervention in Atrial Fibrillation: a randomised trial. Lancet 2000; 356:1789–194.

98. Wyse DG, Waldo AL, DiMarco JP, et al. The Atrial Fibrillation Follow-up Investigation of Rhythm Management (AFFIRM) Investigators. A comparison of rate control and rhythm control in patients with atrial fibrillation. N Engl J Med 2002; 347:1825–33.

Cardioversion of persistent atrial fibrillation

Dwayne S G Conway MRCP

City Hospital, Birmingham, UK

Gregory Y H Lip MD FRCP DFM FACC FESC

City Hospital, Birmingham, UK

DC cardioversion has been developed and refined to become a mainstay in the treatment of both supraventricular and ventricular arrhythmias

Introduction

It is now more than 40 years since Lown and colleagues pioneered the use of a synchronized external electrical current to terminate cardiac arrhythmias.[1] During those intervening years, the practice of direct current (DC) cardioversion has been developed and refined to become a mainstay in the treatment of both supraventricular and ventricular arrhythmias. Modern use of DC cardioversion bridges the clinical spectrum from the emergency resuscitation of life-threatening ventricular arrhythmias in the setting of cardiac arrest (ventricular defibrillation) to the long-term outpatient management of patients with atrial fibrillation (AF). Indeed, with the life-saving potential of DC cardioversion in the setting of ventricular arrhythmias beyond doubt, it is perhaps in AF where we must now carefully consider the clinical evidence behind our current practice.

PATHOPHYSIOLOGY OF AF: POTENTIAL BENEFITS OF DC CARDIOVERSION

As previously discussed, AF leads to substantial morbidity and mortality via hemodynamic disturbances (see Ch. 5) and an increase in thromboembolic stroke. AF leads to abnormal cardiac hemodynamic function by two mechanisms: the loss of atrial systolic function and the rapid, irregular ventricular response.

Both mechanisms reduce effective ventricular filling with a consequent increase in intra-atrial pressure (leading to intra-atrial blood pool stasis, atrial stretch and increased pulmonary venous pressure) and a decrease in stroke volume and cardiac output. Many of the symptoms of AF (e.g. palpitations, dyspnea, dizziness) are related to these hemodynamic changes. Furthermore, the rapid ventricular response increases the metabolic demands of the ventricular myocytes, which may exacerbate the symptoms of ischemic heart disease, if present.

In view of the hemodynamic and thromboembolic consequences of AF, conversion back to sinus rhythm might be expected to reduce or abolish the symptoms, morbidity and mortality associated with AF. However, there is increasing evidence that this theoretical benefit may be difficult to achieve in clinical practice, and that DC cardioversion (and indeed pharmacological attempts to maintain sinus rhythm) may no longer be the goal of treatment for many patients with AF.[2,3]

Following cardioversion, atrial systolic function returns over a few weeks, as evident by the gradual return of the A wave on transmitral Doppler echocardiography. Until full recovery of atrial systolic function, the risk of atrial thrombogenesis remains substantial.

MECHANISM OF DC CARDIOVERSION IN AF

Cardioversion or defibrillation occurs when sufficient electrical current density traverses the muscle of the chamber to be defibrillated.[4] To be successful, a critical muscle mass of the appropriate chamber must be defibrillated.[5] The physical factors (other than the presence of underlying heart disease) which determine the success of cardioversion are those factors which determine current density and the critical muscle mass over which the current passes, in particular, transthoracic impedance, electrode size and electrode placement.

Determinants of transthoracic impedance include patient body habitus, delivered energy, electrode size, interface between electrode and skin, the phase of ventilation, pressure on the electrodes, the distance between electrodes and the effect of previous discharges.[6–10]

Increased body weight is associated with an increased transthoracic diameter, thus greater transthoracic impedance and reduced procedural success rates of DC cardioversion.[9] Larger size electrodes reduce impedance but at the expense of reduced current concentration.[4,6] The optimal electrode size is about 12–13 cm in diameter.[4] The use of gels, paste or pads between electrodes and skin to reduce cutaneous inflammation also affects impedance.[7,11] Firm electrode pressure, with the patient in maximum expiration, reduces transthoracic impedance by improving contact and minimizing air in the lungs.[9] DC shocks themselves lower impedance for subsequent shocks[9,10] and position of the electrodes may influence procedural success by determining the mass of cardiac tissue exposed to the current.

In theory, the anteroposterior position (whereby one electrode is placed over the right sternal edge and the other just below the left scapula) should expose most atrial tissue to the DC current and thus achieve greater success, although randomized prospective studies have failed to consistently demonstrate the superiority of this position in clinical practice.[12]

Key points

Factors determining success of cardioversion

Physical factors
- transthoracic impedance (patient body mass index, energy level, skin resistance)
- electrode size
- electrode placement
- use of biphasic waveform shock

Disease factors
- duration of AF
- underlying etiology

EFFECTS OF DC CARDIOVERSION IN AF

Electrocardiographic changes

The initial effects of a successful DC cardioversion may be seen on a standard 12-lead electrocardiogram (ECG), with almost instantaneous re-emergence of 'p' waves (although frequently of abnormal morphology in the early postcardioversion period) and regular ventricular response indicating that sinus rhythm has been achieved. However, further ECG changes may be observed, including transient ST segment elevation, although the significance of such changes is unclear. These ST changes may be associated with reduced long-term maintenance of sinus rhythm, but this finding may simply be due to the strong association between these ST changes and a history of previous pericardiotomy in the study.[13]

Cutaneous and myocardial damage

Despite occasional transient ST segment changes, DC cardioversion of AF is not associated with myocardial damage. Although a rise in serum creatinine kinase may be observed postcardioversion,[14] there is no rise in troponin-T[15] and no clinical evidence of myocardial injury even following cardioversion at 720 J.[16] However, mild first-degree skin burns are a common complication of external DC cardioversion, which may be more severe at higher peak energies and particularly with greater cumulative energies (i.e. following multiple repeated shocks).[17] Skin burns may be minimized by the use of gel pads between the electrodes and the patient, while the development of biphasic defibrillators (which enhance success of cardioversion at lower energies) might also be expected to reduce the incidence of skin burns associated with DC cardioversion.

Return of atrial mechanical function

Despite the immediate reappearance of 'p' waves and normal sinus rhythm following successful DC cardioversion, atrial mechanical function may not immediately return.

Indeed, when Manning and colleagues[18,19] used pulse wave Doppler evaluation of mitral inflow to assess return of atrial function, they found that up to 3 weeks elapsed before atrial systolic function fully returned to 'normal'. This period of atrial electromechanical dissociation following cardioversion is often referred to as atrial 'stunning', although this may be a misnomer as the phenomenon does not appear to be related to the cardioversion procedure itself, but to the preceding AF. Duration of the preceding AF appears to be the main determinant of the duration of atrial 'stunning',[19] and full atrial systolic function may return within 24 h among those patients with AF of very recent onset. Indeed, atrial 'stunning' appears to be due to electrophysiological remodeling of the atrial myocytes during sustained AF (see Ch. 5).

Adverse effects of DC cardioversion

Local skin burns

Atrial electromechanical dissociation up to 4 weeks

Precipitation of thromboembolic events (1–7%)

Thromboembolic risk of DC cardioversion

Whilst AF itself carries an increased risk of cerebral and peripheral arterial thromboembolism, which might be expected to be reduced by cardioversion, the short-term risk appears to be enhanced in the early postcardioversion period, with thromboembolic complication rates approaching 7% in some series of patients cardioverted without anticoagulation therapy.[20]

Several mechanisms of this phenomenon have been proposed. First, the return of atrial mechanical function may result in the embolization of preformed thrombus within the left atrium or its appendage. In view of the delay in return of atrial systole, this risk may persist for several weeks following successful cardioversion. Furthermore, it is quite possible that the delayed return of atrial systolic function ('stunning') may itself promote the development of new thrombus which may be more prone to subsequent embolism than older, adherent thrombus. Indeed, even in the absence of thrombus detectable by transesophageal echocardiography (TEE) immediately prior to DC cardioversion there remains a small but significant incidence of postcardioversion thromboembolism,[21] supporting the theory of new thrombus formation.

The increased thromboembolic risk associated with cardioversion has led to the routine use of oral anticoagulation to cover this period.[22–24] Although the use of anticoagulation for DC cardioversion has never been subject to a prospective, randomized, placebo-controlled trial, several retrospective studies provide convincing evidence of the efficacy of such practice (Tables 17.1a and 17.1b).[25–30]

Bjerkelund and Orning[20] reported a series of 437 patients undergoing electrical cardioversion for atrial arrhythmias: 228 patients were receiving long-term oral anticoagulants, whilst 209 were not. In those who were successfully cardioverted, only two (1.1%) of 186 patients receiving anticoagulant therapy experienced

Table 17.1a Cardioversion-related thromboembolism without warfarin

Study	n	% Thromboembolism no warfarin
Morris[25]	66	4.5
Bjerkelund[29]	162	6.8
Weinberg[26]	28	7.1
Arnold[27]	115	6.3
Roy[28]	42	4.8

Patients with AF ≥ 2 days are subject to a 5–7% risk of cardioversion-related thromboembolism without warfarin

Table 17.1b Cardioversion-related thromboembolism with warfarin

Study	n	% Thromboembolism no warfarin
Rokseth[29]	274	1.6
Bjerkelund[20]	186	1.1
Weinberg[26]	51	0
Arnold[27]	52	0
Klein[30]	54	1.6

Use of 2–4 weeks warfarin before cardioversion of patients with AF ≥ 2 days reduces thromboembolic risk to ~1.2%.

thromboembolic events, compared to 11 (6.8%) of 162 patients not receiving anticoagulation. The apparent benefit of anticoagulation seen in this study was despite a greater prevalence of additional thromboembolic risk factors in the anticoagulation group, and thus provides strong evidence in favour of anticoagulation. However, the population studied was not 'pure' AF (patients with atrial flutter and other atrial tachycardias were included) and did not sufficiently address issues surrounding the duration of anticoagulant therapy required in the pericardioversion period.

The case for anticoagulation is further supported by two more recently conducted studies. In one retrospective study of 79 patients undergoing DC cardioversion,[26] there were no thromboembolic events in 51 patients receiving anticoagulant therapy, whilst two of 28 (7%) patients who were not anticoagulated suffered an embolic event. More recently, Arnold and colleagues[27] retrospectively assessed 454 elective DC cardioversions for AF or atrial flutter over a 7-year period. In total, 60 patients (1.32%) experienced an embolic complication; of these, all 60 had AF and none was on antithrombotic therapy. Five of the 60 (8%) had AF duration of less than 1 week, emphasizing the risk of cardioversion of AF without anticoagulation, even with a relatively short arrhythmia duration.

Recently, an alternative approach for reducing pericardioversion thromboembolic risk without the need for prior anticoagulation has been proposed, involving the use of TEE to assess the presence or absence of intra-atrial thrombus.[21] TEE is superior to transthoracic echocardiography for detection of intra-atrial thrombus and the sensitivity and specificity of TEE has been reported as over 90%[21] (Table 17.2).[30–41] Initial studies were promising, suggesting that exclusion of intra-atrial thrombus by TEE could allow

Table 17.2a TEE for left atrial thrombi

Study	Probe	n	Sensitivity (%)	Specificity (%)	Accuracy
Mugge[31]	M	12	100	–	100
Olson[32]	M	20	100	100	100
Hwang[33]	M/B	213	93	100	99
Manning[34]	M/B/Mu	231	100	99	99
Fatkin[35]	B	60	100	93	93

M, mono; B, biplane; Mu, multiplane
i.e. Excellent sensitivity and predictive accuracy of TEE for identification and exclusion of left atrial thrombus

Table 17.2b Previous studies documenting resolution of atrial thrombus by serial TEE (From Klein et al[36])

Study	n	Frequency of thrombus	Anticoagulation duration	Atrial thrombus resolved on second TEE
Stoddard[37]	21	NA	5 to 17 weeks	9/21 (43%)
Collins[38]	18	NA	4 weeks (median)	16/18 (89%)
Tsai[39]	8	10%	NA	6/8 (75%)
Klein[30]	7	13%	6 weeks	3/7 (43%)
Jaber[40]	164	NA	6.7 weeks (mean)	131/164 (80%)
Corrado[41]	11	11%	4 weeks (median)	9/11 (82%)

NA, not available; TEE, transesophageal echocardiography.

Table 17.3 Studies of TEE-guided approach to cardioversion of AF (From Klein et al[36])

Study	n	Atrial Thrombi	Embolic Events
Orsinelli[42]	39	9 (23%)	1 (2.56%)
Stoddard[37]	206	37 (18%)	0
Klein[30]	126	7 (13%)	0
Weigner[43]	466	64 (13.9%)	1 (0.21%)
Grimm[44]	417	28 (7%)	0
Corrado[41]	123	11 (9%)	0
ACUTE[45]	619	79 (13.6%)	5 (0.81%)
Total	1,996	235 (11.8%)	7 (0.35%)

ACUTE = Assessment of Cardioversion Using Transesophageal Echocardiography.

safe cardioversion in the absence of oral anticoagulation (but with intravenous heparin for 24 h pericardioversion)[21] (Table 17.3).[30,36,37,42–45]

However, other studies have suggested that the risk of thromboembolism is not sufficiently eliminated by the exclusion of pre-existing atrial thrombus,[46,47] suggesting the possibility of either new thrombus formation in the early postcardioversion procedure or the inability of TEE to accurately detect small but clinically significant thrombi.

The ACUTE study[21] was a large multicenter prospective randomized controlled trial comparing an approach whereby those without thrombus on TEE would be spared the initial period of anticoagulation prior to cardioversion and proceed directly to DC cardioversion, against standard anticoagulant therapy (a minimum of 3 weeks oral anticoagulation prior to cardioversion, with no TEE assessment). The TEE-based approach appeared to successfully reduce hemorrhagic complications and improve initial rates of conversion to sinus rhythm, without a significant increase in embolic complications. However, there was no significant difference in the proportion of patients in sinus rhythm after 8 weeks, and the trial design included anticoagulation for 4 weeks following cardioversion for all patients (including those with no thrombus on TEE) in view of the potential for postcardioversion thromboembolism. Thus, the chief benefits that can be claimed by this approach are a shorter waiting time to DC cardioversion and lower hemorrhagic complications, due to a shorter duration of anticoagulation. Overall, it seems reasonable to consider this approach as an *alternative* to the conventional approach, with *equivalent* effects on thromboembolic risk and procedural success.[23]

A novel, but currently hypothetical, method of assessing thromboembolic risk might be the measurement of plasma markers of thrombosis and the prothrombotic state.[48] Such markers might help to identify those at greatest and least risk of thrombus formation and to stratify patients accordingly, sparing antithrombotic therapy for those at lowest risk.

ASSESSMENT AND WORK-UP OF AF PATIENTS FOR DC CARDIOVERSION

'AF begets AF' – this commonly used phrase among cardiologists refers to the observation that the possibility of successful cardioversion and maintenance of sinus rhythm appears to decrease with a longer preceding arrhythmia duration.[49] Such an observation has encouraged an aggressive approach to treatment of AF, particularly in view of the potential hemodynamic benefits of long-term sinus rhythm maintenance.

However, the results of several recent large-scale randomized controlled trials suggest that aggressive attempts to restore sinus rhythm using currently available methods may not be in the best long-term interest of many AF patients, and may even cause harm.[2,3,50] Indeed, the weight of current evidence would suggest a more conservative approach should be adopted, in which appropriate selection of those AF patients for whom DC cardioversion *is* appropriate will become of even greater importance.

Procedural success rates for DC cardioversion are often excellent and superior to any currently available pharmacological agent, but highly variable, depending upon additional clinical factors (Table 17.1). The highest recorded success rates for cardioversion are seen in patients with AF secondary to hyperthyroidism (particularly once the hyperthyroidism has been treated), whilst the lowest are seen in patients with severe mitral regurgitation.[24] Duration of arrhythmia, increasing age, hypertension, coronary artery disease and other structural heart disease are also associated with a reduced long-term success rate of the procedure.

The RACE study[50] suggests that in patients with a history of prior DC cardioversion who relapse into AF, rate control with anticoagulation may be at least as effective as aggressive rhythm control, with no difference in thromboembolic complication rate or functional parameters between the two groups, but an increased incidence of adverse drug reactions in the rhythm-control group. Therefore, for patients with recurrent AF following cardioversion, rate control may be the better option (except for those patients with hemodynamic compromise or severe symptoms related to their AF, in whom even transient relief from AF may be of benefit). The practice of allowing all failed or relapsed DC cardioversion patients to undergo another attempted cardioversion (albeit with added antiarrhythmics) can no longer be justified on current evidence.

While the RACE study[50] provides insight into the optimal management of patients with recurrent AF, two large prospective randomized controlled trials[2,3] suggest current pharmacological methods of rhythm control (cardioversion and maintenance of sinus rhythm) may be of no greater benefit than rate control alone (which itself may even have advantages due to a lower rate of adverse effects). Meanwhile, there are still no large scale prospective randomized controlled studies of DC cardioversion as a first-line treatment in the setting of new-onset AF. However, it may be the case that, in view of the variable success rate of the procedure and the factors known to associate with a poor long-term outcome, we should be selecting for DC cardioversion only those patients for whom the procedure is likely to provide a long-term 'cure' without the need for repeated attempts or additional pharmacological agents to maintain sinus rhythm. Appropriate selection of patients for DC cardioversion may also help to reduce waiting times for the procedure (due to a reduction in caseload), which may itself increase success rates ('AF begets AF').

Nonetheless, DC cardioversion still has a role in the emergency treatment of 'unselected' hemodynamically unstable patients with AF and may remain a treatment option for acute AF (where the shorter arrhythmia duration may enhance long-term success rates). In patients presenting with a clear history of AF onset < 48 h previously, thromboembolic risk may be sufficiently low to allow cardioversion without anticoagulation, especially if the patient is *in extremis*. However, if the patient is hemodynamically stable, the small risk of thromboembolism may still outweigh the advantages of early DC cardioversion, and unless TEE facilities are available to first exclude the presence of intra-atrial thrombus it may be prudent to delay cardioversion. Furthermore, it may be appropriate to initiate early anticoagulation with unfractionated or low-molecular weight heparin in all acute AF patients where cardioversion may be delayed or arrhythmia duration is unclear.[23]

For patients with a duration of AF > 48 h, once they have been 'selected' as suitable candidates for DC cardioversion, the next decision to be made is whether to initiate 'standard' antithrombotic therapy, or whether to use TEE to exclude left atrial and appendage thrombus and thus to reduce time to DC cardioversion and to reduce the need for a full 3 weeks prior anticoagulation. The evidence from the ACUTE study[21] suggests that both methods are equally efficacious. Thus, it is often the availability of TEE facilities that is the deciding factor in this decision.

PRACTICALITIES OF DC CARDIOVERSION FOR AF

Although DC cardioversion is among the simplest of available therapies for cardiovascular disease, appropriate equipment and suitably trained staff – including a trained anesthetist if general anesthesia is to be used to sedate the patient – must be in place for its routine use.

DC shock energy

In addition to the patient factors which may influence the success rate of DC cardioversion, technique is also important. Traditionally, often influenced by Advanced Life Support guidelines, a step-up approach commencing at 100 J has been employed for treatment of AF. However, such guidelines were in part based upon the findings of Kerber and colleagues,[51] who reported a 40–67% success rate at this energy, depending upon the degree of transthoracic resistance. However, the duration of AF in these patients was not defined and other studies have shown increasing success of cardioversion with energies increasing up to 360 J,[52] with success rates as low as 21–62% even at 200 J for patients with longstanding AF.[52,53] In the only prospective randomized study of initial shock energy, Joglar and colleagues[54] demonstrated that starting with a higher initial energy (360 J vs 200 J or 100 J) resulted in a higher success rate after initial shock. Although differences in overall procedural success rate were not statistically significant, fewer shocks and a lower cumulative shock energy were required to achieve sinus rhythm in the group starting at 360 J, which might potentially reduce the incidence of skin burns related to the procedure. Using troponin-I as an index, no evidence of myocardial damage was found in this group, which is consistent with other studies using energies up to 720 J.[16] It may therefore be both safe and appropriate to commence with an initial shock energy of 360 J (Fig. 17.1).[55]

Paddle position

Another technique that may influence efficacy of DC cardioversion is electrode (or paddle) placement. In theory, the placement of electrodes in an anteroposterior (AP) position places a greater mass of atrium between the electrodes than the traditional anterolateral (AL) position which should improve efficacy of the procedure. Indeed, in pioneering studies, Lown[1] reported an improvement in efficacy using the AP position. However, the results of three subsequent randomized studies comparing AL and AP paddle positions have shown widely differing results.

While Botto and colleagues,[56] using a step-up protocol commencing at 3 J/kg body weight, demonstrated the AP position to be superior, Alp and colleagues[57] found that, using an initial energy of 360 J, the AL position was significantly more successful in attaining sinus rhythm. Finally, Mathew and colleagues,[12] using a step-up protocol starting at 100 J, found no significant

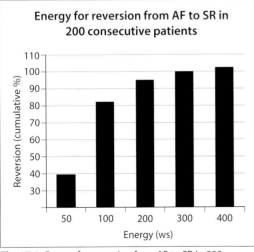

Fig. 17.1 Energy for reversion from AF to SR in 200 consecutive patients. SR, sinus rhythm. Reproduced with permission from Lown.[55]

difference between either paddle position. Despite the lack of consensus, in cases where cardioversion has failed in either AP or AL position at 360 J, it may be worthwhile attempting a final shock in the alternative position before admitting defeat.

In addition to paddle position, differences in electrode type (including size of electrode and the use of self-adhesive versus hand-held electrodes) may be relevant, since transthoracic impedance (a factor in reduction of procedural success) may be minimized by larger electrodes with better skin contact, as discussed earlier.

Antiarrhythmic drugs

One explanation for such a variation between studies could be the use of antiarrhythmic drugs before or at the time of cardioversion. Several antiarrhythmic drugs have been shown to improve the success rates of DC cardioversion, as well as the long-term maintenance of sinus rhythm postcardioversion.[58] Data from a recent meta-analysis are summarized in Figure 17.2,[59–101] demonstrating the benefits of class I and III agents in cardioversion and the prevention of recurrent AF. In general, the drugs suitable for pharmacological cardioversion are similar to those useful for postcardioversion maintenance of sinus rhythm (Fig. 17.3). Nevertheless there is a risk of mortality and morbidity associated with these drugs, as evident by an increased mortality amongst those taking class I agents (e.g. quinidine), but it should be noted that despite antiarrhythmic drugs, only 50% remain in sinus rhythm at 1 year (Fig. 17.4).[102]

New developments: biphasic waveform defibrillation

Finally, the recent development of defibrillators which deliver a biphasic waveform (in contrast to traditional

Absolute treatment differences in proportion of patients with normal sinus rhythm (%) at end of study between class IA drugs and placebo

(a)

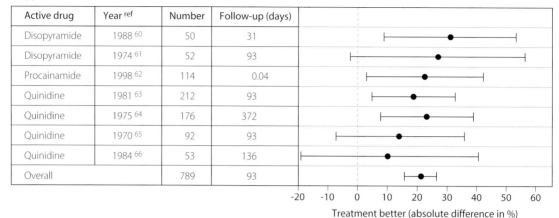

Active drug	Year ref	Number	Follow-up (days)
Disopyramide	1988 [60]	50	31
Disopyramide	1974 [61]	52	93
Procainamide	1998 [62]	114	0.04
Quinidine	1981 [63]	212	93
Quinidine	1975 [64]	176	372
Quinidine	1970 [65]	92	93
Quinidine	1984 [66]	53	136
Overall		789	93

Treatment better (absolute difference in %)

Absolute treatment difference in proportion of patients with normal sinus rhythm (%) at end of study between class IC agents and placebo

(b)

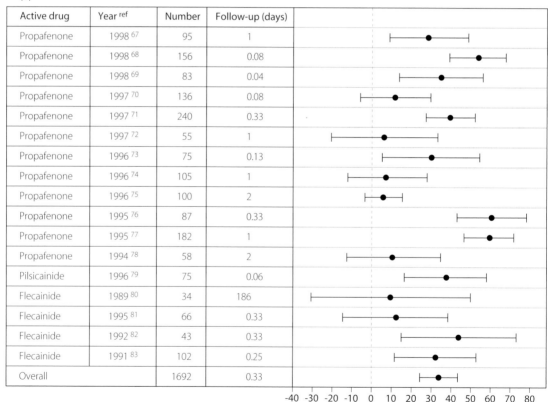

Active drug	Year ref	Number	Follow-up (days)
Propafenone	1998 [67]	95	1
Propafenone	1998 [68]	156	0.08
Propafenone	1998 [69]	83	0.04
Propafenone	1997 [70]	136	0.08
Propafenone	1997 [71]	240	0.33
Propafenone	1997 [72]	55	1
Propafenone	1996 [73]	75	0.13
Propafenone	1996 [74]	105	1
Propafenone	1996 [75]	100	2
Propafenone	1995 [76]	87	0.33
Propafenone	1995 [77]	182	1
Propafenone	1994 [78]	58	2
Pilsicainide	1996 [79]	75	0.06
Flecainide	1989 [80]	34	186
Flecainide	1995 [81]	66	0.33
Flecainide	1992 [82]	43	0.33
Flecainide	1991 [83]	102	0.25
Overall		1692	0.33

Treatment better (absolute difference in %)

Fig. 17.2 Absolute treatment difference in proportion of patients with normal sinus rhythm (%) at end of study between (a) Class IA drugs and placebo, (b) Class IC agents and placebo, and (c) Class III agents and placebo. Reproduced with permission from Nichol et al.[59]

**Absolute treatment difference in proportion of patients with normal sinus rhythm (%)
at end of study between class III agents and placebo**

(c)

Active drug	Year [ref]	Number	Follow-up (days)	
Amiodarone	2000 [84]	208	30	
Amiodarone	2000 [85]	62	0.33	
Amiodarone	1999 [86]	67	30	
Amiodarone	1999 [87]	100	0.33	
Amiodarone	1998 [88]	97	1	
Amiodarone	1996 [89]	64	15	
Amiodarone	1995 [81]	64	0.33	
Amiodarone	1994 [90]	30	1	
Amiodarone	1992 [91]	40	0.33	
Dofetilide	2001 [92]	506	1096	
Dofetilide	2000 [93]	325	0	
Dofetilide	2000 [94]	69	0.04	
Dofetilide	2000 [95]	22	0.12	
Dofetilide	1999 [96]	79	0.12	
Dofetilide	1997 [97]	98	0.12	
Ibutilide	1999 [98]	201	0.06	
Ibutilide	1996 [99]	167	0.06	
Ibutilide	1996 [100]	99	0.04	
Sotalol	1991 [101]	30	186	
Overall		2328	0.33	

Treatment better (absolute difference in %)

Fig. 17.2, cont'd.

sinusoidal monophasic waveform defibrillators) has improved the success rates of DC cardioversion of AF at lower energies. In a prospective randomized study, Ricard and colleagues[103] demonstrated, using initial energies of 150 J, that initial cardioversion success rate was higher in those randomized to cardioversion using a biphasic waveform compared to a monophasic waveform.

More impressive still, in another prospective randomized study Mittal and colleagues[104] demonstrated greater cardioversion efficacy using a biphasic waveform at 70 J than a monophasic waveform at 100 J. Furthermore, the

authors found a greater overall procedural success rate using a step-up protocol of 70–170 J in the biphasic group compared to 100–360 J in the monophasic group. Following multivariate analysis, the use of a biphasic waveform, lower transthoracic impedance and shorter duration of AF were shown to be independent predictors of cardioversion success.

Sedation and anesthesia

Some debate exists over the optimum form of anesthesia or sedation for DC cardioversion. While propofol may be the

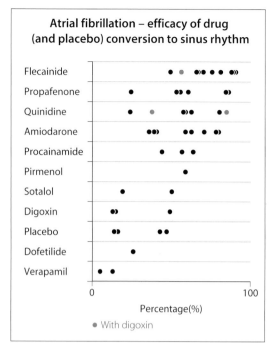

Fig. 17.3 Atrial fibrillation – efficacy of drug (and placebo) conversion to sinus rhythm.

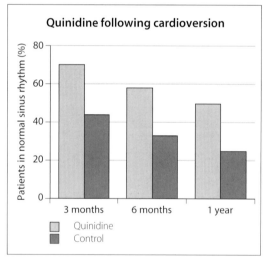

Fig. 17.4 Quinidine following cardioversion. Reproduced with permission from Coplen et al.[102]

closest to 'ideal' in terms of sedative and analgesic effects, the use of this drug is essentially restricted to trained anesthetists.

The use of intravenous midazolam or diazepam by general physicians appears to be a safe and effective alternative,[105,106] providing that adequate monitoring and

resuscitation facilities are available. Furthermore, a randomized comparison of propofol and midazolam has shown fairly equivalent efficacy of the two agents for cardioversion sedation.[107] Such an approach may reduce waiting time to cardioversion (by removing the need for an anesthetist to be present), but some safety concerns may remain. In all cases continuous pulse oximetry, ECG monitoring, equipment for assisted ventilation and flumazenil (for rapid reversal of benzodiazepine-induced respiratory depression) are mandatory, in addition to the presence of staff trained in sedation use and resuscitation, and a trained anesthetist should be available on-site in case of emergency.

MANAGEMENT OF AF PATIENTS FOLLOWING DC CARDIOVERSION

Anticoagulation

The optimal duration of anticoagulation following successful DC cardioversion is unclear. It is well established that the increased risk of thromboembolic events associated with cardioversion may persist for several weeks following the procedure, and this is believed to be a reflection of the delay in return of atrial mechanical function, often taking up to three weeks to fully return on 'normal' levels. The current guidelines from the American College of Chest Physicians reflect this period of increased risk, suggesting a minimum duration of four weeks anticoagulation following successful cardioversion.[22]

Despite these guidelines, no randomized prospective study has been performed to establish whether successful cardioversion alone reduces the risk of thromboembolic events in patients with AF, despite the theoretical benefits. Furthermore, several prospective randomized studies comparing rate-control and rhythm-control strategies in AF have shown no statistically significant difference in thromboembolic events between groups, although anticoagulant therapy was often discontinued in those successfully maintained in sinus rhythm, partly increasing the risk of strokes in this group.[3] It may be the case, therefore, that in certain patients converted to sinus rhythm thromboembolic risk remains high, either due to subsequent recurrence of AF or a persistent thromboembolic risk. Such patients may benefit from lifelong (or long-term) anticoagulation therapy to reduce this risk, although once again there are no randomized placebo-controlled prospective studies to evaluate the risks versus benefits of continued anticoagulation following successful DC cardioversion. In the absence of such studies, it would seem appropriate to continue anticoagulation in patients deemed at high risk of AF recurrence and/or thromboembolic stroke using established risk-stratification criteria.

Anticoagulation and DC cardoversion

Low molecular weight heparin can be used in case of very short AF duration

Duration of AC before DC cardioversion is 4 weeks (3 weeks of stable target international normalized ratio)

Optimal duration of AC duration post-DC is unknown – 4 weeks is minimum

According to newer studies DC cardioversion of persistent AF needs long-term AC

Antiarrhythmic drugs

Without the concomitant and subsequent use of antiarrhythmic drugs to facilitate DC cardioversion and maintenance of sinus rhythm, relapse rate of AF is high, with perhaps only 58% of those successfully cardioverted still remaining in sinus rhythm after 6 months and a continuing risk of relapse resulting in recurrent AF for the majority of patients beyond this timepoint.[108]

Review of available prospective placebo-controlled or comparative studies suggests that quinidine, propafenone and sotalol have approximately equivalent efficacy at maintaining sinus rhythm following cardioversion[24,109] but amiodarone appears to be the most effective agent, maintaining sinus rhythm in 65% of patients at 16 months following DC cardioversion, compared to only 37% receiving sotalol or propafenone[110] (Fig. 17.2). However, the unfavorable side-effect profile of amiodarone may make many physicians wary of its long-term use.

De Simone and colleagues[111] demonstrated that the additional periprocedural administration of verapamil may reduce relapse rates in patients treated with propafenone. Furthermore, Plewan and colleagues[112] demonstrated bisoprolol to be equally efficacious in this setting as sotalol. Indeed, bisoprolol might be safer than sotalol in clinical practice due to the class III effects, QT prolongation and torsade de pointes of the latter drug. Therefore, the choice of antiarrhythmic drug may ultimately depend upon the individual patient and the physician's desire to balance efficacy with safety profile.

Finally, in the RACE study which was a recent study of great clinical importance in patients with recurrent AF,[50] an aggressive policy of repeat DC cardioversion using a step-up regimen of adjuvant antiarrhythmic therapy (sotalol, class Ic drugs, amiodarone) provided no overall clinical benefit compared to a policy of rate control and anticoagulation, but led to significantly more treatment-related adverse events.

Perhaps now the question is no longer 'which antiarrhythmic drug to facilitate DC cardioversion?' but 'is repeat cardioversion truly appropriate?'. Unless there is hemodynamic compromise or failure to suppress symptoms with a rate-control strategy, current methods of rhythm control using DC cardioversion and antiarrhythmic agents appear to offer little advantage over rate control and may, after 40 years as a mainstay of therapy, now begin to assume a marginalized role in the modern management of AF. The implications of the AFFIRM trial on the presumed benefits of rhythm control are summarized in Table 17.4.

Table 17.4 Conclusions

Presumed benefits of maintaining sinus rhythm	Outcome of patients in the rhythm control arm
Fewer symptoms/better exercise tolerance	Functional status no different
Lower risk of stroke	Similar rates of combined secondary endpoints, including stroke
Long-term anticoagulation not needed	Most strokes (65/84) occurred off warfarin or with INR < 2.0.
Better quality of life	Quality of life no different, but more hospitalizations
Better survival	No survival benefit; a trend toward increased late risk

Table 17.5 Predictors of refractoriness to cardioversion of AF or unsuccessful maintenance of sinus rhythm

Author	n	Age	AF duration	LA size	LVdys	Valve
Dethy[113]	50	n	y	y	?	n
Dittrich[108]	65	n	y	n	n	n
Brodsky[114]	43	n	y	y	n	y
Van Gelder[115]	246	y	y	n	?	y
Crijns[116]	127	y	y	?	n	y
Carlsson[117]	1152	n	n	y	y	n

Some uncertainty - probably duration of AF most important

Recent developments

Perhaps now the question is no longer 'which antiarrhythmic drug to facilitate DC cardioversion?' but 'is repeat cardioversion truly appropriate?'

PROGNOSIS FOLLOWING CARDIOVERSION

Predictors of refractoriness to cardioversion or unsuccessful maintenance of sinus rhythm include the following: age, duration of arrhythmia, the presence of hypertension, valve disease and other organic heart disease (Table 17.5).[13,108,113–117] Proper selection of patients who are suitable for the procedure and the use of antiarrhythmic therapy to prevent recurrences of the arrhythmia may allow a successful outcome.

An older age, in combination with a large number of previous episodes of arrhythmia and a long previous duration of arrhythmia, are predictive of the unsuccessful maintenance of sinus rhythm. In addition, the presence of coronary artery disease, hypertension and organic heart disease (such as mitral valve disease, aortic stenosis and cardiomyopathy) are adverse factors for the maintenance of normal sinus rhythm following cardioversion. In a Doppler echocardiographic study, a slow increase (< 10% in first 24 h) in the magnitude of A wave postcardioversion was also predictive for the recurrence of AF.[24]

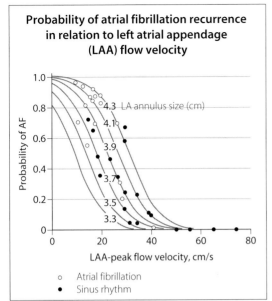

Fig. 17.5 Probability of atrial fibrillation recurrence in relation to left atrial appendage (LAA) flow velocity. Schematic representation of a multivariate analysis relating to LAA peak flow velocity, left atrial (LA) annulus size shown as S curves, and the probability of atrial fibrillation. Open circles represent each patient who reverted to atrial fibrillation and closed circles represent each patient who maintained sinus rhythm. Data from Verhorst et al.[118]
© 1997 The American College of Cardiology Foundation.

The effects of left atrial size are less certain. In a small study (50 patients), a left atrial dimension of ≥ 45 mm was important, and had a positive predictive value of 66% for recurrence of AF (Fig. 17.5).[118] However, the duration of AF was probably the most important predictor for outcome following cardioversion. These studies suggest therefore that atrial size does not strongly influence outcome of cardioversion and patients should not be excluded on these grounds from consideration of cardioversion. The increase in left atrial size may be consequent upon the presence of AF, which may explain why it does not necessarily predict outcome following cardioversion. Even in the presence of a dilated left atrium, long-term sinus rhythm (79% at 12 months) is possible with the use of antiarrhythmic drugs.[24]

The duration of the arrhythmia is also an important factor influencing prognosis following cardioversion of AF. For example, there is a two-fold increase in the proportion remaining in sinus rhythm postcardioversion when patients with a short duration of AF (less than 3 months) are compared with those in whom AF was present for more than 12 months. However, the duration of AF alone should not be the sole basis for exclusion of such patients from cardioversion and many factors, such as the clinical state and the presence of structural heart disease, should be considered.

Full assessment of the patient with AF for cardioversion should therefore include an assessment for the underlying etiological factor(s). For example, patients with specific pathology (such as mitral stenosis and poor left ventricular function) are unlikely to successfully cardiovert. By contrast, a patient with AF secondary to thyrotoxicosis or a chest infection that has since be treated, would have a high success rate if cardioversion was attempted. If the underlying etiology and triggering factor(s) continue to exert an effect, attempts at cardioversion may be unsuccessful.

Another intriguing development is the observation that treatment with the angiotensin receptor antagonist, irbesartan improves prognosis postcardioversion (Fig. 17.6).[119] The mechanisms remain uncertain, and may simply reflect the hemodynamic benefits of treating hypertension and reducing intracardiac pressures by blockade of the renin angiotensin system. However, a beneficial effect on left atrial remodeling cannot be excluded.

DC CARDIOVERSION FOR AF: SUMMARY

DC cardioversion is a simple and often effective treatment of AF, which usually results in sinus rhythm in the short term. However, many factors, including patient comorbidities and procedural technique may reduce the overall long-term success rate in achieving and maintaining sinus rhythm. Therefore, in many AF patients,

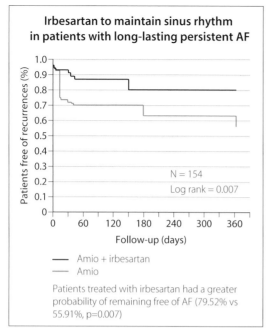

Irbesartan to maintain sinus rhythm in patients with long-lasting persistent AF

N = 154
Log rank = 0.007

— Amio + irbesartan
— Amio

Patients treated with irbesartan had a greater probability of remaining free of AF (79.52% vs 55.91%, p=0.007)

Fig. 17.6 Irbesartan to maintain sinus rhythm in patients with long-lasting persistent AF. Patients treated with irbesartan had a greater probability of remaining free of AF (79.52% vs 55.91%, p=0.007). amio, amiodarone. Reproduced with permission from Madrid et al.[119]

long-term success rates of DC cardioversion may be disappointing without the additional use of antiarrhythmic drugs. Furthermore, the procedure is associated with an increased short-term risk of thromboembolic events that persists for up to 4 weeks afterwards and thus, even in those in whom no thrombus is found to be present by TEE at the time of cardioversion, requires a period of prophylactic anticoagulant therapy in all patients with AF duration longer than 48 h. In addition, recent prospective randomized studies comparing rhythm control (pharmacological and/or using DC cardioversion) with rate-control strategies have shown no convincing benefits from a rhythm-control strategy, in terms of mortality, morbidity and functional parameters. Nonetheless, the observation that 'AF begets AF' suggests that the theoretical benefits of early cardioversion and maintenance of sinus rhythm may remain a goal sufficient for development of new antiarrhythmic strategies.

The recent development of biphasic defibrillators may play a role in improving outcomes from a rhythm-control strategy, but is likely to affect only short-term outcomes unless combined with additional approaches including novel antiarrhythmic drugs and electrophysiological interventions, such as pulmonary vein ablation of focal AF. Until we have further evidence of the benefits of these new approaches, DC cardioversion may be best

- Long-term success rates of DC cardioversion may be disappointing without the additional use of antiarrhythmic drugs
- DC cardioversion may be best reserved for those who stand to gain most benefit, including AF of recent-onset, hemodynamically compromised or highly symptomatic patients, and those free from additional comorbidities known to predispose to recurrent AF

Cardioversion of AF - how to do it:

- Admit patient to hospital for ECG monitoring (e.g. Coronary Care Unit).
- Serum electrolytes (especially potassium) should be normal.
- Ensure anticoagulation adequate, with an INR of 2.0 to 3.0.
- If the patient is taking digoxin, with no evidence of digitoxicity, the drug can be taken up to the day before the procedure. Serum digoxin levels should be checked if digitoxicity is suspected and the procedure delayed.

Pharmacological cardioversion
- Infusion of drug (e.g. flecainide, amiodarone) should be started under continuous ECG monitoring.

Electrical
- Patient should be fasted
- Short general anaesthetic required to eliminate discomfort associated with the transthoracic shock. Resuscitation equipment should be available. ECG and blood pressure monitoring, and pulse oximetry is desirable
- Synchronised DC shock is given, starting at 100 Joules, with intermediate 'step-ups', eventually to 360 Joules.
- After the procedure, the patient is monitored for at least 1 hour to ensure stability of rhythm and blood pressure

reserved for those who stand to gain most benefit, including AF of recent-onset, hemodynamically compromised or highly symptomatic patients, and those free from additional comorbidities known to predispose to recurrent AF.

References

1. Lown B, Amarasingham R, Neuman J. New method for terminating cardiac arrhythmias: use of synchronized capacitor discharge. JAMA 1962; 182:548–555.
2. Hohnloser SH, Kuck KH, Lilienthal J. Rhythm or rate control in atrial fibrillation – pharmacological intervention in atrial fibrillation (PIAF): a randomised trial. Lancet 2000; 356:1789–1794.
3. Wyse DG, Waldo AL, DiMarco JP, et al. The Atrial Fibrillation Follow-up Investigation of Rhythm Management (AFFIRM) Investigators. A comparison of rate control and rhythm control in patients with atrial fibrillation. N Engl J Med 2002; 347:1825–33.
4. Ewy GA. Effectiveness of direct current defibrillation: Role of paddle electrode size: II. Am Heart J 1977; 93:674–675.
5. Ewy GA. Ventricular fibrillation and defibrillation. In: Ewy GA, Bressler R, eds. Cardiovascular drugs and the management of heart disease. 1st edn. New York:, Raven Press; 1982:331–349.
6. Connell PN, Ewy GA, Dahl CF, et al. Transthoracic impedance to defibrillator discharge: Effect of electrode size and chest wall interface. J Echocardiogr 1973; 6:313–317.
7. Ewy GA, Taren D. Comparison of paddle electrode pastes used for defibrillation. Heart Lung 1977; 6:847–850.
8. Ewy GA, Hellman DA, McClung S, et al. Influence of ventilation phase on transthoracic impedance and defibrillation effectiveness. Crit Care Med 1980; 8:164–166.
9. Kerber RE, Grayzel J, Hoyt R, et al. Transthoracic resistance in human defibrillation: Influence of body weight, chest size, serial shocks, paddle size and paddle contact pressure. Circulation 1981; 63:676–682.
10. Dahl CF, Ewy GA, Ewy MD, et al. Transthoracic impedance to direct current discharge: effects of repeated countershocks. Med Instrum 1976; 10:151–154.
11. Aylward PE, Kieso R, Hite P, et al. Defibrillator electrode-chest wall coupling agents: influence on transthoracic impedance and shock success. J Am Coll Cardiol 1985; 6:682–686.
12. Mathew TP, Moore A, McIntyre M, et al. Randomised comparison of electrode positions for cardioversion of atrial fibrillation. Heart 1999; 81(6):576–579.
13. Van Gelder IC, Crijns HJ, Van der Laarse A, et al. Incidence and clinical significance of ST segment elevation after electrical cardioversion of atrial fibrillation and atrial flutter. Am Heart J 1991; 121:51–56.
14. Metcalfe MJ, Smith F, Jennings K, et al. Does cardioversion of atrial fibrillation result in myocardial damage? Br Med J 1988; 296:1364.
15. Greaves K, Crake T. Cardiac troponin-T does not increase after electrical cardioversion for atrial fibrillation or atrial flutter. Heart 1998; 80:226–228.
16. Saliba W, Juratli N, Chung MK, et al. Higher energy synchronized external direct current cardioversion for refractory atrial fibrillation. J Am Coll Cardiol 1999; 34:2031–2034.
17. Pagan-Carlo LA, Stone MS, Kerber RE. Nature and determinants of skin 'burns' after transthoracic cardioversion. Am J Cardiol 1997; 79:689–691.
18. Manning WJ, Leeman DE, Gotch PJ, et al. Pulsed Doppler evaluation of atrial mechanical function after electrical cardioversion of atrial fibrillation. J Am Coll Cardiol 1989; 13:617–623.
19. Manning WJ, Silverman DI, Katz SE, et al. Impaired left atrial mechanical function after cardioversion: relation to the duration of atrial fibrillation. J Am Coll Cardiol 1994; 23:1535–1540.
20. Bjerkelund CJ, Orning OM. The efficacy of anticoagulant therapy in preventing embolism related to D.C. electrical conversion of atrial fibrillation. Am J Cardiol 1969; 23:208–216.
21. Klein AL, Grimm RA, Murray RD, et al. Assessment of cardioversion using transesophageal echocardiography investigators. Use of transesophageal echocardiography to guide cardioversion in patients with atrial fibrillation. N Engl J Med 2001; 344:1411–1420.
22. Albers GW, Dalen JE, Laupacis A, Manning WJ, Petersen P, Singer DE. Antithrombotic therapy in atrial fibrillation. Chest. 2001 Jan; 119(1 Suppl):194S–206S.
23. Fuster V, Ryden LE, Asinger RW, et al. American College of Cardiology/American Heart Association/European Society of Cardiology Board. ACC/AHA/ESC guidelines for the management of patients with atrial fibrillation: executive summary. A Report of the American College of Cardiology/American Heart Association Task Force on Practice Guidelines and the European Society of Cardiology Committee for Practice Guidelines and Policy Conferences (Committee to Develop Guidelines for the Management of Patients With Atrial Fibrillation): developed in Collaboration With the North American Society of Pacing and Electrophysiology. J Am Coll Cardiol 2001; 38:1231–66.
24. Lip GYH. Cardioversion of atrial fibrillation. Postgrad Med J 1995; 71:457–465.
25. Morris JJ, Peter RH, McIntosh HD, et al. Experience with cardioversion of atrial fibrillation and flutter. Am J Cardiol 1964; 14:94–100.

26. Weinberg DM, Mancini J. Anticoagulation for cardioversion of atrial fibrillation. Am J Cardiol 1989; 63(11):745–746.

27. Arnold AZ, Mick MJ, Mazurek RP, et al. Role of prophylactic anticoagulation for direct current cardioversion in patients with atrial fibrillation or atrial flutter. J Am Coll Cardiol 1992; 19(4):851–855.

28. Roy D, Marchand E, Gagne P, et al. Usefulness of anticoagulant therapy in the prevention of embolic complications of atrial fibrillation. Am Heart J 1986; 112:1039–43.

29. Rokseth R, Storstein Q. Quinidine therapy of chronic auricular fibrillation: the occurrence and mechanism of syncope. Arch Intern Med 1963; 111:184–9.

30. Klein AL, Grimm RA, Black IW, et al. Cardioversion guided by transesophageal echocardiography: the ACUTE pilot study: a randomized controlled trial: Assessment of Cardioversion Using Transesophageal Echocardiography. Ann Intern Med 1997; 126:200–9.

31. Mugge A, Daniel WG, Hausmann J, Godke J, Wagenbreth L, Lichtlen PR. Diagnosis of left atrial appendage thrombi by transesophageal echocardiography: clinical implications and follow-up. Am J Card Imaging 1990; 4:173–9.

32. Olson JD, Goldenberg IF, Pedersen W, et al. Exclusion of atrial thrombus by transesophageal echocardiography. J Am Soc Echocardiogr 1992; 5:52–6.

33. Hwang JJ, Chen JJ, Lin SC, et al. Diagnostic accuracy of left atrial appendage thrombi by transesophageal echocardiography for detecting left atrial thrombi in patients with rheumatic heart disease having undergone mitral valve operations. Am J Cardiol 1993; 72:677–81.

34. Manning WJ, Weintraub RM, Waksmonski CA, et al. Accuracy of transesophageal echocardiography for identifying left atrial thrombi: a prospective, intraoperative study. Ann Intern Med 1995; 123:817–822.

35. Fatkin D, Scalia G, Jacobs N, et al. Accuracy of biplane transesophageal echocardiography in detecting left atrial thrombus. Am J Cardiol 1996; 77:321–3.

36. Klein AL, Murray RD, Grimm RA. Role of transesophageal echocardiography-guided cardioversion of patients with atrial fibrillation. JACC 2001;37:691–704.

37. Stoddard MF, Dawkins PR, Prince CR, Longaker RA. Transesophageal echocardiographic guidance of cardioversion in patients with atrial fibrillation. Am Heart J 1995; 129:1204–15.

38. Collins LJ, Silverman DI, Douglas PS, Manning WJ. Cardioversion of nonrheumatic atrial fibrillation: reduced thromboembolic complications with four weeks of precardioversion anticoagulation are related to atrial thrombus resolution. Circulation 1995; 92:160–3.

39. Tsai LM, Lin LJ, Teng JK, Chen JH. Prevalence and clinical significance of left atrial thrombus in nonrheumatic atrial fibrillation. Int J Cardiol 1997; 58:163–9.

40. Jaber WA, Prior DL, Thamilarasan M, et al. Efficacy of anticoagulation in resolving left atrial and left atrial appendage thrombi: a transesophageal echocardiographic study. Am Heart J 2000; 140:150–6.

41. Corrado G, Tadeo G, Beretta S, et al. Atrial thrombi resolution after prolonged anticoagulation in patients with atrial fibrillation. Chest 1999; 115:140–3.

42. Orsinelli DA, Pearson AC. Usefulness of transesophageal echocardiography to screen for left atrial thrombus before elective cardioversion for atrial fibrillation. Am J Cardiol 1993; 72:1337–9.

43. Weigner MJ, Patel U, Thomas LR, et al. Transesophageal echocardiography facilitated cardioversion from atrial fibrillation: short-term safety and implications regarding maintenance of sinus rhythm (abstr.). Circulation 1998; 98 Suppl I:I500.

44. Grimm RA, Agler DA, Vaughn SE, et al. TEE-guided anticoagulation in patients undergoing electrical cardioversion of atrial fibrillation: results from the ACUTE registry (abstr.). J Am Coll Cardiol 1998; 31 Suppl:353A.

45. ACUTE Investigators. Assessment of Cardioversion Using Transesophageal Echocardiography (ACUTE) multicenter study: eight-week clinical outcomes. Presented at the American College of Cardiology Scientific Sessions, Late-Breaking Clinical Trial, 2000.

46. Black IW, Fatkin D, Sagar KB, et al. Exclusion of atrial thrombus by transesophageal echocardiography does not preclude embolism after cardioversion of atrial fibrillation. A multicenter study. Circulation 1994; 89:2509–2513.

47. Moreyra E, Finkelhor RS, Cebul RD. Limitations of transesophageal echocardiography in the risk assessment of patients before nonanticoagulated cardioversion from atrial fibrillation and flutter: an analysis of pooled trials. Am Heart J 1995; 129:71–75.

48. Lip GYH. Does atrial fibrillation confer a hypercoagulable state? Lancet 1995; 346:1313–1314.

49. Wijffels MCEF, Kirchhof CJHJ, Dorland R, et al. Atrial fibrillation begets atrial fibrillation. A study in awake chronically instrumented goats. Circulation 1995; 92:1954–1968.

50. Van Gelder IC, Hagens VE, Bosker HA, et al. Rate Control versus Electrical Cardioversion for Persistent Atrial Fibrillation Study Group. A comparison of rate control and rhythm control in patients with recurrent persistent atrial fibrillation. N Engl J Med 2002; 347(23):1834–40.

51. Kerber RE, Martins JB, Kienzle MG, et al. Energy, current, and success in defibrillation and cardioversion: clinical studies using an automated impedance-based method of energy adjustment. Circulation 1988; 77(5):1038–1046.

52. Ricard P, Levy S, Trigano J, et al. Prospective assessment of the minimum energy needed for external electrical cardioversion of atrial fibrillation. Am J Cardiol 1997; 79:815–16.

53. Dalzell GW, Anderson J, Adgey AA. Factors determining success and energy requirements for cardioversion of atrial fibrillation. Q J Med 1990; 76:903–913.

54. Joglar JA, Hamdan MH, Ramaswamy K, et al. Initial energy for elective external cardioversion of persistent atrial fibrillation. Am J Cardiol 2000; 86:348–350.

55. Lown B. Electrical reversion of cardiac arrhythmias. Br Heart J 1967; 29:469–89.

56. Botto GL, Politi A, Bonini W, et al. External cardioversion of atrial fibrillation: role of paddle position on technical efficacy and energy requirements. Heart 1999; 82:726–730.

57. Alp NJ, Rahman S, Bell JA, et al. Randomised comparison of antero-lateral versus antero-posterior paddle positions for DC cardioversion of persistent atrial fibrillation. Int J Cardiol 2000; 75(2–3):211–216.

58. Capucci A, Villani GQ, Aschieri D, et al. Oral amiodarone increases the efficacy of direct-current cardioversion in restoration of sinus rhythm in patients with chronic atrial fibrillation. Eur Heart J 2000; 21:66–73.

59. Nichol G, McAlister F, Pham B, et al. Meta-analysis of randomised controlled trials of the effectiveness of antiarrhythmics agents at promoting sinus rhythm in patients with atrial fibrillation. Heart 2002; 87:535–543.

60. Karlson BW, Torstensson I, Abjorn C, et al. Disopyramide in the maintenance of sinus rhythm after electroconversion of atrial fibrillation: a placebo-controlled one-year follow-up study. Eur Heart J 1988; 9:284–90.

61. Hartel G, Louhija A, Konttinen A. Disopyramide in the prevention of recurrence of atrial fibrillation after electroconversion. Clin Pharmacol Ther 1974; 15:551–5.

62. Kochiadakis GE, Igoumenidis NE, Solomou MC, et al. Conversion of atrial fibrillation to sinus rhythm using acute intravenous procainamide infusion. Cardiovasc Drugs Ther 1998; 12:75–81.

63. Boissel JP, Wolf E, Gillet J, et al. Controlled trial of a long-acting quinidine for maintenance of sinus rhythm after conversion of sustained atrial fibrillation. Eur Heart J 1981; 2:49–55.

64. Sodermark T, Jonsson B, Olsson A, et al. Effect of quinidine on maintaining sinus rhythm after conversion of atrial fibrillation or flutter: a multicentre study from Stockholm. Br Heart J 1975; 37:486–92.

65. Byrne-Quinn E, Wing AJ. Maintenance of sinus rhythm after DC reversion of atrial fibrillation: a double-blind controlled trial of long-acting quinidine bisulphate. Br Heart J 1970; 32:370–6.

66. Lloyd EA, Gersh BJ, Forman R. The efficacy of quinidine and disopyramide in the maintenance of sinus rhythm after electroconversion from atrial fibrillation: a double-blind study comparing quinidine, disopyramide and placebo. S Afr Med J 1984; 65:367–9.

67. Kochiadakis GE, Igoumenidis NE, Simantirakis EN, et al. Intravenous propafenone versus intravenous amiodarone in the management of atrial fibrillation of recent onset: a placebo-controlled study. Pacing Clin Electrophysiol 1998; 21:2475–9.

68. Ganau G, Lenzi T. Intravenous propafenone for converting recent onset atrial fibrillation in emergency departments: a randomized placebo-controlled multicenter trial. FAPS Investigators Study Group. J Emerg Med 1998; 16:383–7.

69. Bianconi L, Mennuni M. Comparison between propafenone and digoxin administered intravenously to patients with acute atrial fibrillation. PAFIT-3 Investigators. The propafenone in atrial fibrillation Italian trial. Am J Cardiol 1998; 82:584–8.

70. Stroobandt R, Stiels B, Hoebrechts R. Propafenone for conversion and prophylaxis of atrial fibrillation. Propafenone Atrial Fibrillation Trial Investigators. Am J Cardiol 1997; 79:418–23.

71. Boriani G, Biffi M, Capucci A, et al. Oral propafenone to convert recent-onset atrial fibrillation in patients with and without underlying heart disease: a randomized, controlled trial. Ann Intern Med 1997; 126:621–5.

72. Azpitarte J, Alvarez M, Baun O, et al. Value of single oral loading dose of propafenone in converting recent-onset atrial fibrillation: results of a randomized, double-blind, controlled study. Eur Heart J 1997; 18:1649–54.

73. Fresco C, Proclemer A, Pavan A, et al. Intravenous propafenone in paroxysmal atrial fibrillation: a randomized, placebo-controlled, double-blind, multicenter clinical trial. Paroxysmal Atrial Fibrillation Italian Trial (PAFIT)-2 Investigators. Clin Cardiol 1996; 19:409–12.

74. Botto GL, Bonini W, Broffoni T, et al. Conversion of recent onset atrial fibrillation with single loading oral dose of propafenone: is in-hospital admission absolutely necessary? Pacing Clin Electrophysiol 1996; 19:1939–43.

75. Bianconi L, Mennuni M, Lukic V, et al. Effects of oral propafenone administration before electrical cardioversion of chronic atrial fibrillation: a placebo-controlled study. J Am Coll Cardiol 1996; 28:700–6.

76. Boriani G, Capucci A, Lenzi T, et al. Propafenone for conversion of recent-onset atrial fibrillation: a controlled comparison between oral loading dose and intravenous administration. Chest 1995; 108:355–8.

77. Bellandi F, Cantini F, Pedone T, et al. Effectiveness of intravenous propafenone for conversion of recent-onset atrial fibrillation: a placebo-controlled study. Clin Cardiol 1995; 18:631–4.

78. Capucci A, Boriani G, Rubino I, et al. A controlled

study on oral propafenone versus digoxin plus quinidine in converting recent onset atrial fibrillation to sinus rhythm. Int J Cardiol 1994; 43:305–13.

79. Atarashi H, Inoue H, Hiejima K, et al. Conversion of recent-onset atrial fibrillation by a single oral dose of pilsicainide (pilsicainide suppression trial on atrial fibrillation). The PSTAF Investigators. Am J Cardiol 1996; 78:694–7.

80. Van Gelder IC, Crijns HJ, Van Gilst WH, et al. Efficacy and safety of flecainide acetate in the maintenance of sinus rhythm after electrical cardioversion of chronic atrial fibrillation or atrial flutter. Am J Cardiol 1989; 64:1317–21.

81. Donovan KD, Power BM, Hockings BE, et al. Intravenous flecainide versus amiodarone for recent-onset atrial fibrillation. Am J Cardiol 1995; 75:693–7.

82. Capucci A, Lenzi T, Boriani G, et al. Effectiveness of loading oral flecainide for converting recent-onset atrial fibrillation to sinus rhythm in patients without organic heart disease or with only systemic hypertension. Am J Cardiol 1992; 70:69–72.

83. Donovan KD, Dobb GJ, Coombs LJ, et al. Reversion of recent-onset atrial fibrillation to sinus rhythm by intravenous flecainide. Am J Cardiol 1991; 67:137–41.

84. Vardas PE, Kochiadakis GE, Igoumenidis NE, et al. Amiodarone as a first-choice drug for restoring sinus rhythm in patients with atrial fibrillation: a randomized, controlled study. Chest 2000; 117:1538–45.

85. Peuhkurinen K, Niemela M, Ylitalo A, et al. Effectiveness of amiodarone as a single oral dose for recent-onset atrial fibrillation. Am J Cardiol 2000; 85:462–5.

86. Kochiadakis GE, Igoumenidis NE, Solomou MC, et al. Efficacy of amiodarone for the termination of persistent atrial fibrillation. Am J Cardiol 1999; 83:58–61.

87. Cotter G, Blatt A, Kaluski E, et al. Conversion of recent onset paroxysmal atrial fibrillation to normal sinus rhythm: the effect of no treatment and high-dose amiodarone. A randomized, placebo-controlled study. Eur Heart J 1999; 20:1833–42.

88. Kochiadakis GE, Igoumenidis NE, Simantirakis EN, et al. Intravenous propafenone versus intravenous amiodarone in the management of atrial fibrillation of recent onset: a placebo-controlled study. Pacing Clin Electrophysiol 1998; 21:2475–9.

89. Galve E, Rius T, Ballester R, et al. Intravenous amiodarone in treatment of recent-onset atrial fibrillation: results of a randomized, controlled study. J Am Coll Cardiol 1996; 27:1079–82.

90. Cochrane AD, Siddins M, Rosenfeldt FL, et al. A comparison of amiodarone and digoxin for treatment of supraventricular arrhythmias after cardiac surgery. Eur J Cardiothorac Surg 1994; 8:194–8.

91. Capucci A, Lenzi T, Boriani G, et al. Effectiveness of loading oral flecainide for converting recent-onset atrial fibrillation to sinus rhythm in patients without organic heart disease or with only systemic hypertension. Am J Cardiol 1992; 70:69–72.

92. Pedersen OD, Bagger H, Keller N, et al. Efficacy of dofetilide in the treatment of atrial fibrillation-flutter in patients with reduced left ventricular function: a Danish investigations of arrhythmia and mortality on dofetilide (diamond) substudy. Circulation 2001; 104:292–6.

93. Singh S, Zoble RG, Yellen L, et al. Efficacy and safety of oral dofetilide in converting to and maintaining sinus rhythm in patients with chronic atrial fibrillation or atrial flutter: the symptomatic atrial fibrillation investigative research on dofetilide (SAFIRE-D) study. Circulation 2000; 102:2385–90.

94. Lindeboom JE, Kingma JH, Crijns HJ, et al. Efficacy and safety of intravenous dofetilide for rapid termination of atrial fibrillation and atrial flutter. Am J Cardiol 2000; 85:1031–3.

95. Bianconi L, Castro A, Dinelli M, et al. Comparison of intravenously administered dofetilide versus amiodarone in the acute termination of atrial fibrillation and flutter: a multicentre, randomized, double-blind, placebo-controlled study. Eur Heart J 2000; 21:1265–73.

96. Norgaard BL, Wachtell K, Christensen PD, et al. Efficacy and safety of intravenously administered dofetilide in acute termination of atrial fibrillation and flutter: a multicenter, randomized, double-blind, placebo-controlled trial. Danish Dofetilide in Atrial Fibrillation and Flutter Study Group. Am Heart J 1999; 137:1062–9.

97. Frost L, Mortensen PE, Tingleff J, et al. Efficacy and safety of dofetilide, a new class III antiarrhythmic agent, in acute termination of atrial fibrillation or flutter after coronary artery bypass surgery. Dofetilide Post-CABG Study Group. Int J Cardiol 1997; 58:135–40.

98. VanderLugt JT, Mattioni T, Denker S, et al. Efficacy and safety of ibutilide fumarate for the conversion of atrial arrhythmias after cardiac surgery. Circulation 1999; 100:369–75.

99. Stambler BS, Wood MA, Ellenbogen KA, et al. Efficacy and safety of repeated intravenous doses of ibutilide for rapid conversion of atrial flutter or fibrillation. Ibutilide Repeat Dose Study Investigators. Circulation 1996; 94:1613–21.

100. Ellenbogen KA, Clemo HF, Stambler BS, et al. Efficacy of ibutilide for termination of atrial fibrillation and flutter. Am J Cardiol 1996; 78:42–5.

101. Singh S, Saini RK, DiMarco J, et al. Efficacy and safety of sotalol in digitalized patients with chronic atrial fibrillation. The Sotalol Study Group. Am J Cardiol 1991; 68:1227–30.

102. Coplen SE, Antman EM, Berlin JA, Hewitt P, Chalmers TC. Efficacy and safety of quinidine

therapy for maintenance of sinus rhythm after cardioversion. A meta-analysis of randomized control trials. Circulation 1990; 82:1106–16.

103. Ricard P, Levy S, Boccara G, Lakhal E, Bardy G. External cardioversion of atrial fibrillation: comparison of biphasic vs monophasic waveform shocks. Europace 2001; 3:96–9.

104. Mittal S, Ayati S, Stein KM, et al. Transthoracic cardioversion of atrial fibrillation: comparison of rectilinear biphasic versus damped sine wave monophasic shocks. Circulation 2000; 101:1282–1287.

105. Raipancholia R, Sentinella L, Lynch M. Role of conscious sedation for external cardioversion. Heart 2001; 86:571–572.

106. Pugh PJ, Spurrell P, Kamalvand K, Sulke AN. Sedation by physician with diazepam for DC cardioversion of atrial arrhythmias. Heart 2001; 86:572–573.

107. Gale DW, Grissom TE, Mirenda JV. Titration of intravenous anesthetics for cardioversion: a comparison of propofol, methohexital, and midazolam. Crit Care Med 1993; 21:1509–13.

108. Dittrich HC, Erickson JS, Schneidermen T, Blacky AR, Savides T, Nicod PH. Echocardiographic and clinical predictors for outcome of elective cardioversion of atrial fibrillation. Am J Cardiol 1989; 63:193–7.

109. Miller MR, McNamara RL, Segal JB, et al. Efficacy of agents for pharmacologic conversion of atrial fibrillation and subsequent maintenance of sinus rhythm: a meta-analysis of clinical trials. J Fam Pract 2000; 49:1033–46.

110. Roy D, Talajic M, Dorian P, et al. Amiodarone to prevent recurrence of atrial fibrillation. N Engl J Med 2000; 342:913–920.

111. De Simone A, Stabile G, Vitale DF, et al. Pretreatment with verapamil in patients with persistent or chronic atrial fibrillation who underwent electrical cardioversion. J Am Coll Cardiol 1999; 34:810–4.

112. Plewan A, Lehmann G, Ndrepepa G, et al. Maintenance of sinus rhythm after electrical cardioversion of persistent atrial fibrillation; sotalol vs bisoprolol. Eur Heart J 2001; 22:1504–10.

113. Dethy M, Chassat C, Roy D, Mercier LA. Doppler echocardiographic predictors of recurrence of atrial fibrillation after cardioversion. Am J Cardiol 1988; 62:723–6.

114. Brodsky MA, Allen BJ, Capparelli EV, Luckett CR, Morton R, Henry WL. Factors determining maintenance of sinus rhythm after chronic atrial fibrillation with left atrial dilatation. Am J Cardiol 1989; 63:1065–8.

115. Van Gelder IC, Crijns HJ, Van Gilst WH, Verwer R, Lie KL. Prediction of uneventful cardioversion and maintenance of sinus rhythm from direct-current electrical cardioversion of chronic atrial fibrillation and flutter. Am J Cardiol 1991; 68:41–6.

116. Crijns HJ, Van Gelder IC, Van Gilst WH, Hillege H, Gosslink AM, Lie KL. Serial antiarrhythmics drug treatment to maintain sinus rhythm after electrical cardioversion for chronic atrial fibrillation or atrial flutter. Am J Cardiol 1991; 68:335–341.

117. Carlsson J, Tebbe U, Rox J, et al. Cardioversion of atrial fibrillation in the elderly. ALKK-Study Group. Arbeitsgemeinschaft Leitender Kardiologischer Krankenhausaerzte. Am J Cardiol 1996; 78:1380–4.

118. Verhorst PM, Kamp O, Welling RC, Van Eenige MJ, Visser CA. Transesophageal echocardiographic predictors for maintenance of sinus rhythm after electrical cardioversion of atrial fibrillation. Am J Cardiol 1997; 79:1355–9.

119. Madrid AH, Bueno MG, Rebollo JM, Marin I, Pena G, Bernal E, Rodriguez A, Cano L, Cano JM, Cabeza P, Moro C. Use of irbesartan to maintain sinus rhythm in patients with long-lasting persistent atrial fibrillation: a prospective and randomized study. Circulation 2002; 106:331–6.

Antithrombotic therapy in atrial fibrillation: a clinical approach

Dwayne S G Conway MRCP
City Hospital, Birmingham, UK

Gregory Y H Lip MD FRCP DFM FACC FESC
City Hospital, Birmingham, UK

In AF antithrombotic therapy should be administered on the basis of clinical evidence (rather than pharmacological supposition), a thorough risk evaluation, and tailored to the needs of the individual

Introduction

The excess thromboembolic stroke risk conferred by atrial fibrillation (AF),[1] especially in the presence of additional risk factors, has massive implications for public health expenditure. AF itself is notoriously difficult to eradicate: long-term success rates for cardioversion and maintenance of sinus rhythm are poor and evidence is accumulating from randomized controlled trials that such an approach may confer no overall benefit compared to rate control alone and may in certain cases cause harm.[2–4] Consequently, any therapeutic agent or procedure which might cost-effectively reduce the risk of thromboembolism associated with AF would be of vital importance in the prevention of stroke. Of all AF patients, those with additional stroke risk factors would be expected to gain the most benefit from such interventions.

Although the precise mechanisms leading to left atrial (LA) thrombus formation in AF are incompletely understood,[5] examination of LA thrombi reveals a fibrin-rich structure with relatively few platelet aggregates, compared to the arterial thrombi associated with atheromatous plaque rupture (Fig. 18.1). Furthermore, in a large cross-sectional study of participants enrolled in the SPAF III trial, diabetes was the only AF stroke risk factor associated with increased platelet activation (assessed by plasma levels of soluble P-selectin).[6] Other AF stroke risk factors were associated with no change or even lower levels of this platelet marker, while several atherothrombotic risk factors (male sex, peripheral vascular disease, current smoking) were associated with raised soluble P-selectin. Plasma levels of soluble P-selectin did not differ between those AF patients at low, moderate or high risk of future stroke,[6] and did not predict stroke or cardiovascular events among 994 patients treated with aspirin,[7] suggesting platelet activation may be relatively unimportant in determining thromboembolic risk in AF. If

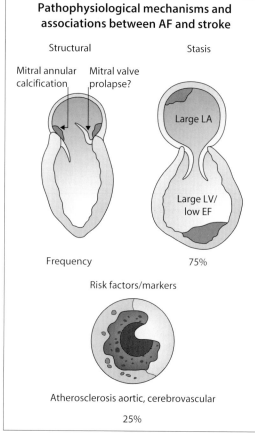

Pathophysiological mechanisms and associations between AF and stroke

Structural   Stasis

Mitral annular calcification   Mitral valve prolapse?

Large LA

Large LV/ low EF

Frequency   75%

Risk factors/markers

Atherosclerosis aortic, cerebrovascular

25%

Fig. 18.1 Pathophysiologic mechanisms and associations between AF and stroke. AF may confer a prothrombotic or hypercoagulable state.

so, while blockade of the coagulation cascade might be expected to reduce LA thrombus formation, platelet inhibition may have a less pronounced effect than seen in the prevention of atherothrombotic disorders such as myocardial infarction.

Nonetheless, despite the likelihood of a lesser role for platelets in the origins of LA thrombosis and embolism, it is difficult to completely exclude such a role, particularly early in the process (where secretion of platelet granule components might provide a stimulus for fibrin production via the coagulation cascade). Furthermore, AF is frequently accompanied by additional cardiovascular disorders which may promote *atherothrombotic* stroke and it is often difficult to identify the etiology of stroke (atherothrombotic versus cardioembolic) in patients with AF.[8] Therefore anticoagulant and antiplatelet drugs may each have separate theoretical advantages in stroke prevention in AF. However, since the potential benefits of antiplatelet or anticoagulant agents must be offset against potential hemorrhagic complications or issues regarding ease of administration, decisions regarding appropriate choice of antithrombotic therapy should be made on the basis of clinical evidence (rather than pharmacological supposition) and tailored to the needs of the individual.

Of the currently available pharmacological agents targeting the coagulation cascade, warfarin and phenindione are the only orally-active agents currently available. Similarly, despite great advances in recent years in the use of intravenous glycoprotein IIb/IIIa inhibitors in the setting of acute coronary syndromes, the disappointing results achieved with oral glycoprotein IIb/IIIa inhibitors mean that only aspirin, dipyridamole, clopidogrel and certain non-steroidal anti-inflammatory drugs (such as indobufen) are available as oral antiplatelet strategies. Several of these available antithrombotic/antiplatelet agents remain untested in the setting of AF and, although there is much research activity in this area with new agents undergoing phase III clinical trials, it is important to first consider the evidence base behind currently available therapies.

STROKE PREVENTION IN AF: EVIDENCE FROM CLINICAL TRIALS

Several large-scale clinical trials have been undertaken over the past 15 years to establish the relative benefits of warfarin and aspirin, against placebo or each other, in prevention of stroke in AF. In addition, smaller studies and substudies have been undertaken to establish the role of other anticoagulant or antiplatelet stategies.

Warfarin

Between 1989 and 1993, five primary prevention trials[9–13] and one secondary prevention trial[14] evaluated the use of adjusted dose warfarin compared to placebo in AF. Despite differences in trial design and target INR ranges (see Table 18.1),[12–17] four of the trials showed statistically significant benefits of warfarin therapy (with the other two trials showing non-significant trends in favor of warfarin) in reducing the incidence of 'all stroke' (ischemic and hemorrhagic combined). The CAFA trial[12] was stopped early due to publication of other trial results, and showed a non-significant trend towards a beneficial effect of warfarin. Pooling the results from all trials (including data from AF subgroups from other published trials) suggests that adjusted-dose warfarin reduces stroke by 62% [95% confidence interval (CI) 48–72%], with absolute risk reductions of 2.7% per year for primary prevention and 8.4% per year for secondary prevention (Fig. 18.2).[18] In contrast, aspirin reduced stroke by 22% (95% CI 2–38%), with absolute risk reductions of 1.5% per year for primary prevention and 2.5% per

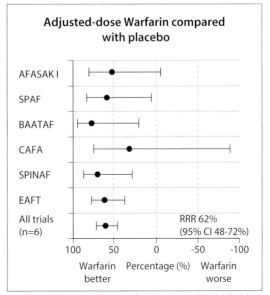

Fig. 18.2 Adjusted-dose Warfarin compared with placebo. Relative risk reduction of stroke (95% CI). (From Hart et al[18])

Table 18.1 Adjusted-dose warfarin compared with placebo. (Reproduced with permission from Hart et al[18])

Study (Reference)	Year	Type of Prevention	Total Participants	Target International Normalized Ratio	Warfarin Group			Placebo Group			Relative Risk Reduction (95% CI)†	Absolute Risk Reduction per Year
					Strokes	Participants	Person-Years	Strokes	Participants	Person-Years		
			n		n			n			%	
AFASAK[15]	1989	Primary	671	2.8–4.2	9	335	413	19	336	398	54	2.6
SPAF[16]	1991	Primary	421	2.0–4.5‡	8	210	263	19	211	245	60§	4.7
BAATAF[13]||	1990	Primary	420	1.5–2.7‡	3	212	487	13	208	435	78§	2.4
CAFA[12]	1991	Primary	378	2.0–3.0	6	187	237	9	191	241	33	1.2
SPINAF[17]	1992	Primary	571	1.4–2.8‡	7	281	489	23	290	483	70§	3.3
EAFT[14]¶	1993	Secondary	439	2.5–4.0	20	225	507	50	214	405	68§	8.4
All trials**	–		2900	–	53	1450	2396	133	1450	2207	62 (48–72)	3.1

AFASAK, Copenhagen Atrial Fibrillation, Aspirin, and Anticoagulation Study; BAATAF, Boston Area Anticoagulation Study for Atrial Fibrillation; CAFA, Canadian Atrial Fibrillation Anticoagulation Study; EAFT, European Atrial Fibrillation Trial; SPAF, Stroke Prevention in Atrial Fibrillation Study; SPINAF, Stroke Prevention in Nonrheumatic Atrial Fibrillation.

† For combined ischemic and hemorrhagic stroke by intention-to-treat analysis; trials of primary prevention included 3%–8% of participants with previous stroke or transient ischemic attack. In EAFT, a variety of coumarins were used, not only warfarin.

‡ Prothrombin time ratios were used; international normalized ratios were estimated by the investigators.

§ $P < 0.05$, two-sided.

|| 46% of exposure in the control group occurred during self-selected use of varying doses of aspirin.

¶ Various types of coumarin were used.

** Weighted estimates of relative risk reduction ($P > 0.2$ for homogeneity) and absolute risk reduction ($P > 0.2$ for homogeneity) year for secondary prevention (Fig. 18.3).[18]

In addition to the placebo-controlled trials, warfarin has been studied in 'head-to-head' comparison trials versus aspirin therapy.[9,14,19–21] Pooling the results from these trials appears to confirm the superiority of warfarin over aspirin (relative risk reduction 36% (95% CI 14–52%),[18] although much of the observed effect in this meta-analysis was exerted by the large secondary prevention EAFT trial[14] (Fig. 18.4). A subsequent systematic review

of 'aspirin versus warfarin' trials claimed the benefits of warfarin may be overstated,[22] but this review did not include all trials and, most notably, excluded EAFT from the review (Fig. 18.5).[22]

The reduction in relative risk with warfarin applies equally to primary and secondary prevention but, as the absolute risk of stroke is higher in those with a prior stroke (12% per annum versus 4.5% per annum if no prior cerebral ischemia), the absolute risk reduction achievable with warfarin is greater for secondary prevention. Thus, the number of patients with AF needing treatment (NNT) with warfarin to prevent one stroke is therefore approximately three times greater in primary prevention (NNT=37) than in secondary prevention (NNT=12).[18]

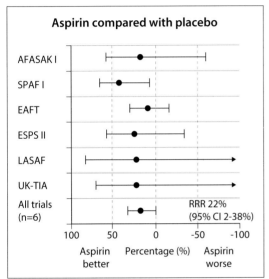

Fig. 18.3 Aspirin compared with placebo. Relative risk reduction of stroke (95% CI). (From Hart et al[18])

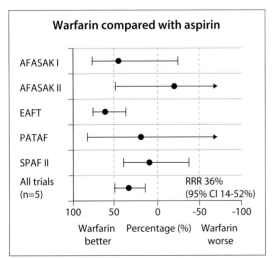

Fig. 18.4 Warfarin compared with aspirin. Relative risk reduction of stroke (95% CI). (From Hart et al[18])

'Mini-dose' warfarin

Treatment with full-dose anticoagulation carries the potential risk of major bleeding, including intracranial hemorrhage. Meta-

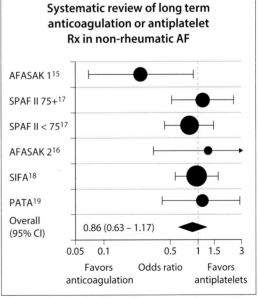

Fig. 18.5 Systematic review of long term anticoagulation or antiplatelet Rx in non-rheumatic AF. Comparison of fatal vascular outcomes in trials of anticoagulation versus antiplatelet treatment. (From Taylor et al[22])

analysis of the six major trials suggests the risk of hemorrhagic stroke is only marginally increased from 0.1 to 0.3% per year,[18] although many might argue that the conditions of a clinical trial are far different from the reality of everyday patient care, where hemorrhage rates may be expected to be higher. Nonetheless, there is evidence that the risk/benefit ratios of the clinical trials can be achieved in clinical practice.[23]

In the clinical trials, the highest rates of major hemorrhage were seen amongst elderly subgroups and those with higher

Table 18.2 Adjusted-dose warfarin compared with other antithrombotic regimens (Reproduced with permission from Hart et al[18])

Study (Reference)	Year	Type of Prevention	Total Participants	Target International Normalized Ratio	Target Dosage
			n		*mg/d*
Adjusted-dose warfarin compared with aspirin					
AFASAK[15]	1989	Primary	671	2 to 3	75
SPAF II[19]	1994	Primary	–	2.0 to 4.5	325
		Age ≤75	715	–	
		Age >75	385	–	
EAFT[14]	1993	Secondary	455	2.5 to 4.0	300
AFASAK II[20]	1998	Primary	339	2 to 3	300
PATAF[21]	1997	Primary	272	2.5 to 3.5	150
All trials		–	2837		
Adjusted-dose warfarin compared with low- or fixed-dose warfarin plus aspirin					
SPAF III[26]	1996	Primary and Secondary	1044††	2 to 3	1 to 3 plus 325
AFASAK II[20]	1998	Primary	341	2 to 3	1.25 plus 300
Adjusted-dose warfarin compared with indobufen					
SIFA[27]	1997	Secondary	916	2.0 to 3.5	400
Adjusted-dose warfarin compared with low- or fixed-dose warfarin					
AFASAK II[20]	1998	Primary	337	2 to 3	1.25
MWNAF[25]	1998	Primary	303	2 to 3	1.25
PATAF[21]	1997	Primary	253	2.5 to 3.5	1.1 to 1.6‡‡
All trials			893		

AFASAK, Copenhagen Atrial Fibrillation, Aspirin, and Anticoagulation Study; EAFT, European Atrial Fibrillation Trial; MWNAF, Minidose Warfarin in Nonrheumatic Atrial Fibrillation; PATAF, Prevention of Arterial Thromboembolism in Atrial Fibrillation; SIFA, Studio Italiano Fibrillazione Atriale; SPAF, Stroke Prevention in Atrial Fibrillation.

† For combined ischemic and hemorrhagic strokes by intention-to-treat analysis.

‡ Various types of coumarin were used.

§ Total patient-years of exposure were estimated from mean duration of follow-up because total exposure was not published.

intensity anticoagulation (especially in the SPAF-II trial, using an international normalized ratio (INR) range of 2.0–4.5).[24] In the quest for a 'low-risk' alternative, three studies compared the effect of fixed low dose warfarin to adjusted dose warfarin,[20,21,25] but these low-dose regimens failed to provide equivalent protection (see Table 18.2).[14,15,19–21,25–27] Furthermore, the SPAF III trial clearly demonstrated that even with the addition of aspirin therapy to fixed low doses of warfarin the result remains inferior to adjusted-dose warfarin (INR 2–3) alone (Fig. 18.6).[26]

Table 18.2 cont'd

Warfarin Group			Other Treatment Groups			Relative Risk Reduction (95% CI)†	Absolute Risk Reduction per Year
Strokes	Participants	Patient-Years	Strokes	Participants	Patient-Years		
n			*n*			%	
9	335	413	16	336	409	45	1.7
19	358	1099	21	357	1083	10	0.2
20	197	394	21	188	377	10	0.5
20	225	507	52	230	477§	67‖	7.0
11	170	355	9	169	365	−23	−0.6
3	131	401	4	141	392	20	0.3
82	1416	3169	123	1421	3103	36 (14 to 52)¶	0.8**
14	523	581	48	521	558	73‖	6.2
11	170	355	11	171	377	−1	−0.2
18	454	450§	23	462	460§	21 (−54 to 60)	1.0
11	170	355	14	167	363	24	0.8
1	153	182§	5	150	183§	81	2.2
3	131	401	4	122	361	31	0.4
15	454	938	23	439	907	38 (−20 to 68)¶	1.0**

‖ P < 0.05, two-sided.
¶ Weighted estimates (*P* = 0.09 for homogeneity for comparisons with aspirin and *P* > 0.2 for comparisons with low-dose warfarin).
** Weighted estimates (*P* = 0.2 for homogeneity for comparisons with aspirin and *P* > 0.2 for comparisons with low-dose warfarin).
†† Preselected as those with high rates of stroke during aspirin therapy.
‡‡ International normalized ratio.

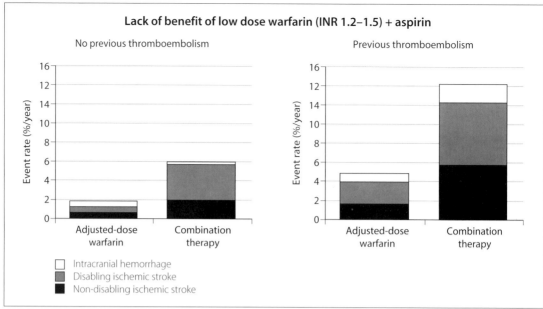

Fig. 18.6 SPAF-III: lack of benefit of low dose warfarin (INR 1.2–1.5)+ aspirin. (From SPAF Investigators[26])

Heparin

Unfractionated or low molecular weight heparins are unlikely to play important roles in long-term chronic stroke prevention due to the practical difficulty of intravenous and subcutaneous routes of administration, but in view of the inevitable delay in achieving target INR, heparin is sometimes employed provide a temporary alternative whilst initiating warfarin.

There are currently no long-term prospective randomized controlled trials demonstrating a significant reduction in thromboembolic events with unfractionated or low molecular weight heparins compared to placebo in patients with AF. However, one study demonstrated a small non-significant trend towards stroke reduction over 6 months using low molecular weight heparin in chronic AF but sample sizes were small and there was poor standardization of the control group.[28] For secondary prevention of stroke, the HAEST (Heparin in Acute Embolic Stroke) study compared dalteparin (100 IU/kg subcutaneous twice daily) with aspirin (160 mg oral once daily) commenced within 30 h of ischemic stroke in patients with AF,

but again failed to show any difference in outcome between the two groups during the following 14 days, despite a relatively high occurrence of endpoints in both groups.[29]

Regardless of the absence of conclusive prospective data, the consensus view from the American College of Chest Physicians is that heparin may still have a role to play in acute AF (and immediately prior to cardioversion) in patients not already commenced on warfarin, due to the cluster of thromboembolic events witnessed in these situations when no anticoagulant therapy is used.[30,31] Furthermore, low molecular weight heparins may be successfully used to cover the pericardioversion period in those undergoing 'TEE-guided' (transesophageal echocardiography) cardioversion.[32]

Antiplatelet therapy in AF

Five large prospective randomised placebo-controlled trials[11,14,15,33,34] have compared the use of aspirin and placebo in AF, although trial designs have varied widely, with doses ranging from 25 mg twice daily to 1200 mg per day (see Table 18.3). Taking

Table 18.3 Antiplatelet agents compared with placebo. (Reproduced with permission from Hart et al[18])

Study (Reference)	Year	Type of Prevention[†]	Total Participants	Dosage	Antiplatelet Treatment Group			Placebo Group			Relative Risk Reduction (95% CI)[†]	Absolute Risk Reduction per Year
			n		Strokes	Participants	Person-Years	Strokes	Participants	Person-Years	%	
						n			n			
Aspirin compared with placebo												
AFASAK[15]	1989	Primary	672	75 mg/d	16	336	409	19	336	398	17	0.9
SPAF[16]	1991	Primary	1120	325 mg/d	25	552	723	44	568	734	44	2.5
EAFT[14]	1993	Secondary	782	300 mg/d	88	404	853	90	378	734	11	1.9
ESPS II[35]	1997	Secondary	211	25 mg twice per day	17	104	123	23	107	111	29§	6.9
LASAF[34]	1996	Primary	195	125 mg/d	4	104	145	3	91	135	-17	-0.5
			181	125 mg every other day	1	90	148	3	91	135	67	1.6
UK-TIA[36]	1999	Secondary	28	300 mg/d	3	13	52||	4	15	60||	17	0.9
			36	1200 mg/d	5	21	84||	4	15	60||	14	0.7
All aspirin trials	–	–	3119	–	159	1624	2539	190	1601	2363	22 (2 to 38)	1.7
Dipyridamole compared with placebo												
ESPS II[35]	1997	Secondary	221	200 mg twice per day	20	114	133	23	107	111	22 (−60 to 62)§	5.7
Dipyridamole and aspirin compared with placebo												
ESPS II[35]	1997	Secondary	211	Dipyridamole, 200 mg twice per day, plus aspirin, 25 mg twice per day	14	104	127	23	107	111	43 (−24 to 74)§	9.7
All antiplatelet trials[¶]	–	–	3337	–	193	1842	2799	236	1815	2585	24 (7 to 39)	1.9

AFASAK, Copenhagen Atrial Fibrillation, Aspirin, and Anticoagulation Study; ESPS II, European Stroke Prevention Study II; LASAF, Low-Dose Aspirin, Stroke, and Atrial Fibrillation Pilot Study; SPAF, Stroke Prevention in Atrial Fibrillation Study; UK-TIA, United Kingdom TIA Study; † In trials of primary prevention, 6%–8% of participants had previous stroke or transient ischemic attack; ‡ For combined ischemic and hemorrhagic stroke by intention-to-treat analysis unless otherwise specified; § Only results of efficacy (that is, results of participants receiving therapy) were reported; || Total patient-years of exposure were estimated from mean duration of follow-up because total exposure was not published; ¶ Weighted estimates of relative risk reductions (P > 0.2 for homogeneity for all aspirin trials and for all antiplatelet trials) and absolute risk reductions (P > 0.2 for homogeneity for all aspirin trials and P > 0.2 for all antiplatelet trials).

all the major placebo-controlled trials together, aspirin reduces the relative risk of stroke by about 22% (with no apparent benefit of increasing aspirin dose).[18] It should be noted, however, that despite the inclusion of 3119 participants, the figure of 22% only marginally reaches statistical significance (with 95% CI, from 2–38%). Furthermore, aspirin seems to carry greatest benefit in reducing smaller non-disabling strokes, rather than the disabling strokes particularly common in AF, which may be due to an effect primarily on carotid and cerebral artery platelet thrombus formation rather than on formation of intra-atrial thrombus.[8] However, in the warfarin versus aspirin trials, in which adjusted dose warfarin reduced the risk of stroke by 36% ((95% CI 14–52%) compared to aspirin, the relative risk reduction was similar for both disabling and non-disabling strokes.[18] In acute onset stroke, subgroup analyses of the International Stroke Trial and the Chinese Acute Stroke Trial do not show any significant benefits of aspirin in AF patients, in contrast to non-AF patients.[37–39]

Other antiplatelet agents

While the ESPS-II study suggests the combination of aspirin and dipyridamole following stroke may be superior to either agent alone,[33] this effect did not reach statistical significance in the AF subgroup, although this may be due to lack of statistical power rather than a lack of effect. Furthermore, despite the apparent superiority of warfarin above aspirin for stroke prevention (especially secondary prevention) in AF, one well conducted secondary prevention study comparing the antiplatelet agent indobufen (a reversible cyclo-oxygenase inhibitor) with warfarin (INR 2–3.5) suggested relative similarity between the two treatment arms,[27] although the event rate in the warfarin group was perhaps a little higher than observed in other studies. Further studies of recently developed antiplatelet agents

(including clopidogrel) and combination antiplatelet therapies are lacking in the setting of AF, but are needed to fully evaluate the potential role of antiplatelet therapy in AF.

New agents

Promising news for the prevention of thromboembolism in AF is the development of drugs such as the oral thrombin and factor Xa inhibitors.[40] Recent data from a Phase III clinical trial (SPORTIF III, n = 3407) comparing the oral direct thrombin inhibitor, ximelagatran, to warfarin, demonstrated a similar efficacy in stroke reduction of both treatments (Event rates: 2.3% per year on warfarin vs 1.62% per year on ximelagatran), with lower bleeding rates on ximelagatran (25.5% per year vs 29.5% on warfarin, p=0.007). Potential advantages over warfarin include fixed dosage and abolition of the need for INR monitoring. If the safety and efficacy profiles are found to be superior or equivalent to warfarin, anticoagulant service provision for AF may be set to change beyond recognition.

ANTITHROMBOTIC THERAPY IN AF: PRACTICE GUIDELINES

Key points

Using risk stratification, we may target anticoagulant therapy at those at greatest stroke risk and avoid anticoagulant therapy in those for whom the benefits of warfarin treatment may be no greater than the potential risk of hemorrhage

Risk stratification

The major epidemiological studies of AF (including the Framingham study) and the major clinical trials have all identified similar additional risk factors which, when present in patients with AF, further increase

Table 18.4 Relative risk for development of AF in the presence of associated conditions

	Men	Women
Diabetes	1.4	1.6
Hypertension	1.5	1.4
Heart failure	4.5	5.9
Valvular heart disease	1.8	3.4
Myocardial infarction	1.4	NS

the risk of stroke (see Table 18.4). In fact, as AF is commonly associated with additional cardiovascular risk factors,[41] true 'lone AF' (that is, AF in the absence of additional risk factors) is relatively rare and (probably) carries a lower risk of thromboembolism compared to AF patients as a whole. As a result, we may effectively stratify the thromboembolic risk of AF patients according to presence or absence of these risk factors.[42,43] This is important when considering the absolute risk reductions achievable by warfarin therapy (or the number of patients requiring treatment to prevent one stroke). Using risk stratification, we may target anticoagulant therapy at those at greatest stroke risk and avoid anticoagulant therapy in those for whom the benefits of warfarin treatment may be no greater than the potential risk of hemorrhage. Many evidence-based risk stratification schemes have been suggested and validated (Table 18.5).[35,44–46] A simple, practical guide based upon the evidence available to date is presented in Table 18.6.[42]

Nearly all of the additional risk factors can be assessed easily and clinically. Echocardiographic assessment is therefore not mandatory for risk stratification of every patient with AF. However, echocardiography may be useful to refine

Table 18.5 Risk stratification schemes for primary prevention of stroke in non-valvular atrial fibrillation

Criteria (year)	High risk	Intermediate risk	Low risk
Atrial Fibrillation Investigators (1994)[44]	Age < 65 years History of hypertension Diabetes mellitus	Age ≥ 65 years No high-risk features	
American College of Chest Physicians Consensus (1998)[45]	Age >75 years History of hypertension Left ventricular dysfunction† > 1 moderate risk factor	Age 65–75 years Diabetes mellitus Coronary disease (Thyrotoxicosis)*	Age < 65 years No risk factors
Stroke Prevention in Atrial Fibrillation (1995)[46]	Women >75 years Systolic blood pressure > 160 mHg Left ventricular dysfunction‡	History of hypertension No high-risk features	No high-risk features No history of hypertension
Lip GYH (1999)[42]	Patients ≥ 75 years and with diabetes or hypertension Patients with clinical evidence of heart failure, thyroid disease, and /or impaired left ventricular function on echocardiography§	Patients < 65 years with clinical risk factors: diabetes, hypertension, peripheral arterial disease, ischemic heart disease Patients over 65 not in high risk group	Patients < 65 years with no risk factors

* Patients with thyrotoxicosis were excluded from participation in the test cohort

† Moderate to severe left ventricular dysfunction on echocardiography

‡ Recent congestive heart failure or fractional shortening ≤ 25% by M-mode echocardiography

§ Echocardiography not needed for routine risk assessment but refines clinical risk stratification in case of impaired left ventricular function and valve disease

Table 18.6 Risk stratification and anticoagulation in non-valvular AF (NVAF) (From Lip[42])

ASSESS RISK:

1. *High risk*   (annual risk of CVA = 8–12%)
   - All patients with NVAF and previous TIA or CVA
   - All patients aged 75 and over with NVAF and diabetes and/or hypertension
   - All patients with NVAF and clinical evidence of valve disease, heart failure, thyroid disease and/or impaired LV function on echocardiography*.

2. *Moderate risk*   (annual risk of CVA = 4%)
   - All patients under 65 with NVAF and clinical risk factors:- diabetes, hypertension, peripheral arterial disease, ischemic heart disease.
   - All patients over 65 with NVAF who have not been identified in high risk group.

3. *Low risk*   (annual risk of CVA = 1%)
   - All other patients under 65 with NVAF with no history of embolism, hypertension, diabetes or other clinical risk factors.

*ECHOCARDIOGRAM - not needed for routine risk assessment but refines clinical risk stratification in case of impaired LV function and valve disease (see 1 above). A large left atrium per se is not an independent risk factor on multivariate analysis.
REASSESS RISK FACTORS AT REGULAR INTERVALS

TREATMENT:
High risk: use WARFARIN (target INR 2.0–3.0) if no contraindications and possible in practice.
Moderate risk: Either WARFARIN or ASPIRIN. In view of insufficient clearcut evidence, treatment may be decided on individual cases. Referral and ECHOCARDIOGRAPHY may help.
Low risk: use ASPIRIN 75–300 mg daily

risk status in those patients who fall in the moderate or low risk groups clinically, as LV dysfunction in such patients would indicate high risk of thromboembolism and warfarin would be the drug of choice. An increase in left atrial size is strongly associated with subsequent thromboembolic risk, but this feature has been shown to be linked to many of the underlying clinical risk factors and is not in itself independently predictive.[47]

Elderly patients are often denied anticoagulant therapy by their physician due to fears of increased hemorrhage risk yet paradoxically the benefits of anticoagulant therapy are greater for patients with advanced age due to the increased underlying thromboembolic risk. Although the available data from clinical trials so far does not extend much beyond the age of 80 years, the increased benefit appears to be consistent up to this age and further ongoing trials are examining more closely the use of anticoagulant therapy in patients over the age of 80 years. Conversely, young patients may have such a low risk of stroke that the hemorrhagic complication rate may outweigh the minimal reduction in thromboembolism that warfarin therapy would convey in such patients.

Despite the superiority of warfarin in the clinical trials, aspirin still has a role to play in the thromboprophylaxis of patients unsuitable for warfarin therapy, whether due to contraindications to warfarin or a low inherent stroke risk. However, some may argue that where the risk of thromboembolism is very low (such as lone AF in patients under the age of 60 years), aspirin may provide only minute reductions in absolute risk and may not be necessary at all. The process of risk stratification should be repeated regularly for every patient with AF not on warfarin as the clinical and echocardiographic features are not static and may develop at any time.

> Echocardiographic assessment is not mandatory for risk stratification of every patient with AF – it may be useful to refine risk status in patients in the moderate- or low-risk groups clinically

Hemorrhagic risk of anticoagulant therapy

The risk of hemorrhagic complications itself varies from patient to patient. In the clinical trials an overall small increase in intracranial hemorrhage rates from 0.1% in controls to 0.3% per year with warfarin therapy seems a small price to pay for the benefits of warfarin,[18] but many factors may adversely influence the risk of bleeding to a higher rate. Amongst these, an INR greater than 3.0, poor control of the INR, uncontrolled hypertension and age >75 years are clinically important when considering warfarin therapy in AF. The SPAF-II trial reported a relatively high hemorrhagic complication rate, but this was mainly in elderly patients in whom the INR range was allowed to be maintained as high as 4.5.[8,24] The evidence from meta-analyses of the major AF trials suggests that INR levels greater than 3 may result in an excess rate of hemorrhage whereas low-dose warfarin regimens (with INR maintained below 1.5) do not achieve the desired reductions in thromboembolic stroke.[18] An INR range of 2 to 3 (target 2.5) appears to be highly effective without leading to excessive hemorrhage and is therefore recommended for all patients with AF treated with warfarin, unless they have another indication for higher levels of anticoagulation (such as a mechanical heart valve).[30]

> An INR range of 2–3 (target 2.5) appears to be highly effective without leading to excessive hemorrhage and is therefore recommended for all patients with AF treated with warfarin, unless they have another indication for higher levels of anticoagulation (such as a mechanical heart valve)

Some concern over increased hemorrhagic risk in the elderly has led to the suggestion that the INR range for patients over 75 years of age be reduced to 1.6 to 2.5 with a target of 2.0 (Fig. 18.7).[48] However, such a practice is based on extrapolation of data from the clinical trials

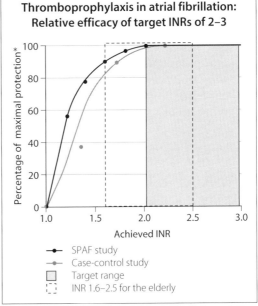

Fig. 18.7 Thromboprophylaxis in atrial fibrillation: relative efficacy of target INRs of 2–3. INR, international normalized ratio. * presumes maximal protection with INRs > 2.0

and has never been proven effective in a prospective randomized study. Furthermore, despite the strict conditions of the clinical trials, similarly low hemorrhage rates have been achieved in clinical practice,[23] and thus fears that the hemorrhage risk from the trial data may be unrealistically low are probably overstated. Nonetheless, a target INR of 2.0 may provide a reasonable compromise between toxicity and efficacy for elderly patients at high-risk of hemorrhagic complications, in the absence of additional thromboembolic risk factors, pending further data about the safety of warfarin in elderly patients with AF.[31,48]

Given the high prevalence of AF in an increasingly elderly population, the burden on traditional anticoagulant monitoring resources is likely to continue to increase as more physicians become aware of the importance of correct anticoagulant therapy in AF. Although the role of INR monitoring is often co-ordinated by hospital-based anticoagulant clinics, family practitioners may need to play an increasingly involved role, in order to meet the increased demands on anticoagulant services which will result from improved preventative management of AF. This change in practice may be facilitated by the development of near-patient INR testing,[49] which appears to be achievable and may improve anticoagulant management and prove more convenient for patients themselves.

ANTITHROMBOTIC THERAPY IN AF: SPECIAL SITUATIONS

Key points

The process of risk stratification should be repeated regularly for every patient with AF not on warfarin as the clinical and echocardiographic features and hence the thromboembolic risk are not static and may develop at any time

Paroxysmal AF

Patients with paroxysmal AF appear to carry the same risk as those with persistent AF,[14,18] and the same criteria should therefore be used to identify and treat high-risk patients (Fig. 18.8).[30,31,42,43] Whether the risk is dependent upon the frequency and duration of the paroxysms themselves remains unclear, although the clustering of thromboembolic events witnessed around the time of onset of AF[9,50] and following cardioversion back to sinus rhythm[51] may indicate potential dangers of paroxysmal AF that are not seen in permanent AF.

Acute stroke

Evidence supporting the benefit of aspirin following acute stroke is lacking among patients with AF. The mortality benefits of aspirin therapy following acute stroke seen in the International Stroke Trial and Chinese Acute Stroke Trial[37,38] were less marked among patients with AF. This may be due to the embolization of preformed intra-atrial thrombus rather than newly formed platelet thrombus adhering to

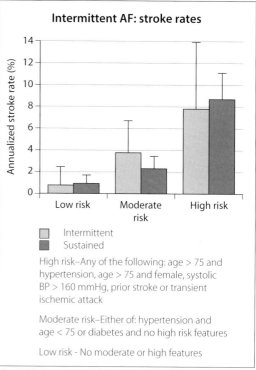

Fig. 18.8 Intermittent AF:stroke rates. The annualized rate of ischemic stroke was similar for those with intermittent (3.2%) and sustained AF (3.3%). (From Hart et al. JACC 2000; 35:183) © 2000 The American College of Cardiology Foundation.

carotid and cerebral artery atheroma, or may be a reflection of a lesser role of platelets in AF-related stroke. Furthermore, while warfarin is superior to aspirin for the secondary prevention of stroke in AF,[14] there is uncertainty about the optimal timing of administration of anticoagulants following acute stroke. Indeed, one must be sure that there is no ongoing intracerebral hemorrhage (or risk of new intracerebral hemorrhage within an area of recent infarction) before commencing anticoagulation. The HAEST study failed to show any difference in outcome between AF patients treated with dalteparin or aspirin within 30 h of ischemic stroke.[29]

Consensus guidelines from the ACCP[30] state that before commencing any antithrombotic agent, a computerized tomography (CT) or magnetic resonance imaging (MRI) scan should be obtained to confirm the absence of intracranial hemorrhage and to assess the size of any cerebral infarction. In AF patients with no evidence of hemorrhage and small infarct size (or no evidence of infarction) warfarin (INR 2–3) can be commenced with minimal risk, provided the patient is normotensive. In AF patients with large areas of cerebral infarction, the initiation of warfarin therapy should be delayed for 2 weeks due to the potential risk of hemorrhagic transformation. The presence of intracranial hemorrhage is an absolute contraindication to the immediate and future use of anticoagulation for stroke prevention in AF.

Acute AF

There is good epidemiological evidence to suggest that the onset of AF is associated with a cluster of thromboembolic events.[50] However, the development of intra-atrial thrombus, and thus the *immediate* risk of thromboembolism, is thought to be minimal if the arrhythmia has been present for less than 48 h.[52] Thus, in patients presenting de novo with AF, a clear history of arrhythmia onset is necessary in order to guide appropriate antithrombotic therapy and safety of direct current (DC) cardioversion.

Although no randomized trials have specifically addressed the issue, there is evidence that cardioversion may be safely performed without anticoagulation if the arrhythmia has been present for less than 48 h.[52] However, in one series intra-atrial thrombus was detected by TEE in approximately 15% of patients presenting with acute AF (apparent duration < 3 days),[53] raising the possibility that the development of intra-atrial thrombus may be more rapid than previously suspected or that many apparent cases of acute AF have developed the arrhythmia asymptomatically more that 48 h before. Thus, in cases of uncertainty, anticoagulation is warranted. Again, no randomized prospective studies have addressed the use of intravenous unfractionated heparin or subcutaneous low molecular weight heparin derivatives, but both have been used with good results in the acute and pericardioversion periods.

Although there are no prospective data showing a reduction in AF-related thromboembolism with heparin, this may be due to a lack of studies rather than a lack of effect. In this case, it is often prudent to initiate anticoagulation with heparin whilst the INR remains subtherapeutic in the initiating phase of warfarin.[30] Furthermore, acute AF often confers a fast ventricular response, which may require urgent DC cardioversion. The initiation of heparin sooner rather than later may therefore provide a 'bridge' to safer DC cardioversion, especially if commenced within 48 h of onset of AF, or combined with a 'TEE-guided' approach.[32] It should be noted, however, that in certain cases of acute AF where the patient is *in extremis* (for example cardiogenic shock) DC cardioversion may need to be performed rapidly and the initiation of anticoagulation should not be allowed to delay this emergency procedure.[30,42,54]

Cardioversion of chronic (persistent) AF

It is well proven that AF increases the risk of thromboembolic stroke, but it is less clear whether this risk can be reduced by cardioversion (by electrical or pharmacological means) to normal sinus rhythm. Despite the theoretical antithrombotic benefits of normalizing left atrial blood flow and evidence that some elevated levels of markers of thrombogenesis can be normalized by cardioversion,[55] there is no strong prospective data demonstrating reduced incidence of stroke after cardioversion. Indeed, there is increasing evidence to suggest that many patients may fare better with rate control and anticoagulation than with attempts to restore sinus rhythm.[2–4] Nonetheless, certain patients may still be considered for DC cardioversion and appropriate thromboprophylactic measures are essential.

Cardioversion itself is known to increase the short-term (pericardioversion) risk of thromboembolism[51] and thus, unless the arrhythmia has been present for less than 48 h,[52] thromboprophylactic measures are required.[30] The precise mechanism behind pericardioversion thromboembolism is complex and incompletely understood, but is likely to be associated with the return of atrial systole, temporary 'stunning' of the left atrium prior to return of systolic function,[56] and possibly an increase in thrombotic tendency due to the procedure itself.[55] The increase in thromboembolic risk may be present up to 3 weeks after successful cardioversion as atrial function may take this time to fully return.

There have been no prospective randomized controlled trials testing the efficacy of warfarin (versus placebo) in prevention of pericardioversion thromboembolism, but several retrospective studies have shown convincing evidence of the benefit of warfarin in this setting. Consequently, it would be ethically difficult to propose a randomized trial in which patients may be allocated no thromboprophylaxis. As a result of the available evidence, the Sixth American College of Chest Physicians (ACCP) recommendations for pericardioversion anticoagulation are for a minimum of 3 weeks of warfarin (INR 2–3) prior to cardioversion, followed by a minimum of 4 weeks postcardioversion (Table 18.7).[30] The recent ACUTE study found that, by excluding thrombus on TEE examination prior to cardioversion, the need for prior anticoagulation could be safely avoided,[57] although a full 4 weeks postcardioversion anticoagulation was given in the study as a normal TEE does not remove the risk of thromboembolism arising de novo. In fact, although thromboembolism rates were similar with this technique and the standard antithrombotic regimen, hemorrhage rates were reduced. The TEE-guided technique

Table 18.7 Recommendations for anticoagulation for cardioversion (From Albers et al [30])

The administration of warfarin for 3 weeks before elective cardioversion of AF of ≥ 48 h duration; continuation of warfarin therapy for 4 weeks after cardioversion

Administration of intravenous heparin followed by warfarin if cardioversion cannot be postponed for 3 weeks; and treat atrial flutter similarly

No anticoagulant therapy for SVT or atrial fibrillation of < 48 h duration

also allowed more rapid cardioversion of cases and resulted in higher initial success rates, although by 8 weeks there was no significant difference in death rates, maintenance of sinus rhythm or functional status between the two groups. TEE-guided cardioversion is now recognized as an alternative to 'standard practice' by the ACCP,[30] but limited resources for TEE mean that 'standard practice' will continue to be practiced in many centers.

SUMMARY

AF is a major cause of stroke due to embolism of thrombus formed in the left atrium and its appendage. The factors leading to thrombus formation are complex and, although left atrial blood-pool stasis secondary to the arrhythmia itself is a major factor, it is likely that abnormalities of atrial endocardium and blood constituents also play a part. These factors may explain the variation in thromboembolic risk in AF according to the presence or absence of other clinical and echocardiographically identifiable factors.

The strong evidence for current guidelines for antithrombotic therapy in AF is derived from several large-scale clinical trials. Both warfarin and aspirin have been shown to reduce thromboembolic risk in AF, but the benefits of warfarin are far greater than aspirin (despite a higher hemorrhagic risk with warfarin) perhaps because platelets may not play a major role in left atrial thrombosis. Using data derived from clinical trials and epidemiological studies of stroke in AF, risk stratification schemes have been developed to target warfarin at those at greatest risk and aspirin to those at least risk. Warfarin is now the thromboprophylactic treatment of choice for most patients in AF.

Although certain clinical situations require deviation from treatment guidelines for chronic AF, paroxysmal AF is not one of these situations and thromboprophylactic therapy should be based upon the same criteria as for sustained AF. The requirement for anticoagulation prior to DC cardioversion may be safely removed by exclusion of intra-atrial thrombus on TEE, but all patients require 4 weeks postcardioversion anticoagulation. Cardioversion of patients in whom the arrhythmia has been present for less than 48 h may be relatively safe without antithrombotic cover but, as some risk remains, early antithrombotic therapy is recommended in all patients presenting acutely with AF.

> Warfarin is the thromboprophylactic treatment of choice for most patients in AF

References

1. Wolf PA, Abbott RD, Kannel WB. Atrial fibrillation as an independent risk factor for stroke: the Framingham Study. Stroke 1991; 22:983–988.
2. Hohnloser SH, Kuck KH, Lilienthal J. Rhythm or rate control in atrial fibrillation—Pharmacological Intervention in Atrial Fibrillation (PIAF): a randomised trial. Lancet 2000; 356:1789–1794.
3. Wyse DG, Waldo AL, Di Marco JP, et al. The Atrial Fibrillation Follow-up Investigation of Rhythm Management (AFFIRM) Investigators. A comparison of rate control and rhythm control in patients with atrial fibrillation. N Engl J Med 2002; 347:1825–1833.
4. Van Gelder IC, Hagens VE, Bosker HA, et al. Rate Control versus Electrical Cardioversion for Persistent Atrial Fibrillation Study Group. A comparison of rate control in patients with recurrent persistent atrial fibrillation. N Engl J Med 2002; 347:1834–1840.
5. Hart RG, Halperin JL. Atrial fibrillation and stroke : concepts and controversies. Stroke 2001; 32:803–808.
6. Conway DS, Pearce LA, Chin BS, et al. Plasma von Willebrand factor and soluble p-selectin as indices of endothelial damage and platelet activation in 1321 patients with nonvalvular atrial fibrillation: relationship to stroke risk factors. Circulation 2002; 106:1962–1967.
7. Conway DSG, Pearce LA, Chin BSP, et al. High plasma von Willebrand factor levels predict future stroke, myocardial infarction and vascular death in 994 patients with atrial fibrillation. Eur Heart J 2002; 23(Suppl):239 (abstract 1292).
8. Hart RG, Pearce LA, Miller VT, et al. Cardioembolic vs. noncardioembolic strokes in atrial fibrillation: frequency and effect of antithrombotic agents in the stroke prevention in atrial fibrillation studies. Cerebrovasc Dis 2000; 10:39–43
9. Petersen P, Godtfredsen J. Embolic complications in paroxysmal atrial fibrillation. Stroke 1986; 17:622–626.
10. Ezekowitz MD, Bridgers SL, James KE, et al. Warfarin in the prevention of stroke associated with nonrheumatic atrial fibrillation. Veterans affairs stroke prevention in nonrheumatic atrial fibrillation investigators. N Engl J Med 1992; 327:1406–1412.
11. SPAF Investigators. Stroke Prevention in Atrial Fibrillation Study. Final results. Circulation 1991; 84:527–539.
12. Connolly SJ, Laupacis A, Gent M, et al. Canadian Atrial Fibrillation Anticoagulation (CAFA) Study. J Am Coll Cardiol 1991; 18:349–355.
13. BAATAF Investigators: The effect of low-dose warfarin on the risk of stroke in patients with nonrheumatic atrial fibrillation. The Boston Area Anticoagulation Trial for Atrial Fibrillation Investigators. N Engl J Med 1990; 323:1505–1511.
14. EAFT Study Group: Secondary prevention in non-rheumatic atrial fibrillation after transient ischaemic attack or minor stroke. EAFT (European Atrial Fibrillation Trial) Study Group. Lancet 1993; 342:1255–1262.
15. Petersen P, Boysen G, Godtfredsen J, et al. Placebo-controlled, randomised trial of warfarin and aspirin for prevention of thromboembolic complications in chronic atrial fibrillation. The Copenhagen AFASAK study. Lancet 1989; 1:175–179.
16. Stroke Prevention in Atrial Fibrillation Study. Final results. Circulation 1991; 84:527–539.
17. Ezekowitz MD, Bridgers SL, James KE, et al. Warfarin in the prevention of stroke associated with nonrheumatic atrial fibrillation. Veterans Affairs Stroke Prevention in Nonrheumatic Atrial Fibrillation Investigators. N Engl J Med 1992; 327:1406–1412.
18. Hart RG, Benavente O, McBride R, et al. Antithrombotic therapy to prevent stroke in patients with atrial fibrillation: a meta-analysis. Ann Intern Med 1999; 131:492–501.
19. SPAF Investigators. Warfarin versus aspirin for prevention of thromboembolism in atrial fibrillation: Stroke Prevention in Atrial Fibrillation

II Study. Lancet 1994; 343:687 SPAF Investigators 691.

20. Gullov AL, Koefoed BG, Petersen P, et al. Fixed minidose warfarin and aspirin alone and in combination vs adjusted-dose warfarin for stroke prevention in atrial fibrillation: Second Copenhagen Atrial Fibrillation, Aspirin, and Anticoagulation Study. Arch Intern Med 1998; 158:1513–1521.

21. Hellemons BS, Langenberg M, Lodder J, et al. Primary prevention of arterial thromboembolism in nonrheumatic atrial fibrillation: the PATAF trial study design. Control Clin Trials 1999; 20:386–393.

22. Taylor FC, Cohen H, Ebrahim S. Systematic review of long term anticoagulation or antiplatelet treatment in patients with non-rheumatic atrial fibrillation. Br Med J 2001; 322:321–326.

23. Kalra L, Yu G, Perez I, et al. Prospective cohort study to determine if trial efficacy of anticoagulation for stroke prevention in atrial fibrillation translates into clinical effectiveness. Br Med J 2000; 320:1236–1239.

24. SPAF Investigators. Bleeding during antithrombotic therapy in patients with atrial fibrillation. The Stroke Prevention in Atrial Fibrillation Investigators. Arch Intern Med 1996; 156:409–416.

25. Pengo V, Zasso A, Barbero F, et al. Effectiveness of fixed minidose warfarin in the prevention of thromboembolism and vascular death in nonrheumatic atrial fibrillation. Am J Cardiol 1998; 82:433–437.

26. SPAF Investigators. Adjusted-dose warfarin versus low-intensity, fixed-dose warfarin plus aspirin for high-risk patients with atrial fibrillation: Stroke Prevention in Atrial Fibrillation III randomised clinical trial. Lancet 1996; 348:633–638.

27. Morocutti C, Amabile G, Fattapposta F, et al. Indobufen versus warfarin in the secondary prevention of major vascular events in nonrheumatic atrial fibrillation. SIFA (Studio Italiano Fibrillazione Atriale) Investigators. Stroke 1997; 28:1015–1021.

28. Harenberg J, Weuster B, Pfitzer M, et al. Prophylaxis of embolic events in patients with atrial fibrillation using low molecular weight heparin. Semin Thromb Hemost 1993; 19 (suppl 1):116–121.

29. Berge E, Abdelnoor M, Nakstad PH, et al. Low molecular-weight heparin versus aspirin in patients with acute ischaemic stroke and atrial fibrillation: a double-blind randomised study. HAEST Study Group. Heparin in acute embolic stroke trial. Lancet 2000; 355:1205–1210.

30. Albers GW, Dalen JE, Laupacis A, et al. Antithrombotic therapy in atrial fibrillation. Chest 2001; 119(1 suppl):194S–206S.

31. Fuster V, Ryden LE, Asinger RW, et al American College of Cardiology/American Heart Association Task Force on Practice Guidelines. European Society of Cardiology Committee for Practice Guidelines and Policy Conferences (Committee to Develop Guidelines for the Management of Patients With Atrial Fibrillation).; North American Society of Pacing and Electrophysiology. ACC/AHA/ESC Guidelines for the Management of Patients With Atrial Fibrillation: Executive Summary A Report of the American College of Cardiology/American Heart Association Task Force on Practice Guidelines and the European Society of Cardiology Committee for Practice Guidelines and Policy Conferences (Committee to Develop Guidelines for the Management of Patients With Atrial Fibrillation) Developed in Collaboration With the North American Society of Pacing and Electrophysiology. Circulation 2001; 104:2118–2150.

32. Murray RD, Deitcher SR, Klein AL. Use of low-molecular-weight heparin as bridge anticoagulation therapy in patients with atrial fibrillation undergoing transoesophageal echocardiography guided cardioversion. Eur Heart J 2001; 22:712–713

33. Diener HC, Cunha L, Forbes C, et al. European Stroke Prevention Study 2. Dipyridamole and acetylsalicylic acid in the secondary prevention of stroke. J Neurol Sci 1996; 143:1–13.

34. Posada IS, Barriales V. Alternate-day dosing of aspirin in atrial fibrillation. LASAF Pilot Study Group. Am Heart J 1999; 138:137–143.

35. Diener HC, Lowenthal A. Antiplatelet therapy to prevent stroke: risk of brain hemorrhage and efficacy in atrial fibrillation. J Neurol Sci 1997; 153:112.

36. Benavente O, Hart R, Koudstaal P, et al. Antiplatelet therapy for preventing stroke in patients with nonvalvular atrial fibrillation and no previous history of stroke or transient ischemic attacks. In: Warlow C, Van Gijn J, Sandercock P, eds. Stroke Module of the Cochrane Database of Systematic Reviews. Oxford: The Cochrane Collaboration; 1999.

37. CAST collaborative group: Randomised placebo-controlled trial of early aspirin use in 20,000 patients with acute ischaemic stroke. CAST (Chinese Acute Stroke Trial) Collaborative Group. Lancet 1997; 349:1641–1649.

38. IST Collaborative Group: The International Stroke Trial (IST): a randomised trial of aspirin, subcutaneous heparin, both, or neither among 19435 patients with acute ischaemic stroke. International Stroke Trial Collaborative Group. Lancet 1997; 349:1569–1581

39. Lip GYH, Beevers DG. Interpretation of IST and CAST stroke trials. Lancet 1997; 350:443–444.

40. Li Saw Hee FL, Lip GYH. Melagatran (Astra). Curr Opinion Invest Drugs 2001; 1:88–92.

41. Kannel WB, Abbott RD, Savage DD, et al. Epidemiologic features of chronic atrial fibrillation: the Framingham study. N Engl J Med 1982; 306:1018–1022.

42. Lip GY. Thromboprophylaxis for atrial fibrillation. Lancet 1999; 353:4–6.

43. Pearce LA, Hart RG, Halperin JL. Assessment of three schemes for stratifying stroke risk in patients with nonvalvular atrial fibrillation. Am J Med 2000; 109:45–51.

44. Atrial Fibrillation Investigators. Risk factors for stroke and efficacy of antithrombotic therapy in atrial fibrillation: analysis of pooled data from five randomised clinical trials. Arch Intern Med 1999; 131:688–695.

45. Laupacis A, Albers G, Dalen J, et al. Antithrombotic therapy in atrial fibrillation. Chest 1998; 114:579S–589S.

46. Stroke Prevention in Atrial Fibrillation Investigators. Risk factors for thromboembolism during aspirin therapy in patients with atrial fibrillation: the stroke prevention in atrial fibrillation study. J Stroke Cerebrovasc Dis 1995; 5:147–157.

47. SPAF Investigators. Transesophageal echocardiographic correlates of thromboembolism in high-risk patients with nonvalvular atrial fibrillation. The Stroke Prevention in Atrial Fibrillation Investigators Committee on Echocardiography. Ann Intern Med 1998; 128:639 SPAF Investigators 647.

48. Hart RG, Benavente O. Primary prevention of stroke in patients with atrial fibrillation. Proc R Coll Physicians Edinb 1999; 29:20–26.

49. Fitzmaurice DA, Hobbs FD, Murray ET, et al. Oral anticoagulation management in primary care with the use of computerized decision support and near-patient testing: a randomised controlled trial. Arch Intern Med 2000; 160:2343–2348.

50. Wolf PA, Kannel WB, McGee DL, et al. Duration of atrial fibrillation and imminence of stroke: the Framingham study. Stroke 1983; 14:664–667.

51. Bjerkelund CJ, Orning OM. The efficacy of anticoagulant therapy in preventing embolism related to DC electrical conversion of atrial fibrillation. Am J Cardiol 1969; 23:208–216.

52. Weigner MJ, Caulfield TA, Danias PG, et al. Risk for clinical thromboembolism associated with conversion to sinus rhythm in patients with atrial fibrillation lasting less than 48 hours. Ann Intern Med 1997; 126:615–620.

53. Stoddard MF, Dawkins PR, Prince CR, Ammash NM. Left atrial appendage thrombus is not uncommon in patients with acute atrial fibrillation and a recent embolic event: a transesophageal echocardiographic study. J Am Coll Cardiol 1995; 25:452–459.

54. Lip GYH. How would I manage a 60-year-old woman presenting with atrial fibrillation? Proc R Coll Physicians Edinb 1999; 29:301–306.

55. Lip GY, Rumley A, Dunn FG, Lowe GD. Plasma fibrinogen and fibrin D-dimer in patients with atrial fibrillation: effects of cardioversion to sinus rhythm. Int J Cardiol 1995; 51:245–251.

56. Fatkin D, Kuchar DL, Thorburn CW, et al. Transesophageal echocardiography before 'atrial stunning' as a mechanism of thromboembolic complications. J Am Coll Cardiol 1994; 23:307–316.

57. Klein AL, Grimm RA, Murray RD, et al. Use of transesophageal echocardiography to guide cardioversion in patients with atrial fibrillation. N Engl J Med 2001; 344:1411–1420.

Ventricular tachycardias

Audrius Aidietis PhD
Vilnius University Hospital, Vilnius, Lithuania

Germanas Marinskis PhD
Vilnius University Hospital, Vilnius, Lithuania

> **Ventricular tachycardias include a broad group of rhythm disturbances varying from single premature contractions to life-threatening ventricular tachycardias (VT) and ventricular fibrillation (VF)**

Introduction

Ventricular arrhythmias are single or repetitive impulses originating distally to the His bundle bifurcation that do not depend on atrial or atrioventricular AV junctional tissues.[1] They can arise in the ventricular conduction system or ventricular myocardium, or sometimes both structures.[2]

Ventricular arrhythmias include broad group of rhythm disturbances varying from single premature contractions to life-threatening ventricular tachycardias (VT) and ventricular fibrillation (VF). Their etiology, clinical presentation and morphology are different and make uniform classification hardly possible. For these reasons, many classifications do exist, including basic electrophysiological mechanisms, etiology, duration, QRS complex morphology, etc. (see Table 19.1).[3] Differentiation between premature ventricular contractions (PVCs) and VTs is difficult in some patients in whom both single PVCs and sustained VT of the same QRS morphology are seen.

Division of VTs into idiopathic and structure-related is somewhat provisory, because it depends on currently available investigations which may or may not reveal underlying disease related to arrhythmia.

Below the most common and clinically relevant forms of VTs are presented with the principles of their management.

Table 19.1 Classification of ventricular arrhythmias

Duration	1. Premature ventricular contractions: single or paired
	2. Ventricular tachycardias (VT) - more than three consecutive beats[3]
	a. Salvos (3–5 consecutive impulses)
	b. Non-sustained VT (≥ 6 impulses, < 30 s)
	c. Sustained VT (≥ 30 s), including ventricular flutter
	d. Ventricular fibrillation (VF)
Morphology	1. Monomorphic (shapes of consecutive QRS complexes are similar)
	2. Polymorphic (beat-to-beat QRS shape and possibly, R-R intervals do differ)
	3. Torsades
	4. Bidirectional
Etiology	1. Monomorphic ventricular tachycardia
	a. Structural heart disease
	i. Coronary artery disease
	ii. Idiopathic dilated cardiomyopathy
	iii. Bundle branch reentry
	iv. Arrhythmogenic right ventricular dysplasia
	2. No structural heart disease
	a. Right ventricular outflow tract VT
	b. Left ventricular outflow tract VT
	c. Idiopathic left ventricular VT
	3. Polymorphic ventricular tachycardia
	a. Normal QT interval
	i. Ischemia
	ii. Hypertrophic cardiomyopathy
	iii. Torsades
	iv. Catecholaminergic VT
	v. Right bundle branch block with elevated ST segment
	b. Long QT interval
	i. Congenital long QT syndrome
	ii. Acquired long QT syndrome

VENTRICULAR TACHYCARDIA RELATED TO ISCHEMIC MYOCARDIAL DISEASE

Key points

Ischemic scar-related VTs are the most frequent type of arrhythmic emergency and if untreated may lead to hemodynamic collapse, degeneration into ventricular fibrillation and sudden cardiac death

Ischemic heart disease is the most common form of VT substrate. After myocardial infarction (MI), some muscle fibers surrounded by interweaving fibrotic tissues survive at the border between scar and myocardium. In this non-homogeneous transitional zone, connections between myocardial fibers may lead to tortuous impulse propagation (Fig. 19.1). Impulse propagation in these areas leads to appearance of late (fragmented) electrical activity, and electrograms are often of small amplitude (single fibers of myocardium surrounded by scars). These signals can be recorded non-invasively as late potentials using signal-averaged electrocardiography. Prolonged conduction time and refractory periods different from that of neighboring myocardium (because of different cell-to-cell coupling and possible residual ischemia) can form the basis for unidirectional conduction block and slow

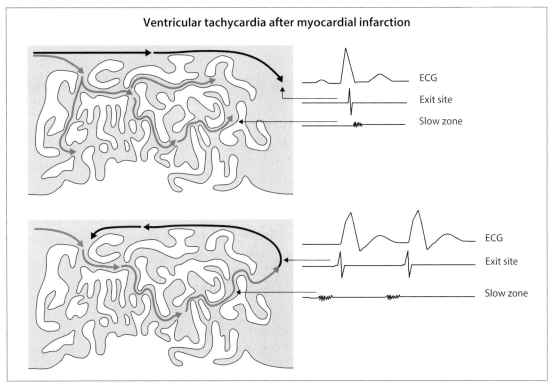

Ventricular tachycardia after myocardial infarction

ECG
Exit site
Slow zone

ECG
Exit site
Slow zone

Fig. 19.1 Initiation of VT related to scar after myocardial infarction. In transitional zone adjacent to infarct area, interconnected and isolated areas of myocardium (gray) exist and are surrounded by scar tissue (white). *(Top panel)* During sinus rhythm, excitation wanders in randomly interconnected myocardial fibers, and because of a tortuous pathway, late (fragmented) activity is recorded in these areas. *(Bottom panel)* After initiating ventricular premature beat(s), conduction in transitional zone slows even more (block in some areas, necessary for tachycardia initiation, can occur in some areas of the transitional zone making conduction time longer), and retrogradely enters the myocardium that has just recovered from refractoriness. This may give rise to re-entrant VT. Stylized ECGs during sinus rhythm and ventricular tachycardia are presented with electrograms from the exit from the slow zone (with possible far-field slow zone potentials), and slow zone critical for tachycardia perpetuation (with early presystolic or continuous mid-diastolic activity), are presented on the right side.

conduction – the prerequisites for re-entrant arrhythmias.[4-6]

Electrocardiographic and electrophysiological recognition of these arrhythmias (most often sustained monomorphic VT) is discussed in Chapter 8.

Therapy for ischemic scar-related VTs may be subdivided into tachycardia termination and long-term prevention (or elimination) of arrhythmia. These VTs are most often encountered form of cardiac arrhythmic emergency and if untreated lead to hemodynamic collapse, degeneration into ventricular fibrillation and sudden cardiac death. An approach to this situation is presented in Chapter 8. These patients often have compromised hemodynamics and require immediate direct current (DC) shock, and in case of stable hemodynamics, amiodarone and sotalol may be used. Class I antiarrhythmics as procainamide are also effective in these patients, but caution is necessary because of possible hypotension. Because flecainide and moricizine were shown to increase mortality in MI survivors, class IC antiarrhythmic drugs should be avoided.[7,8]

Transitional zones between the scar and viable myocardium can be wide; therefore multiple forms of VTs are often possible in this cohort of patients. Because of depressed left ventricular function and possible residual ischemia, risk of sudden death is always present. The following considerations should be kept in mind when deciding about the optimal treatment:

Antiarrhythmic drug treatment showed high probability of recurrences (up to 40% in one year) that often are synonyms of sudden cardiac death in these patients.

Catheter ablation of sustained monomorphic VT is challenging because of thick ventricular wall and several possible circuits, including subepicardial ones (see Ch. 20). It may be a useful adjunct to implantable cardioverter-defibrillator (ICD) implantation.

If revascularization is indicated, coronary bypass surgery may be combined with antiarrhythmic surgery (endocardial resection, encircling ventriculotomy) directed to removal of transitional zones.

There is an opinion supported by several trials that the most efficient method for reducing sudden cardiac death is implantation of ICD (see Ch. 21).

Re-entrant ventricular arrhythmias can also arise due to re-entry circuits formed by differences in tissue electric properties because of acute ischemia. This gives the highest number of sudden cardiac (SCD) deaths in apparently healthy people. Risk stratification in this cohort (primary prevention) and proper prophylaxis could have the most prominent impact on SCD rate. The number of ICD implants rises – from about 50 000 ICDs worldwide in 1997 to more than 80 000 in year 2000. Between 40 and 70% of ICD patients experience one or more ICD discharges during the first 2 years after implantation.[9] More than 50% of these patients require additional treatment because of frequent VT recurrences and heart failure.

> Re-entrant ventricular arrhythmias may arise due to re-entry circuits formed by differences in tissue electric properties because of acute ischemia. This type of VT leads to a large number of sudden cardiac deaths in apparently healthy people

VENTRICULAR TACHYCARDIA ASSOCIATED WITH NON-ISCHEMIC STRUCTURAL HEART DISEASE

Non-ischemic dilated cardiomyopathy is another group of heart muscle diseases often leading to the appearance of re-entry substrate. In these patients, VT can be related to intramyocardial re-entry (transitional zones emerge because of patchy myocardial fibrosis) or bundle branch re-entry related to muscle dilatation and slowing the conduction in His-Purkinje

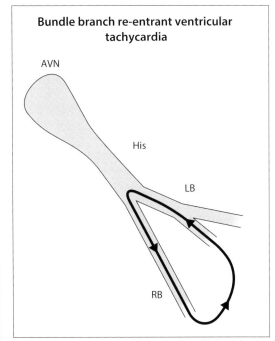

Bundle branch re-entrant ventricular tachycardia

Fig. 19.2 Schematic representation of bundle branch re-entrant VT. These patients often have widened QRS complexes and HV interval prolongation. If slowing of conduction is enough for sustained re-entry, repetitive circulation of impulse leads to VT that is usually fast and poorly tolerated hemodynamically. A common form of bundle branch re-entrant VT is shown, with anterograde conduction over the right bundle branch thus showing LBBB ECG pattern (see Ch. 20 for other details).

system (Fig. 19.2). Approach to treatment of these patients is similar to that in post-MI patients: tachycardia termination by DC shock or class I, III drugs, catheter ablation (that has moderate success, and substantial risk of recurrences, see Ch. 20), ICD implantation. The latter is becoming more common since it gives the biggest decrease in SCD. Overall prognosis, however, depends on severity of muscle involvement, and these patients often require concomitant medical treatment to alleviate heart failure symptoms. Heart transplantation is sometimes the only effective method.

Arrhythmogenic right ventricular dysplasia (ARVD) described by Fontaine et al in 1977[10] is a disease of unknown origin in which RV myocardium is progressively displaced by fatty and fibrous tissue. Three areas of the right ventricle (the so-called triangle of dysplasia) are predominantly involved: the anterior infundibulum, the apex and the basal inferior wall.[11] Left ventricular involvement in this process was also reported.[12–16] Isles of interconnected myocytes surrounded by fibro-fatty tissues often form substrate for re-entry. In these patients, late potentials can be detected not only during intracardiac electrophysiological study and signal-averaged electrocardiogram (ECG),[17–18] but also on surface ECG in some patients. The diagnosis of ARVD may be suggested by ECG features (incomplete or complete right bundle branch block (RBBB)) in 50% of cases, inverted T waves in leads V_1–V_3 in 90% of cases, 'epsilon' waves as manifestation of slow conduction (late potentials) in the anterior precordial leads in 15-60% of cases.[13,19–21] Echocardiography and magnetic resonance imaging (MRI) can confirm the diagnosis,[22–27] but in equivocal cases, RV angiography is the gold standard for diagnosis verification. VT in ARVD may be treated both by antiarrhythmics and catheter ablation. However, 5-year recurrence of VT approaches 40%, depending of the extent of ARVD. SCD was reported in some patients, and ICD implantation is an option, because VT may be initiated and terminated by ventricular pacing.

VT associated with repaired tetralogy of Fallot

Tetralogy of Fallot (infundibular stenosis, an overriding aorta, a ventricular septal defect and right ventricular hypertrophy) comprises 6% of congenital cardiac births and is the most common cyanotic congenital heart lesion.[28] Complete repair is associated with an excellent long-term prognosis,[29] however, retrospective data analysis suggest a 1–6% incidence of sudden death, probably due to malignant ventricular arrhythmias.[30–32]

Complete repair involves ventricular septal defect patching and a right ventriculotomy or infundibulotomy. Resulting scarring and fibrosis can give anatomic substrate for macro re-entrant VT, most often associated with the right ventriculotomy or infundibulotomy scar (with a slow conduction zone between the ventriculotomy scar and pulmonary valve), and less commonly – with the septal patch.

Several QRS morphology variants are possible:

- VT of inferior axis [either of left bundle branch block (LBBB) or RBBB shape] during clockwise rotation around the ventriculotomy scar;
- VT of superior axis (LBBB-shaped) during counterclockwise rotation around the ventriculotomy scar;
- VT of superior axis and usually of RBBB shape (patch-related).

Catheter ablation is possible in these patients, and an electroanatomical approach may be necessary to create line of block connecting scars to anatomical obstacles (usually pulmonary valve).

VT related to infiltrative myopathies

Heart involvement in sarcoidosis patients is relatively low (5–13%), but if myocardial infiltration with granulomas or fibrotic areas is present, both bradyarrhythmias (as heart block) and tachyarrhythmias (as re-entrant VT) may be present. If cardiac involvement is severe and extensive fibrosis is present, patients are at higher risk of sudden death, and ventricular tachyarrhythmias were reported in sarcoid patients.[33–37] In rare instances, congestive heart failure and sustained VT may be the only manifestations of systemic sarcoidosis.[38] Because of the generalized character of this disease, various VT morphologies and cycle lengths of VT can be seen. No systemized data or recommendations on VT treatment specific to this disease are known.

Chagas' disease is an important cause of cardiac dysfunction in Latin America, with up to 20 million people infected and about 100 million at risk. Increasing migration with possible spread through blood products leads to an increasing rate of this pathology in other regions of the world. After an acute infection caused by *Trypanosoma cruzii*, a parasite spread by bug vector, myocarditis and other organ involvement may develop. In the chronic phase of the disease that can emerge 20 years after the acute infection, cardiomyopathy of poorly understood mechanism (possibly autoimmune) develops, with high prevalence of rapidly progressing heart failure, thromboembolism, re-entrant VTs and sudden death.[39–41] Treatment includes amiodarone, catheter ablation and ICD implantation, but overall prognosis in full-blown Chagas' cardiomyopathy is poor.

Cardiac tumors

Rate of primary cardiac tumors is low – 0.002–0.08% of cases in three autopsy series.[42–44] Most frequently associated with cardiac arrhythmias disturbances are rhabdomyomas, fibromas, histiocytoid tumors; rarer are hemangiomas, teratomas and primary malignant cardiac tumors.

VT is frequent in rhabdomyomas[42,45–47] that usually are multiple and involve the ventricular septum, but may occur in the ventricular free wall, papillary muscles and atrial wall.[47] Fibromas are usually single, occur most commonly in the LV free wall, or ventricular septum, and have been associated with VT and SCD. Malignant VTs are often seen in myocardial hamartomas. Rhythm and conduction disturbances can be seen also in primary cardiac malignant tumors and metastases. Drug treatment of VTs associated with cardiac tumors is often unsuccessful, and surgery is the only option. Prognosis depends on tumor size and is poor in malignant tumors.

VENTRICULAR TACHYCARDIAS WITHOUT EVIDENT STRUCTURAL HEART DISEASE

Some VTs can occur in the absence of anatomical or functional abnormalities, and are least detectable by currently available diagnostic techniques. These so-called 'idiopathic' VTs represent about 10% of all VTs and may be classified according to:

- site of origin (RV or LV): RV origin shows LBBB pattern, LV origin – RBBB pattern (with some exclusions of LV outflow tract tachycardias showing LBBB);

- clinical presentation (salvos, non-sustained or sustained);
- precipitating factors (exercise);
- response to pacing and antiarrhythmic drugs (adenosine, verapamil or propranolol).

The mechanisms of idiopathic VTs include re-entry, triggered activity due to delayed afterdepolarizations, or catecholamine-mediated automaticity.

The group of idiopathic VTs include a number of entities of diverse properties, therefore several classifications have been developed. The classification proposed by Lerman et al[48] is often referred to and is based on response of the arrhythmia to programmed pacing and to adenosine, verapamil and propranolol. This classification includes nearly all forms of idiopathic VT (Table 19.2).

Table 19.2 Classification of idiopathic monomorphic ventricular tachycardias (Modified from Lerman et al[48])

	Adenosine Sensitive	Verapamil sensitive	Propranolol sensitive	Undifferentiated
Characterization	A. Paroxysmal exercise induced B. RMVT[a]	Paroxysmal	Exercise induced	Paroxysmal exercise induced
Induction	PS[b] ± CA[c]	PS ± CA	CA	PS ± CA
Morphology	LBBB[d], inf. axis	RBBB, LAD[e] RBBB, RAD[f]	LBBB; RBBB (polymorphic)	LBBB, RAD
Origin	RVOT[g] or LVOT[h]	LV[i]	RV, LV	RVOT
Mechanism	cAMP-mediated TA	Re-entry	Automatic	Re-entry
Propranolol	Terminates	No effect	Terminates	No effect
Adenosine	Terminates	No effect suppression	Transient	No effect
Verapamil	Terminates	Terminates	No effect	No effect

[a] RMVT, repetitive monomorphic ventricular tachycardia; [b] PS, programmed stimulation; [c] CA, catecholamines; [d] LBBB, left bundle branch block; [e] LAD, left axis deviation; [f] RAD, right axis deviation; [g] RVOT, right ventricular outflow tract; [h] LVOT, left ventricular outflow tract; [i] LV, left ventricle; [j] RV, right ventricle; [k] cAMP, cyclic adenosine monophosphate; [l] TA, triggered activity

Right ventricular outflow tract (RVOT) tachycardia

Gallavardin[49] was the first to describe this form of VT in 1922. These tachycardias account for 70% of idiopathic VTs[50] and arise from the RV outflow region. Other known names include: exercise induced VT, adenosine sensitive VT and repetitive monomorphic VT. In a substantial number of patients, PVCs with ECGs similar to that of tachycardia may exist.

Several closely spaced foci with slight variations of QRS shape are seen in some patients. The more leftward the axis, the more posterior the origin of tachycardia. Conversely, the more rightward the axis, the closer the origin to the anterior LV and pulmonary valve. Lead V_1 during tachycardia is negative in RVOT VTs, and it has been reported that the presence of an R wave in lead V_1, or V_2, suggests a left septal origin of VT.[51]

According to current data, the basic electrophysiological mechanism of exercise-induced RVOT VT is catecholamine-mediated triggered activity due to delayed afterdepolarizations (DADs). Stimulation of the beta-adrenergic receptor leads to sequential activation of the stimulatory guanine nucleotide binding protein (G_S), adenylate cyclase, cyclic adenosine monophosphate (cAMP), protein kinase A, and phosphorylation of multiple ion channels, in particular the L-type calcium current, $I_{Ca(L)}$.[52] The resultant increase in intracellular calcium ($[Ca^{2+}]_i$) leads to an oscillatory release of calcium from the sarcoplasmic reticulum and an inward transient current (I_{Ti}) due to Na^+–Ca^{2+} exchange.[53] I_{Ti} is associated with a DAD, which follows the repolarization phase of the action potential.[54]

Repetitive monomorphic RVOT tachycardia, unlike the exercise-induced form, typically occurs at rest and is usually non-sustained. Its mechanism is also cAMP-mediated, and transient increases in sympathetic tone have been shown to occur before tachycardia initiation.[55] Both exercise-induced (sustained) and repetitive monomorphic non-sustained forms probably are manifestations of the same cAMP-mediated triggered activity mechanism.[48,49,56]

Catecholamine-enhanced automaticity (due to change of phase 4 depolarization slope) can also be responsible for some of these tachycardias.[49]

It is not clear if arrhythmia can progress from ectopy to non-sustained and sustained forms of the same morphology. Prognosis of RVOT VT is considered benign even if not treated;[57–61] however, rare cases of sudden deaths have been reported.[62]

Idiopathic RVOT arrhythmias have to be differentiated from the ARVD, especially if multiple forms are encountered. RVOT tachycardias show no abnormalities in the right precordial ECG leads in sinus rhythm, no late potentials are detected by signal-averaged ECG, and local electrograms at the site of origin of tachycardia in sinus rhythm are not fractionated.

For acute termination of RVOT tachycardias, the following measures may be attempted:

- increasing of vagal tone (Valsalva maneuver, carotid sinus pressure);
- adenosine i.v. bolus (6–24 mg);
- i.v. verapamil (10 mg over 1 min);
- lidocaine (lignocaine)

The need to treat RVOT tachycardia depends on the severity of symptoms. If the patient experiences presyncope or syncope, radiofrequency catheter ablation of the arrhythmogenic focus is the treatment of choice.[48,49,63] (See Ch. 20).

Pharmacological treatment is usually the first option in mildly symptomatic patients. RVOT tachycardia is responsive to all classes of antiarrhythmic agents, and effectiveness is far higher than in structural-related VTs and left ventricular idiopathic VTs.

For long-term therapy, the following medications may be used:

- Beta-blockers are the first choice drugs. Their effectiveness varies from 25 to

50%, and they are usually well tolerated.[64,65]

- Calcium channel blockers may also be used. Their effectiveness is 25–30%,[66] verapamil and diltiazem being equally effective.
- Combinations of beta-blocker and calcium channel blockers.[48]
- Class IA (procainamide, quinidine), with effectiveness of 25–50%.[64]
- Class III (sotalol, amiodarone), with effectiveness of 25–50%.
- Class IC drugs may also be used in the absence of structural heart disease.

Long-term antiarrhythmic treatment, however, is seldom used because of the high effectiveness of catheter ablation.

Idiopathic left ventricular tachycardias

Idiopathic left ventricular tachycardias (ILVT), first described by Blanchot and Warin in 1973,[67] differ from idiopathic RVOT tachycardias in respect to mechanism and pharmacological sensitivity. Features of ILVTs are:[68–70]

- induction with atrial pacing;
- RBBB pattern with left-axis deviation;
- relatively narrow QRS complexes (about 150 ms);
- presence in patients without structural heart disease (usually in young male patients);
- responsiveness to verapamil but usually not to adenosine or vagal maneuvers;
- inducibility and terminated by programmed stimulation;
- benign course (unless incessant tachycardia).

Re-entry is likely to be the underlying mechanism, and it is possible to terminate tachycardia by pacing.

ILVT may be categorized into three subgroups:

1. verapamil-sensitive intrafascicular tachycardia:
   - originates in the region of left posterior fascicle of the left bundle (common form);
   - originates in the region of left anterior fascicle of the left bundle;
2. adenosine-sensitive LV tachycardia:
   - originates in the region of LV outflow tract;
   - originates in other regions of LV;
3. automatic (propranolol-sensitive).

Verapamil-sensitive intrafascicular tachycardia

This is the most common form of ILVT. Its mechanism has attracted the interests of many electrophysiologists. Entrainment pacing studies and other observations have demonstrated that the mechanism of ILVT is re-entry. The relatively narrow QRS with pattern typical for bifascicular block (RBBB and left anterior fascicular block in 90–95% of patients) suggests that VT may arise in the left posterior fascicle and the specialized conduction system (Fig. 19.3). This is supported by the fact that radiofrequency catheter ablation is usually successful at the posterior inferior apical septal region – the site of posterior fascicle. Purkinje potential is often seen at the successful ablation site during sinus rhythm and tachycardia, and fascicular block is often seen after successful ablation (see Ch. 20). This together with retrograde His bundle activation 20–40 ms after the QRS onset, suggests the origin of the tachycardia in the fascicle, possibly due to re-entry in the fascicular branches (Fig. 19.3).

The remaining 10–15% of patients (uncommon form of verapamil-sensitive fascicular ILVT) present with an RBBB and left posterior fascicular block pattern, ILVT originating in the region of the left anterior fascicle, near the anterosuperior left ventricular septum.[59]

Participation of false tendon (fibromuscular band that extends from the posteroinferior left ventricle to the basal septum) in the tachycardia circuit is

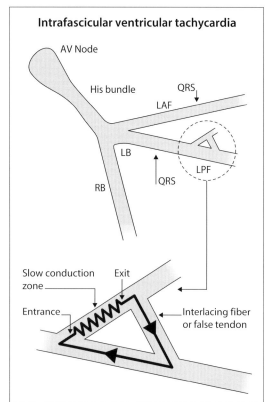

Intrafascicular ventricular tachycardia

Fig. 19.3 Schematic representation of the conduction system and postulated circuit of a common type of intrafascicular (verapamil-sensitive) idiopathic VT. The part of left posterior fascicular (LPF) system is magnified on the right. Tachycardia possibly arises between the fascicular branches because of conduction slowing in one of them. Then, after PVC or SVT, unidirectional block in one of branches with slow conduction and retrograde penetration into the blocked branch causes re-entrant VT. A typical form originating in the LPF system gives upward-directed QRS axis (arrow), while the uncommon form originating from the left anterior fascicle (LAF) – downward-directed QRS axis.

discussed,[71–73] but according to one study, this structure was seen not only in 17 of 18 patients with intrafascicular tachycardia, but also in 35 of 40 control patients.[74]

Although intravenous verapamil is effective in ILVT, chronic effects differ from good results in mildly symptomatic patients to almost no effect in patients with tachycardia that was difficult to suppress when treatment began.[59] The response to other antiarrhythmics including amiodarone is usually less satisfactory. These points together with excellent results of catheter ablation, have led to evaluating catheter ablation as the treatment of choice, especially in highly symptomatic patients.

Interfascicular tachycardia is an electrophysiologically distinct entity that involves reentry between two fascicles of the left branch. Its recognition is somewhat difficult (requires simultaneous recording of the His bundle and left fascicular components), and its clinical relevance (regarding difference in prognosis) is not yet determined, although RBBB or left fascicular block presenting during sinus rhythm suggests conduction defects that could be due to some underlying disease. This tachycardia can be cured by ablating either anterior or posterior fascicle.

Left ventricular outflow tract tachycardia (adenosine-sensitive VT)

Some tachycardias with LBBB morphology typical for RVOT origin cannot be approached from the right ventricle. About 10% of patients with adenosine-sensitive VT have left ventricular origin of tachycardia that can be ablated either below of above the aortic valve. This form of VT also responds to verapamil and is thought to be due to cAMP-mediated triggered automatic activity. A morphological feature distinguishing RVOT and LVOT origin could be early precordial R-wave transition (in lead V_2). Pharmacological features of this tachycardia are similar to that of RVOT, but catheter ablation is more difficult because the nearby presence of coronary arteries.

THE LONG QT SYNDROME AND OTHER CASES OF IDIOPATHIC VENTRICULAR FIBRILLATION

Patients with congenital or acquired long QT syndrome (LQTS) can experience polymorphic ventricular tachycardia and sudden death. Several forms of this syndrome are encountered in clinical practice.

Congenital long QT interval syndrome

Congenital long QT interval syndrome for a long time has been considered as a consequence of cardiac sympathetic imbalance with abnormally low right-sided sympathetic activity, or abnormally high left-sided sympathetic activity.[75,76] This opinion was partly supported by a fact that ablation of the left stellate ganglion reduced the incidence of arrhythmia.[77] It was also shown that beta-blocking agents are a mainstay for LQTS treatment.

Contemporary diagnostic techniques have revealed several chromosome mutations leading to potassium (LQT1, chromosome 11, LQT2, chromosome 7) or sodium (LQT3, chromosome 3) channel anomalies that make possible early depolarizations manifesting as polymorphic ventricular tachycardia leading to palpitations, syncope, and sometimes to sudden cardiac death. These variants can be distinguished electrocardiographically and/or clinically, and optimal treatment differs. To date, no genetic pattern specific to Jervell-Lange-Nielsen syndrome has been found.

Several diagnostic criteria and LQTS and grades of QT interval prolongation have been proposed.[78] Main diagnostic criteria not to be missed in patients with syncope and familial history of SCD are presented in Table 19.3.

In some patients, 'torsade de pointes' polymorphic VT may be seen with normal QT intervals[79] and also has congenital basis. Yet another syndrome described by Brugada[80] is idiopathic ventricular fibrillation associated with RBBB and ST-segment elevation in the anterior precordial leads. The pathophysiology of these syndromes is to be elucidated.

Acquired long QT interval syndrome

Some patients may experience QT interval prolongation and life-threatening ventricular arrhythmias associated with use of antiarrhythmics and other drugs. QT interval prolongation is intrinsic to the action of class IA and III antiarrhythmic drugs, and concomitant bradycardia, hypokalemia, and hypomagnesemia increase the risk.[81–83] Other compounds reportedly associated with QT prolongation and polymorphic ventricular tachycardia include the phenothiazines, some antibiotics (erythromycin), pentamidine, terfenadine and cocaine.

Management

Long-term therapy of congenital LQTS includes beta-blockers and/or left cardiac sympathetic denervation.[77] In emergency settings, intravenous beta-blockers, magnesium, lidocaine (lignocaine) and mexiletine may be used. Cardiac pacing is reported to be a useful adjunct when early depolarizations tend to occur on bradycardia. Specific therapy can depend

Table 19.3 Diagnostic criteria of long QT syndrome

Major	Minor
Prolonged Q-T interval (Q-Tc > 440 ms)	Congenital deafness
Stress-induced syncope	Episodes of T wave alternans
Family members with LQTS	Low heart rate (in children) Abnormal ventricular repolarization

on the genetic variant and other clinical features.

ICD should be considered for patients with resistant arrhythmias; although it has been shown that some patients experience multiple shocks because of enhanced sympathetic activity caused by ICD discharge. Genetic verification of specific types and development of channel-specific antiarrhythmics seem to be promising.

Therapy for acquired LQTS usually requires withdrawal of offending drugs, correction of ischemia and electrolyte imbalance. Emergency therapy is similar to that of congenital LQTS. In the absence of correctable cause, and in other cases of idiopathic ventricular fibrillation, ICD implantation may be considered.

SUMMARY

Ventricular tachycardias are a heterogeneous group of rhythm disturbances characterized by various etiologies, clinical courses and prognoses. Advances in clinical diagnostic techniques and evaluation of catheter ablation results help us to better understand tachycardia mechanisms and choose optimal treatment.

The treatment of VT relies on the hemodynamic status of the patient, and in emergency cases hemodynamic instability often requires immediate DC cardioversion. Drug choice is not big and depends on the underlying heart disease. Simultaneous use of several antiarrhythmic drugs is nowadays discouraged because of the high probability of hypotension and proarrhythmia. Other issues that should be kept in mind are the presence of acute ischemia, and other detectable and possibly correctable conditions such as electrolyte disbalance and so on. Long-term treatment options are discussed in other chapters.

Key points

Treatment of VT depends on the hemodynamic status of the patient, and in emergency cases hemodynamic instability often requires immediate DC cardioversion

References

1. Myerburg RJ, Castellanos A, Huikuri HV. Origins, classification, and significance of ventricular arrhythmias. In: Spooner PM, Rosen MR, eds. Foundations of cardiac arrhythmias. Basic concepts and clinical approaches. New York: Marcel Dekker; 2001:547–569.
2. Shenasa M, Borggrefe M, Haverkamp W, et al. Ventricular tachycardia. Lancet 1993; 341:512.
3. Myerburg RJ, Kessler KM, Castellanos A. Recognition, clinical assessment and management of arrhythmias and conduction disturbances. In: Alexander RW, Schlart RC, Fuster V, eds. Hurst's 'The heart'. New York: McGraw Hill; 1998:873–941.
4. De Bakker JMT, van Capelle FJL, Janse MJ, et al. Reentry as a cause of ventricular tachycardia in patients with chronic ischemic heart disease: Electrophysiologic and anatomic correlates. Circulation 1988; 77:589.
5. Gardner PI, Ursell PVC, Fenoglio JJ Jr, et al. Electrophysiologic and anatomic basis for fractionated electrograms recorded from healed myocardial infarcts. Circulation 1985; 72:596.
6. Spear JS, Michelson EL, Moore EN. Cellular electrophysiologic characteristics of chronically infarcted myocardium in dogs susceptible to sustained ventricular tachyarrhythmias. J Am Coll Cardiol 1983; 14:1090.
7. The Cardiac Arrhythmia Suppression Trial (CAST) Investigators: CAST mortality and morbidity. Treatment versus placebo. N Engl J Med 1991; 324:781–788.
8. The Cardiac Arrhythmia Suppression Trial II Investigators: Effect of the antiarrhythmic agent moricizine on survival after myocardial infarction. N Engl J Med 1992; 327:227–233.
9. Zipes DP, Roberts D. Results of the international study of the implantable pacemaker cardioverter-defibrillator. Circulation 1995; 92:59–65.
10. Fontaine G, Guiradon G, Frank R, et al. Stimulation studies and epicardial mapping in VT: study of mechanisms and selection for surgery. In: Kulbertus HE, ed. Reentrant arrhythmias. Lancaster: MTP Publishers; 1977:334–350.
11. Marcus FI, Fontaine GH, Guiradon G, et al. Right ventricular dysplasia: a report of 24 adult cases. Circulation 1982; 65:384–398.
12. Cherrier F, Floquet J, Cuilliere M, et al. Les dysplasies ventriculaires droites: apropos de 7 observations. Arch Mal Coeur 1979; 72:766–773.
13. Halphen CH, Beaufils PL, Azancot I, et al. Tachycardies ventriculaires recidivantes par dysplasie ventriculaire droite: association a des anomalies du ventricule gauche. Arch Mal Coeur 1981; 74:1113–1118.
14. Pinamonti B, Salvi A, Silvestri F, et al. Left ventricular involvement in right ventricular cardiomyopathy. Eur Heart J 1989; 10(suppl D):20–21.

15. Manyari DE, Klein GH, Gulamhusein S, et al. Arrhythmogenic right ventricular dysplasia: a generalized cardiomyopathy? Circulation 1983; 68: 251–257.

16. Webb JG, Kerr CR, Huckell VF, et al. Left ventricular abnormalities in arrhythmogenic right ventricular dysplasia. Am J Cardiol 1986; 58:568–570.

17. Blomstrom-Lundqvist C, Hirsch I, Olsson SB. Quantitative analysis of the signal-averaged QRS in patients with arrhythmogenic right ventricular dysplasia. Eur Heart J 1988; 9:301–312.

18. Kinoshita O, Kamakur S, Ohe T, et al. Frequency analysis of signal-averaged electrocardiogram in patients with right ventricular tachycardia. JAm Coll Cardiol 1992; 20:1230–1237.

19. Reiter MI, Smith WM, Gallagher JI. Clinical spectrum of ventricular tachycardia with left bundle branch morphology. Am J Cardiol 1983; 51:113–1121.

20. Okano Y, Kamkura S, Katayama K, et al. Electrocardiographic features and their significance in arrhythmogenic right ventricular dysplasia [abstract] Circulation 1992; 86:857.

21. Manyari DE, Duff HJ, Kostuk WJ, et al. Usefulness of noninvasive studies for diagnosis of right ventricular dysplasia. Am J Cardiol 1986; 57:1147–1153.

22. Robertson JH, Bardy GH, German LD, et al. Comparison of two-dimensional echocardiographic and angiographic findings in arrhythmogenic right ventricular dysplasia. Am J Cardiol 1985; 55:1506–1508.

23. Kisslo J. Two-dimensional echocardiography in arrhythmogenic right ventricular dysplasia. Eur Heart J 1989; 10(suppl D):22–26.

24. Casolo GC, Poggese L, Boddi M, et al. ECG-gated magnetic resonance imaging and right ventricular dysplasia. Am Heart J 1989; 113:1245–1248.

25. Blake LM, Scheinman MM, Higgins CB. MR features of arrhythmogenic right ventricular dysplasia. Am J Radiol 1994; 162:809–812.

26. Gill JS, Rowland E, De Belder M, et al. Cardiac abnormalities not visualized by echocardiography are detected by magnetic resonance imaging in patients with idiopathic ventricular tachycardia [abstract]. Eur Heart J 1993; 14:7A.

27. Auffermann W, Wichter T, Breithardt G, et al. Arrhythmogenic right ventricular disease: MR imaging versus angiography. Am J Radiol 1993; 161: 549–555.

28. Mitchell SC, Korones SB, Berendes HW. Congenital heart disease in 56109 births: incidence and natural history. Circulation 1971; 43:323.

29. Waien SA, Liu PP, Robb BL, et al. Serial follow-up of adults with repaired tetralogy of Fallot. J Am Coll Cardiol 1992; 20:295–300.

30. Wolf MD, Landtman B, Neill CA, et al. Total correction of tetralogy of Fallot: follow-up study of 104 cases. Circulation 1965; 31:385–393.

31. James FW, Kaplan S, Chou T. Unexpected cardiac arrest in patients after surgical correction of tetralogy of Fallot. Circulation 1975; 52:691–695.

32. Gillette PC, Yeoman MA, Mullins CE, et al. Sudden death after repair of tetralogy of Fallot: electrocardiographic and electrophysiologic abnormalities. Circulation 1977; 56:566–571.

33. James TN. Clinicopathologic correlations. De subitaneis mortibus XXV: Sarcoid heart disease. Circulation 1977; 56:320–326.

34. Matsui Y, Iwai K, Tachibana T, et al. Clinicopathological study on fatal myocardial sarcoidosis. Ann NY Acad Sci 1976; 278:455–469.

35. Mayock RL, Bertrand P, Morrison CE, et al. Manifestations of sarcoidosis: analysis of 145 patients, with a review of nine series selected from the literature. Am J Med 1963; 35:67–88.

36. Silverman KJ, Hutchins GM, Bulkley BH. Cardiac sarcoid: a clinico-pathologic study of 84 unselected patients with systemic sarcoidosis. Circulation 1978; 58:1204–1211.

37. Paz HL, McCormick DJ, Kutalek SP, et al. The automated implantable cardiac defibrillator: prophylaxis in cardiac sarcoid. Chest 1994; 106:1603–1607.

38. Lopez JA, Hogan PJ, Capek P, et al. Cardiac sarcoidosis: an unusual form of acute congestive cardiomyopathy. Tex Heart Inst J 1995; 22:265–267.

39. Filho MM, Sosa E, Nishioka S, et al. Clinical and electrophysiologic features of syncope in chronic heart disease. J Cardiovasc Electrophys 1994; 5:563–570.

40. Andrade ZA. Mechanisms of myocardial damage in *Trypanosoma cruzi* infection. Ciba Foundation Symposium 99: Cytopathology of parasitic diseases. London: Pitman Books; 1983:214–233.

41. Bestetti RB, Santos CRF, Machado-Junion OB, et al. Clinical profile of patients with Chagas' disease before and during sustained ventricular tachycardia. Int J Cardiol 1990; 29:39–46.

42. Garson A, Gillette PC, Titus JL, et al. Surgical treatment of ventricular tachycardia in infants. N Engl J Med 984; 310:1443–1445.

43. Nadas AS, Ellison RC. Cardiac tumors in infancy. Am J Cardiol 1968; 21:363–366.

44. Simcha A, Wells BG, Tynan MJ, et al. Primary cardiac tumors in childhood. Arch Dis Child 1971; 46:508–514.

45. Case CL, Gillette PC, Crawford FA. Cardiac rhabdomyoma causing supraventricular and lethal ventricular arrhythmias in an infant. Am Heart J 1991; 122:1484–1486.

46. Ott DA, Garson A, Cooley DA, McNamara DG. Definitive operation for refractory cardiac tachyarrhythmias in children. J Thorac Cardiovasc Surg 1985; 90:681–689.

47. Arcinegus E, Hakimi M, Farooki ZQ, et al. Primary cardiac tumors in children. J Thorac Cardiovasc Surg 1980; 79:582–591.

48. Lerman BB, Stein KM, Markowitz SM. Idiopathic right ventricular outflow tract tachycardia: A clinical approach. PACE 1996;19: 2120–2137.

49. Gallavardin L. Extrasystolie ventriculaire a paroxysmes tachycardiques prolonges. Arch Mal Coeur Vaiss 1922; 15:298–306.

50. Varma N, Josephson ME. Therapy of 'idiopathic' ventricular tachycardia. J Cardiovasc Electrophysiol 1997; 8:104–116.

51. Callans DJ, Menz V, Gotlieb CD, et al. Repetitive monomorphic tachycardia from left ventricular outflow tract – ECG criteria for a new clinical entity. (abstract) PACE 1996; 19:599.

52. Yamada KA, Corr PB. Effects of beta-adrenergic receptor activation on intracellular calcium and membrane potential in adult cardiac myocytes. J Cardiovasc Electrophysiol 1992; 3:209–224.

53. Xinqiang H, Ferrier G. Contribution of Na^+–Ca^{2+} exchange to stimulation of transient inward current by isoproterenol in rabbit cardiac Purkinje fibers. Circ Res 1995; 76:664–674.

54. Lerman BB, Stein K, Markowitz S. Adenosine-sensitive ventricular tachycardia: A conceptual approach. J Cardiovasc Electrophysiol 1996; 7:559–569.

55. Lerman BB, Stein K, Engelstein ED, et al. Mechanism of repetitive monomorphic ventricular tachycardia. Circulation 1995; 92:421–429.

56. Shibuya T, Kimura M, Oda E, et al. Ventricular arrhythmia with postural dependency. J Electrocardiol 1985; 18:303–308.

57. Koch DM, Rosenfeld LE. Tachycardias of right ventricular origin. Cardiol Clin 1992; 10:151–164.

58. Coggins DL, Lee RJ, Sweeney J, et al. Radiofrequency catheter ablation as a cure for idiopathic tachycardia of both left and right ventricular origin. J Am Coll Cardiol 1994; 23:1333–1341.

59. Ohe T, Aihara N, Kamakura S, et al. Long-term outcome of verapamil-sensitive sustained left ventricular tachycardia in patients without structural heart disease. J Am Coll Cardiol 1995; 25:54–58.

60. Bhandari AK, Hong RA, Rahimtoola SH. Triggered activity as a mechanism of recurrent ventricular tachycardia. Br Heart J 1988; 59:501–505.

61. DeLacey WA, Nath S, Haines DE, et al. Adenosine and verapamil-sensitive ventricular tachycardia originating from the left ventricle: Radiofrequency catheter ablation. PACE 1992; 15:2240–2244.

62. Tada H, Ohe T, Yutani C, et al. Sudden death in a patient with apparent idiopathic ventricular tachycardia. Jpn Circ J 1996; 60:133–136.

63. Silka MJ, Kron J. Radiofrequency catheter ablation for idiopathic right ventricular tachycardia: First, last or only therapy—who decides? Editorial. J Am Coll Cardiol 1996; 27:875–876.

64. Buxton AE, Waxman HL, Marchlinski F, et al. Right ventricular tachycardia: clinical and electrophysiologic characteristics. Circulation 1983; 65:917–927.

65. Mont L, Seixas T, Brugada P, et al. Clinical and electrophysiologic characteristics of exercise-related idiopathic ventricular tachycardia. Am J Cardiol 1991; 68:897–900.

66. Gill JS, Blaszyk K, Ward DE, et al. Verapamil for the suppression of idiopathic ventricular tachycardia of left bundle branch block-like morphology. Am Heart J 1993; 126:1126–1133.

67. Blanchot P, Warin JF. Un nouveau cas de tachycardie ventriculaire par reentree. Arch Mal Coeur 1973; 66:915–923.

68. Zipes DP, Foster PR, Troup PJ, et al: Atrial induction of ventricular tachycardia: Reentry versus triggered activity. Am J Cardiol 1979; 441–448.

69. Belhassen B, Rotmensch HH, Laniado S. Response of recurrent sustained ventricular to verapamil. Br Heart J 1981; 46:679–682.

70. Lin FC, Finley CD, Rahimtoola SH, et al. Idiopathic paroxysmal ventricular tachycardia with a QRS pattern of right bundle branch block and left axis deviation: a unique clinical entity with specific properties. Am J Cardiol 1983; 52:95–100.

71. Gallagher JJ, Selle JG, Sevenson RH, et al. Surgical treatment of arrhythmias. Am J Cardiol 1988; 61:27A–44A.

72. Suwa M, Yoneda Y, Nagao H, et al. Surgical correction of idiopathic paroxysmal ventricular tachycardia possibly related to left ventricular false tendon. Am J Cardiol 1989;64:1217–1220.

73. Thakur RK, Klein GJ, Sivaram CA, et al. Anatomic substrate for idiopathic left ventricular tachycardia. Circulation 1996; 93:497–501.

74. Lin PC, Wen MS, Wang CC, et al. Left ventricular fibromuscular band is not a specific substrate for idiopathic left ventricular tachycardia. Circulation 1996; 93:525–528.

75. Schwartz PJ, Periti M, Malliani A. The long Q-T syndrome. Am Heart J 1975; 89:378–390.

76. Schwartz PJ, Locati E. The idiopathic long QT syndrome. Pathogenetic mechanisms and therapy. Eur Heart J 1985;6:103–114.

77. Schwartz PJ, Locati EH, Moss AJ, et al. Left cardiac sympathetic denervation in the therapy of congenital long QT syndrome: A worldwide report. Circulation 1991; 84:503–511.

78. Schwartz PJ, Moss AJ, Vincent GM, et al. Diagnostic criteria for the long QT syndrome: An update. Circulation 1993; 88:782–784.

79. Leenhardt L, Glaser E, Burguera M, et al. Short-coupled variant of torsade de pointes: A new electrocardiographic entity in the spectrum of idiopathic ventricular tachyarrhythmias. Circulation 1994; 89:206–215.

80. Brugada P, Brugada J. Right bundle branch block, persistent ST segment elevation, and sudden cardiac death: A distinct clinical and electrocardiographic syndrome – a multicenter report. Am Coll Cardiol 1992; 20:1391–1396.

81. Krikler DM, Curry PVL. Torsades de pointes, an atypical ventricular tachycardia. Br Heart J 1976; 38:117–120.

82. Smith WM, Gallagher JJ. 'Les torsades de pointes': An unusual ventricular arrhythmia. Ann Intern Med 1980; 93:578–584.

83. Keren A, Tzivoni D, Gavish D, et al. Etiology, warning signs and therapy of torsades de pointes – a study often patients. Circulation 1981; 64:1167–1174.

Non-pharmacological treatment of arrhythmias

Audrius Aidietis PhD
Vilnius University Hospital, Vilnius, Lithuania

Germanas Marinskis PhD
Vilnius University Hospital, Vilnius, Lithuania

Non-pharmacological treatment offers a curative approach and allows avoidance of lifelong drug therapy in a considerable number of arrhythmia patients. In others, a combination of both methods is necessary. Device therapy (pacemakers, implantable cardioverter-defibrillators) is often the only lifesaving option in life-threatening conduction and rhythm disturbances

Introduction

Non-pharmacological treatment offers a curative approach and allows lifelong drug therapy to be avoided in a considerable number of arrhythmia patients. In others, a combination of both methods is necessary. Device therapy [pacemakers, implantable cardioverter-defibrillators (ICDs)] is often the only lifesaving option in life-threatening conduction and rhythm disturbances. The purpose of this chapter is to review widely used non-pharmacological treatment modalities of various tachycardias.

Since many tachycardias either are of local origin or use some area critical for impulse propagation, these spots can be targets for ablative therapy. Any action taken to destroy this substrate therefore eliminates arrhythmia and often cures the patient.

Non-pharmacological treatment of arrhythmias was started by cardiac surgeons; the first case of surgical division of an accessory pathway (AP) in Wolff-Parkinson-White (WPW) syndrome was reported by Sealy et al in 1969.[1] Then results of surgical treatment for ischemic ventricular tachycardias (VT) were published.[2] It was realized later, that in some cases, action or energy destroying arrhythmia substrate might be applied without opening the chest and direct access to the heart. First reports on catheter ablation of the atrioventricular (AV) junction by high-energy direct current (DC) shocks in drug-refractory atrial fibrillation were reported in 1982.[3,4] Successful catheter DC shock ablation of accessory pathways[5–7] and ventricular tachycardias[8,9] followed these pioneering steps in a new field of catheter ablation.

Wide clinical application of DC shock ablation was not possible because of the high potential of complications related to barotrauma, danger of cardiac perforation and the impossibility of titrating energy.[10] A search for alternative energy sources showed that radiofrequency (RF) energy applied to the catheter tip is an excellent substitute for high-energy DC shocks.[11] The first report of a successful ablation of AP in humans was made by Borggrefe et al.[12] This technique was then greatly improved by understanding the possibility of regulating lesion volume by titrating the energy,[13] monitoring catheter tip temperature,[14] and increasing lesion volume by using 4 mm tip electrodes instead of a standard 2 mm tip.[15]

During RF catheter ablation, energy is not radiated, but conducted from the catheter tip to contacting cardiac tissue towards a large external back electrode. As a result, resistive heating occurs in the tissues surrounding the electrode–tissue interface (Fig. 20.1). The heat is then conducted to neighboring tissue layers (conductive heating). The electrode tip is also cooled by circulating blood (convective heat loss). Experimental work has shown that irreversible tissue damage occurs at temperatures exceeding 50°C. The volume of the lesion depends on several factors

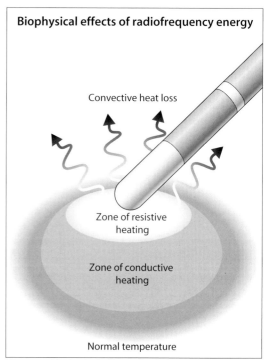

Biophysical effects of radiofrequency energy

Convective heat loss

Zone of resistive heating

Zone of conductive heating

Normal temperature

Fig. 20.1 Biophysical effects of radiofrequency energy. At the electrode–tissue interface, resistive heating due to electrical energy dissipation occurs and is conducted to surrounding tissue areas (conductive heating). This results in tissue damage. The electrode tip is cooled by circulating blood (convective heat loss).

including the stability of the electrode–tissue contact, supplied power (or preset temperature), and duration. It was shown that ablation using a preset temperature (or constant temperature mode, using thermocouple or thermistor integrated into the catheter tip) is more effective than constant power mode because it results in a more predictable effect. Usual parameters of ablation are as follows: preset temperature 50–65°C (depending on desirable lesion size: lower temperatures are usually used for carefully watched ablation of AV nodal tachycardia or avoiding stenosis during pulmonary vein isolation, higher ones – to ablate more tissue in atrial flutter or ventricular tachycardias). The duration or focal ablation is also variable – starting from 10–15 s for AV nodal tachycardia to 60–90 s for atrial flutter and ventricular tachycardias.

To increase lesion volume (necessary for thick trabeculated right atrial isthmus or left ventricular muscle), large-tip electrodes (5–8 mm tip) are useful. In some cases of poor heat dissipation (areas of low flow as right atrial isthmus pouch), low energy is enough to reach preset tip temperature, and inadequate deeper tissue heating is seen. To avoid this problem, so-called 'cooled tip' ablation may be used: a specially designed electrode with tip holes is flushed with room temperature saline (at a rate of 3–5 ml/min to maintain catheter tip holes open to 15–30 ml/min during RF energy application). Catheter tip flushing decreases temperature sensor heating and allows more energy to be delivered into tissues.

ABLATION OF ACCESSORY CONDUCTION PATHWAYS

Accessory conduction pathways (usually referred to as substrate of WPW syndrome) form connections between atria and ventricles and can be found across the tricuspid, mitral rings or in the septum.

They usually consist of working myocardium and do not have decremental conduction properties. Rare variants of APs are those having decremental conduction properties (Mahaim fibers or slow pathways in the region of coronary sinus ostium), and APs related to the coronary sinus anomalies (diverticuli).

Regarding to conduction properties and search for optimal ablation site, APs may be subdivided into those:

- showing bidirectional (anterograde and retrograde) conduction;
- capable only of anterograde conduction;
- capable only of retrograde conduction (concealed APs).

A scheme of APs located in the atrioventricular groove is presented in Figure 20.2.

Ablation of accessory conduction pathways is a highly effective technique and

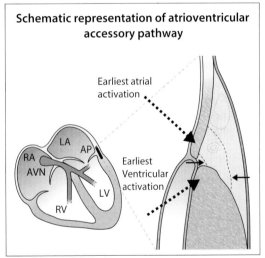

Schematic representation of atrioventricular accessory pathway

Earliest atrial activation

Earliest Ventricular activation

LA AP
RA
AVN
LV
RV

Fig. 20.2 Schematic representation of atrioventricular accessory pathway. In the left part, a scheme of four heart chambers is presented, and left-sided AP is shown by a solid arrow. In the right, cross-section of left atrioventricular groove is presented, with variants of APs connecting LA and LV closer to the endocardial or epicardial surfaces (solid arrows). The ventricular insertion site shows the earliest ventricular activation during pre-excitation; the atrial insertion site shows earliest atrial activation during ventricular pacing or orthodromic tachycardia (correspondingly lower and upper open arrows). AP, accessory pathway; AVN, atrioventricular node; LA, left atrium; LV, left ventricle; RA, right atrium; RV, right ventricle.

complete cure is achieved in most patients. Analysis of electrograms from successful ablation sites provides refining criteria for finding the successful ablation site and interrupts conduction via AP by a median of 1–3 RF energy applications in 99% of cases.[16]

The following criteria may be used to choose appropriate ablation site (see also Table 20.1):

- direct AP potential recording;[16]
- early local ventricular activation (~0 ms in left-sided APs, at least -10 to -20 ms in right-sided) if anterograde conduction over AP is present;
- ventriculoatrial interval of 70–90 ms registered by the ablation electrode during orthodromic tachycardia or ventricular pacing. This criterion has to be used in concealed APs or as an alternative to the earliest ventricular activation in manifest APs.

Diagnosis of AP presence, its participation in tachycardia mechanism, and ablation procedure are usually carried out as a single procedure.[17] Under local anesthesia, three or four multipolar electrode catheters are introduced via femoral veins and positioned in the right atrium, right ventricle, coronary sinus (CS), and His bundle areas. Diagnostic atrial and ventricular pacing is performed to assess the properties of the normal conduction system and AP. Tachycardia is usually initiated, site of the earliest retrograde atrial activation is determined, and pacing maneuvers are performed to examine tachycardia and AP properties. Then the ablation electrode is introduced through the venous system (if AP localization is confined to the right atrioventricular groove) or femoral artery (in case of left-sided APs). Right-sided ablation is usually more technically challenging because of the less stable position of the ablation electrode. Changing electrode loop or using long preformed sheaths is useful in these cases (Fig. 20.3). For left-sided ablation, the electrode enters the LV using a retrograde transaortic approach (Fig. 20.4). This approach in some cases is unsuccessful,

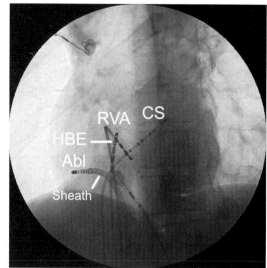

Fig. 20.3 Left anterior oblique 45 degree fluoroscopic view of electrodes positioned for ablation of right-sided AP. This fluoroscopic view represents the tricuspid valve and mitral valve as open faces, with the His bundle electrogram catheter directed toward the investigator. Electrodes in the right ventricular apex (RVA), coronary sinus (CS), His bundle area (HBE), and ablation catheter (Abl) contacting the right free wall atrioventricular groove are shown. A long venous sheath is used to stabilize the ablation catheter against the TV.

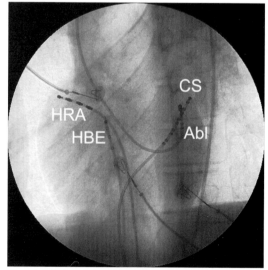

Fig. 20.4 Left anterior oblique 45 degree fluoroscopic view of electrodes positioned for ablation of left-sided AP. Electrodes in the high right atrium (HRA), coronary sinus (CS), His bundle area (HBE) are shown. Ablation catheter (Abl) enters into the LV via aorta and is positioned beneath the mitral valve contacting the left free wall atrioventricular groove.

Table 20.1 Principles of catheter ablative approaches for various tachycardia substrates

Arrhythmia substrate	Verification of ablation target	Ablation technique and remarks
Accessory conduction pathways	Direct accessory potential recording (more important in Mahaim-type pathways) Earliest ventricular activation during sinus rhythm or atrial pacing, rarely during AF[a] or antidromic tachycardia paroxysm Earliest atrial activation during ventricular pacing or orthodromic tachycardia paroxysm (concealed pathways)	Focal ablation in target sites. Endpoint: disappearance of ventricular pre-excitation or anomalous retrograde conduction
Atrioventricular nodal tachycardias	'Slow' AV[b] nodal pathway: -indirect: fragmented or spiked potentials in posteroseptal area, with A:V amplitude ratio < 1 -earliest retrograde atrial activation if 'slow' pathway conduction is identifiable during ventricular pacing (rarely) 'Fast' AV nodal pathway: -indirect: site proximal to His bundle recording, with A:V amplitude ratio ~1 -direct: earliest retrograde atrial activation during typical AVNRT or ventricular pacing	Focal ablation in SP[c] area. Non-inducibility of tachycardia is usually due to disappearance of dual AV nodal physiology, decreasing of AV conduction or increasing AV ERP[d], or impairment of VA[e] conduction in forms other than 'slow–fast' Focal ablation in FP[f] area Non-inducibility of tachycardia is due to impairment of VA conduction, often accompanied by prolongation of AH[g] (PQ) interval
Atrial focal (automatic, triggered activity-mediated) tachycardias	Earliest atrial activation during tachycardia, negative monopolar electrograms Pace mapping can be useful if P wave is not masked by ventricular activation	Focal ablation in target sites, sometimes isolation of focus area
Atrial fibrillation	Focally triggered: search for rapidly firing triggers that induce AF (earliest atrial activation during initiating APB[h]) Without identifiable triggers Palliative technique: AV block creation and implantation of VVIR or DDDR pacemaker	Focal ablation in culprit sites (rarely enough) Pulmonary vein isolation Catheter 'maze' procedures still investigational Modifying of AV conduction without creating III° AV block ('slow' AV nodal pathway ablation) and need for pacemaker implantation is possible in some patients
Atrial re-entrant tachycardias and flutters	Determination of tachycardia circle, 'slow' conduction area and isthmuses necessary for impulse propagation and amenable to ablation Pace and entrainment mapping is useful. 3D-anatomical activation and propagation maps during tachycardia	Ablation between anatomical obstacles: -TV[i] and IVC[j], TV and CS[k] in typical atrial flutter -between surgical scars or fibrotic areas and closest anatomical structures (RA[l]: TV, IVC[m], SVC[n], FO[o]; LA: MV[r], pulmonary vein ostia), depending on tachycardia circle; -focal ablation of 'slow' conduction area is enough in some cases Multiple applications may be necessary because of several circuits possible in one patient

Table 20.1 Principles of catheter ablative approaches for various tachycardia substrates (*cont'd*)

Arrhythmia substrate	Verification of ablation target	Ablation technique and remarks
Ventricular focal (automatic, triggered activity-mediated) tachycardias	Earliest ventricular activation during tachycardia, negative monopolar electrograms Pace-mapping is important	Focal ablation in target sites Match of spontaneous and paced QRS complexes (pace-mapping) is not always perfect in successful sites (LV tachycardias with Purkinje system participation)
Ventricular re-entrant tachycardias	Earliest ventricular activation (exit from 'slow' conduction area) during tachycardia Pace- and entrainment-mapping is useful 3D-anatomical activation and propagation maps during tachycardia	Focal ablation of 'slow' conduction area is enough in some cases Ablation of His bundle branch (usually right) in bundle branch reentrant tachycardias Ablation between scars, scar isolation, or ablation between scars and anatomic obstacles (mitral or tricuspid valve) using conventional or 3D-electroanatomic mapping techniques Multiple circuits may exist in post-infarction tachycardias

[a]AF, atrial fibrillation; [b]AV, atrioventricular; [c]SP, slow pathway; [d]ERP, effective refractory period; [e]VA, ventriculoatrial; [f]FP, fast pathway; [g]AH, atrio-Hisian; [h]APB, atrial premature beat; [i]TV, tricuspid valve; [j]VC, inferior vena cava; [k]CS, coronary sinus; [l]RA, right atrium; [m]IVC, inferior vena cava; [n]SVC, superior vena cava; [o]FO, fossa ovalis; [p]LA, left atrium; [r]MV, mitral valve

and a trans-septal approach may be used (Fig. 20.5). Retrograde and trans-septal approaches are almost equally effective,[18] although some authors report that the crossover from retrograde to trans-septal approach is more frequent.[19]

Using the aforementioned criteria for AP localization, AP often can be ablated by a single or a few RF energy applications (Fig. 20.6). The overall success rate depends on AP localization and is 92–100%.[20,21] Significant complications were reported in 2.1–4.4%, with a procedure-related mortality of 0.13–0.28%.[22,23]

ATRIOVENTICULAR NODAL RE-ENTRANT TACHYCARDIAS (AVNRT)

Before the era of catheter ablation it was thought that the entire circle of AVNRT is intranodal. However, surgical techniques of perinodal tissue dissection with elimination of AVNRT and preservation of normal AV conduction allowed postulation of the participation of perinodal atrial tissues in the AVNRT mechanism.[24–26] After introducing the technique of RF catheter ablation into clinical practice, successful attempts at AVNRT ablation were reported.

The AV node lies at the apex of the Koch triangle (the latter having as boundaries the tricuspid annulus, the tendon of Todaro, and the CS ostium). Experimental, morphological and clinical studies have shown that the 'fast' pathway is located proximally to the His bundle cephalad to the interatrial septum, and the 'slow' pathway - near the ostium of the CS. There can be more atrial insertions into the AV node, including so-called leftward AV nodal extension. The mechanism of AVNRT is re-entrant, and several tachycardia circuits can exist using the above-mentioned pathways. Despite the high effectiveness of catheter treatment of AVNRT, controversy still exists regarding

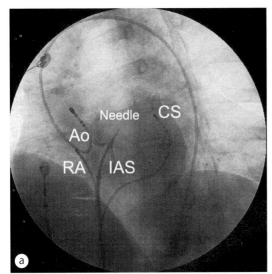
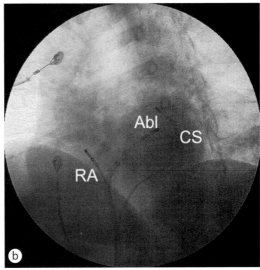

Fig. 20.5 Left anterior oblique 45 degree fluoroscopic views of electrodes positioned for ablation of left-sided AP (crossover from unsuccessful transaortic approach to trans-septal approach). (*Panel A*) Trans-septal puncture. An ablation electrode was withdrawn from the left ventricle and looped above the aortic valve (Ao) to establish an anatomical landmark. The puncture needle inside a long sheath has been pressed against interatrial septum in the fossa ovalis area, and contrast media injected. Interatrial septum was opacified, and panel A shows tenting of this structure (angle-shaped shadow) before introducer entering the left atrium (puncture needle is already inside the LA). (*Panel B*): Ablation catheter (Abl) enters into the LA via the long sheath and is positioned above the mitral valve, contacting the left free wall atrioventricular groove.

the question of whether AVNRT circuit is intranodal, or if participation of perinodal tissues is necessary. Typical AVNRT uses the 'slow' pathway for anterograde conduction and the 'fast' pathway for retrograde conduction (Fig. 20.7).

To eliminate the tachycardia, either ablation of the 'fast' or 'slow' AV nodal pathway may be attempted (some ablation details are presented in Table 20.1). It was shown however, that the 'fast' pathway ablation is more frequently complicated by complete AV block. Another shortcoming of this approach is prolongation of the AH (PQ) interval with subsequent changes in atrioventricular timing and ventricular filling. For these reasons and because of high effectiveness, 'slow' pathway ablation is now the preferable technique for AVNRT treatment. Theoretically 'fast' pathway ablation has to be performed if the patient has a prolonged baseline PQ interval, but it is still possible to perform 'slow' pathway ablation with the low risk of AV block.[27,28]

Several investigators have shown that electrograms from successful 'slow'

pathway ablation sites differ from those recorded in unsuccessful sites: successful sites more often show either sharp spikes recorded in the posteroseptal area, or slow potentials following atrial potentials, or the atrial electrogram is more fragmented or shows double spikes.[29–31] All these characteristics predict a higher success rate, but are not absolutely specific. As an alternative to searching for a particular electrogram pattern, an atomical technique for 'slow' pathway ablation was proposed: the electrode is slowly withdrawn from the ventricle in the posteroseptal area (below the CS ostium) until small atrial deflection is seen. Ablation is performed in this area, and if it is not successful, another application is performed after slightly straightening the electrode and positioning it a bit higher. The sites that are most often successful are located between the ostium of the CS and tricuspid valve, or just above and below the CS. However, in some cases individual peculiarities of AV conduction system require RF energy applications close to the His bundle, or inside the CS, or from

Successful ablation of left-sided accessory pathway

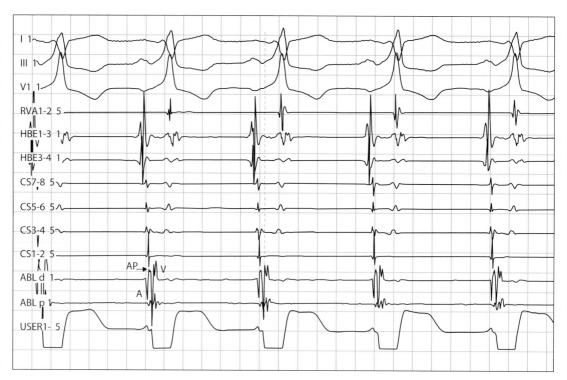

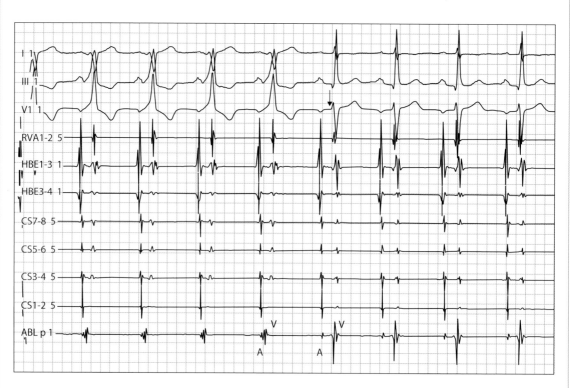

Fig. 20.6 Successful ablation of left-sided accessory pathway. (*Upper panel):* Electrograms before successful ablation. Surface ECG leads I, II and V$_1$ are presented together with right ventricular apex (RVA), distal (HBE1-3) and proximal (HBE 3–4) His bundle electrograms, proximal (CS 7–8) to distal (CS 1–2) coronary sinus electrograms, distal (ABLd) and proximal (ABL p) bipolar electrograms from the ablation electrode, and monopolar electrogram from the ablation electrode (USER1-). Electrograms show presumable accessory pathway (AP) potential between atrial (A) and ventricular (V) potentials (solid arrow), early ventricular activation onset (0 ms to the 'delta' wave, dashed line), and fairly stable negative ventricular potential on the monopolar electrogram (open arrow). *(Lower panel):* Radiofrequency energy delivery results in disappearance of ventricular pre-excitation (solid arrow) and prolongation of the A-V interval on proximal electrode pair of ablation catheter.

the mitral annulus (Fig. 20.7). This combined (anatomical–electrophysiological) approach is reported to be as successful as previously mentioned electrogram analysis-based approaches.[32] Fluoroscopic image and the above-mentioned electrogram patterns that are more often associated with ablation success are presented in Figure 20.8. Successful ablation is often accompanied by junctional rhythm (Fig. 20.9), and if the latter is fast, irregular, or shows VA block (markers of impending complete AV block), RF energy application is stopped immediately.

Difficulties encountered during the 'slow' pathway ablation procedure are lack of criteria for searching the 'slow' pathway ablation sites and less clear procedure endpoint. In rare cases of demonstrable retrograde conduction over the 'slow' pathway (and in 'fast–slow' form of AVNRT), the ablation target is clearer, and single RF energy application can be effective. Subthreshold pacing in the presumed 'slow' pathway area can be useful to find an appropriate ablation site, if tachycardia stops when applying subthreshold stimulus.[33]

Catheter ablation of AVNRT is a highly successful procedure, with effectiveness exceeding 95%, low procedure-related morbidity and no reported procedure-related deaths. The major complication is AV block, seen in 0.8–1.0% of 'slow' pathway ablation and 7–9% of 'fast' pathway ablation procedures.[22,23] Recurrences can be treated by another ablation attempt.

ATRIAL TACHYCARDIAS

The spectrum of atrial tachycardias is broad, including tachycardias of various etiology, mechanisms and localizations. The purpose of this text is to briefly highlight electrophysiological properties of most common atrial tachycardias pertinent to catheter ablation.

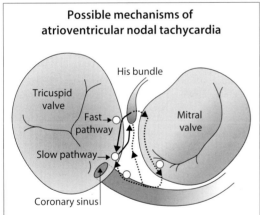

Possible mechanisms of atrioventricular nodal tachycardia

Fig. 20.7 Schematic representation of atrioventricular junction showing possible mechanisms of atrioventricular nodal reciprocal tachycardia and its ablation. Thicker dashed arrows represent mechanism of typical ('slow–fast') AVNRT. Reversal of impulse propagation would represent atypical ('fast–slow') AVNRT. Tachycardia may also use two 'slow' pathways or circulate deeper in the interatrial septum (thinner dashed lines). In some cases the tachycardia circuit can be displaced even deeper (leftward). For these reasons, 'slow' pathway ablation sometimes has to be performed not in typical area (such as between CS ostium and TV, or just below or above CS, lower solid circle), but inside the CS or from the mitral annulus (dashed circles). 'Fast' pathway ablation site is close to the His bundle area (upper solid circle).

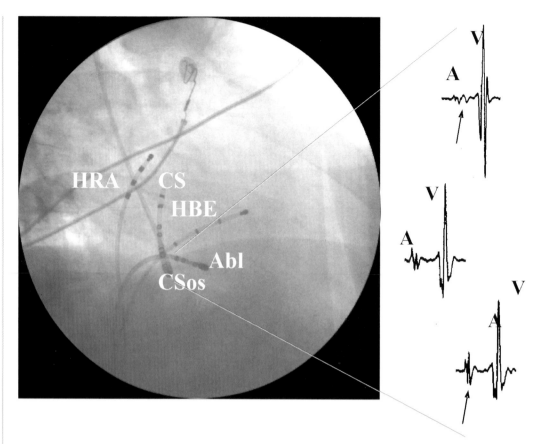

Fig. 20.8 Right anterior oblique 45 degree fluoroscopic view of electrodes positioned for 'slow' AV nodal pathway ablation. This fluoroscopic projection shows the heart from the side, tricuspid and mitral valve orifices being rotated to 'closed' view. Diagnostic electrodes are positioned in the high right atrium (HRA), coronary sinus (CS), and His bundle recording (HBE). Ablation electrode (Abl) is withdrawn from the right ventricle to the posteroseptal portion and is positioned between the coronary sinus ostium and tricuspid annulus. Any tracing presented on the right side is appropriate for an ablation attempt. Upper tracing shows a low-frequency signal after atrial potential (arrow), middle shows fragmented atrial activity, and lower – sharp spike (arrow). See text for discussion.

Atrial focal tachycardias and focally induced atrial fibrillation

Until the importance of focal ectopic electrical activity in induction of atrial fibrillation was realized, ectopic atrial tachycardias were thought to be a clinical problem in a small number of patients. Their course can vary starting from short bursts of tachycardia to incessant, leading to tachycardia-related cardiomyopathy, or very fast focal electrical activity causing atrial electrical remodeling and atrial fibrillation.

The basic electrophysiological mechanism of focal atrial tachycardias (enhanced automaticity or triggered activity) is difficult to differentiate in clinical settings. The main feature of this tachycardia group is early atrial activity preceding the P wave. This is often difficult to evaluate because P waves are obscured by QRS complexes or T waves. Negative monopolar electrograms from the distal electrode of the ablation catheter may also be useful. Mapping of focal atrial tachycardias is difficult in some cases because of the non-sustained character of arrhythmia and individual peculiarities of atrial anatomy. Nevertheless, if the point

Junctional rhythm during ablation of the 'slow' pathway

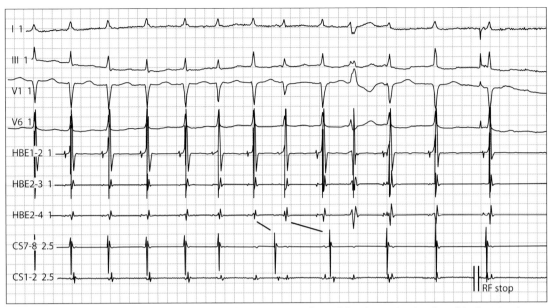

Fig. 20.9 Junctional rhythm during ablation of the 'slow' atrioventricular nodal pathway. Acceleration of the junctional rhythm is accompanied by prolongation of the retrograde conduction time (arrows), and radiofrequency energy application is stopped.

of early electrical activity is identified during atrial ectopic beat or ongoing tachycardia, ablation is often successful (Fig. 20.10). In the right atrium, tachycardia focus is most often found along the crista terminalis, but other localizations, such as the interatrial septum, right atrial appendage and muscle fibers in the superior vena cava, do exist. Left atrial focal tachycardias are most often found in the pulmonary veins and left atrial appendage. Haissaguerre et al[34] has shown that in most cases, rapidly firing foci are located in the pulmonary veins, and pulmonary vein isolation can eliminate atrial fibrillation paroxysms or decrease their rate.[34,35] Different techniques have been established for this purpose, including specially shaped (spiral or circular) multipolar catheters for pulmonary vein ostial mapping, and electrophysiological maneuvers for recognizing the completeness of pulmonary vein isolation. It has been shown that firing foci may be found in all four pulmonary veins and that

the anatomy of those vessels and their branches vary from patient to patient, including a single large ostium and other variants. Major complications have been encountered such as pulmonary vein stenosis, accompanied by pulmonary infectious processes. During the procedure, tachycardia may not show up for some time, and then a single ectopic beat is followed by atrial fibrillation. It was also recognized that up to 30% of the foci are not of pulmonary vein origin. To overcome this, a multielectrode array balloon system with computer analysis has been built (EnSite™, Medtronic Inc.), allowing an activation map to be collected during the single beat and the site of ectopic focus to be established. Another innovation proposed by Pappone et al.[36] is the isolation of all pulmonary veins using a three-dimensional electroanatomic mapping system (CARTO™, Biosense-Webster). Despite all these improvements, ablation of focally triggered atrial fibrillation is still under investigation.

Ablation of focally induced atrial fibrillation

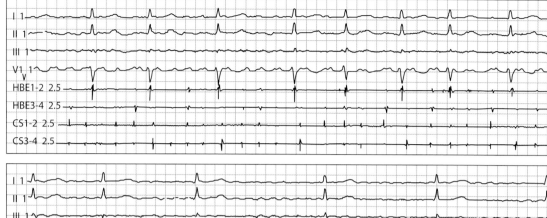

Fig. 20.10 Ablation of left atrial focal tachycardia degenerating into atrial fibrillation in 28-year-old patient. (a) Fast focal atrial tachycardia degenerates into atrial fibrillation. Two ECG strips with a 2 min interval are presented. (b) During tachycardia, the earliest atrial activation (56 ms to P wave onset) is in the orifice of right inferior pulmonary vein. Note shape of P wave (positive in lead V_1, characteristic of left atrial origin, the same as in the upper part of the upper panel). (c) Ablation at this place leads to termination of tachycardia and restoration of stable sinus rhythm.

Atrial flutters and other re-entrant tachycardias

Electrophysiological studies performed in patients with typical atrial flutter showed that the mechanism is impulse rotation in the right atrium around the tricuspid annulus, with activation of right atrial free wall from top to bottom, and septal wall – from bottom to top (counterclockwise rotation). Flutter with opposite impulse rotation (clockwise) is a rare form. Crista terminalis serves as anatomical barrier preventing the fast spread of activation from the septum to the anterior wall, the latter being refractory. The slow conduction zone in low posteroseptal right atrium is a prerequisite for perpetuation of this arrhythmia.[37,38] Attempts to cure atrial flutter by ablating this slow conduction zone were performed, with a considerable number of recurrences. An anatomical approach offered by Cosio et al[39] led to a higher success rate. According to this approach, the complete line of block must be created between the tricuspid annulus and inferior vena cava (or crista terminalis), blocking the impulse propagation from the anterior to septal part of the RA.[39] The recurrence rate is approaching 10–20%, and the main reason for this is an incomplete line of block. Several electrophysiological criteria were proposed for confirming completeness of the ablation line. These criteria require pacing from the CS ostium and lateral free wall. After completing the line of block, changes in right atrial activation occur and may be verified (Table 20.2).

Difficulties encountered during atrial flutter ablation may be related to isthmus anatomy (concave shape, sometimes with aneurysmatic pouches; long isthmus),

(b)

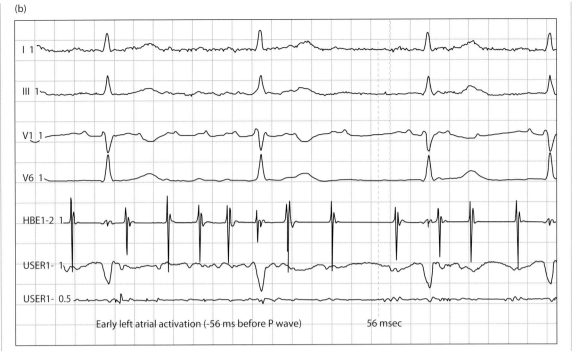

I 1

III 1

V1 1

V6 1

HBE1-2 1

USER1- 1

USER1- 0.5

Early left atrial activation (-56 ms before P wave)   56 msec

(c)

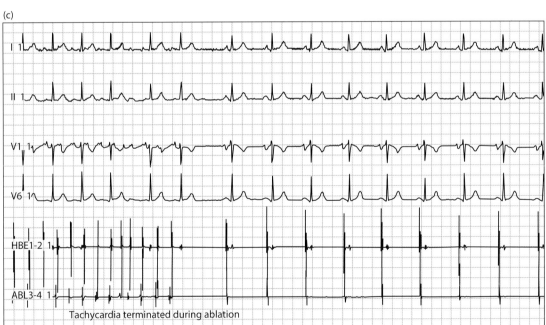

I 1

II 1

V1 1

V6 1

HBE1-2 1

ABL3-4 1

Tachycardia terminated during ablation

Fig. 20.10, cont'd

unstable electrode position, and thick muscular wall in this area. Recurrences are common, and second (or third) procedures may be more complicated due to scars after ablation. There are other forms of flutter that mimic typical atrial flutter on 12-lead electrocardiograms (ECGs), but are not isthmus-dependent. In these cases, entrainment mapping may be used to verify the need for the isthmus for the tachycardia mechanism and to prove that further attempts of isthmus ablation are

Table 20.2 Verification of typical atrial flutter ablation (line of block between tricuspid annulus and inferior vena cava)

Pacing maneuver	Incomplete line of block	Complete line of block
Pacing in the coronary sinus ostium	Multipolar electrode in the RA free wall shows activation sequence from *bottom to top* (conduction via isthmus)	Multipolar electrode in the RA free wall shows activation sequence from *top to bottom* (no conduction via isthmus)
	Low lateral (free wall) RA activation *precedes* atrial activation in the His bundle area	Low lateral (free wall) RA activation *follows* atrial activation in the His bundle area
Pacing in the low lateral (free wall) RA sequence	Multipolar electrode in the septal RA shows activation sequence from *bottom to top*	Multipolar electrode in the septal RA shows activation from *top to bottom*
	Atrial activation in the coronary sinus ostium *precedes* atrial activation in the His bundle area	Atrial activation in the coronary sinus ostium *follows* atrial activation in the His bundle area
Pacing either the coronary sinus ostium or low lateral (free wall) RA	When examining the ablation line, ablation electrode shows *single* atrial potential or *fragmented, narrowly-spaced double* atrial potentials with various distances between components	Examining the ablation line shows *widely spaced double* potentials with constant distance between them (usually > 60 ms)

necessary (Fig. 20.11). In difficult cases ablation can be performed using a three-dimensional electroanatomical mapping system (CARTO), which shows impulse propagation details (Fig. 20.12) and allows the ablation line to be constructed outside the problematic area, or finds 'gaps' in the ablation line by careful analysis of activation sequence in the isthmus area.

Catheter ablation of other re-entrant atrial tachycardias like atypical atrial flutters (right atrial or left atrial, rotating around the zones of fibrosis not related to cardiac surgery) or incisional atrial tachycardias (rotating around the scar after cardiac surgery) is hardly possible using conventional mapping techniques. Three-dimensional electroanatomical systems like CARTO are very useful in these cases and can be used to build activation and propagation maps, mark scar areas and construct ablation lines. The ablation line (a single ablation spot is unusual in these cases) is constructed to connect two anatomical obstacles bordering the corridor necessary for arrhythmia propagation. This is usually scar to tricuspid annulus or inferior vena cava in the RA, scar to scar (or fibrosis area) to mitral valve or pulmonary venous orifice in the LA. The so-called left atrial isthmus (between the MV and left inferior pulmonary vein) may be the ablation site for some forms of left atrial flutter. The ultimate problem is coexistence of several tachycardia mechanisms, including atrial fibrillation, especially in severely fibrosed and enlarged atria. Sinus node dysfunction is an additional problem destabilizing the atria. In these cases curative ablation is either unsuccessful or has to be used with antiarrhythmic drugs and permanent pacing. Ablation of the atrioventricular junction with pacemaker implantation is not unusual in this subset of patients.

Catheter ablation of atrial tachycardias (excluding focally triggered AF) has a success rate of about 75%, with no reported procedure-related deaths and a complication rate of 0.8–5%.[22,23] Ablation of AF triggers has a success rate of up to 60%, with the possibility of pulmonary vein stenosis. Long-term results are not clear yet.

Atrial fibrillation without identifiable triggers, persistent/chronic atrial fibrillation

As mentioned in previous sections discussing atrial tachycardias, atrial fibrillation often coexists with other atrial tachycardias. In many cases however, AF persists despite drug treatment, atrial pacing or ablation of coexistent tachycardias. The surgical 'maze' procedure proposed by Cox[40] is an effective method for converting even chronic AF to sinus rhythm, and may be performed together with valve replacement. The purpose of this operation is to create a 'maze' for sinus impulse propagation, and resulting narrower propagation pathways preclude persistence of sustained atrial fibrillation rotors. An additional measure during this operation is surgical isolation of pulmonary veins, by far the most common site generating rapid focal atrial activity. The drawback of this operation is its traumaticity, precluding widespread use in 'lone' atrial fibrillation. Atrial pacemaker implantation is quite often (up to 40%) necessary after the 'maze' operation. Catheter analogs of the 'maze' procedure are being sought, but it is extremely difficult to make continuous lines of transmural lesions. The thrombogenicity of massive RF lesions is also an important factor.

In some patients atrial fibrillation is accompanied by a rapid ventricular rate and resulting deterioration of ventricular function (tachycardia-related cardiomyopathy). If other treatment measures for maintaining sinus rhythm or appropriate ventricular rate fail, catheter modification of the AV junction with subsequent pacemaker implantation is the method of preserving failing ventricular function and improving the patient's functional status.[3] For this approach, the ablation catheter has to be positioned at the region of compact AV node (usually with small His bundle deflection seen). In a small number of patients, a right-sided approach is unsuccessful, and high AV block may be created by ablation in the upper septal part of the left ventricle. Possible symptoms of lacking atrial activity and embolic risk are not affected by this method. Dual-chamber pacing is preferable in these cases if there is a hope of maintaining sinus rhythm, and rate-adaptive ventricular pacing is indicated in cases of chronic atrial fibrillation. In a small percentage of patients, it is possible to modify AV conduction without the need for pacemaker implantation (Fig. 20.13). The rationale for this method is 'slow' AV nodal pathway ablation with resulting decrease of AV conduction. Risks of significant bradycardia and inadequately high heart rate on exertion have to be ruled out before deciding not to implant a pacemaker. Some patients come back because of high heart rate on exertion, and treatment usually involves creating a complete AV block with pacemaker implantation.

Successful creation of an AV block is achieved in about 95% of patients, with a complication rate of 1.3–3.2% and procedure-related death in 0.1%.[22,23]

VENTRICULAR TACHYCARDIAS

Etiology and mechanisms of ventricular tachycardias are discussed in other chapters of this book. This section deals with principles of focal and re-entrant VT ablation in detail not discussed elsewhere.

Ablation of typical atrial flutter

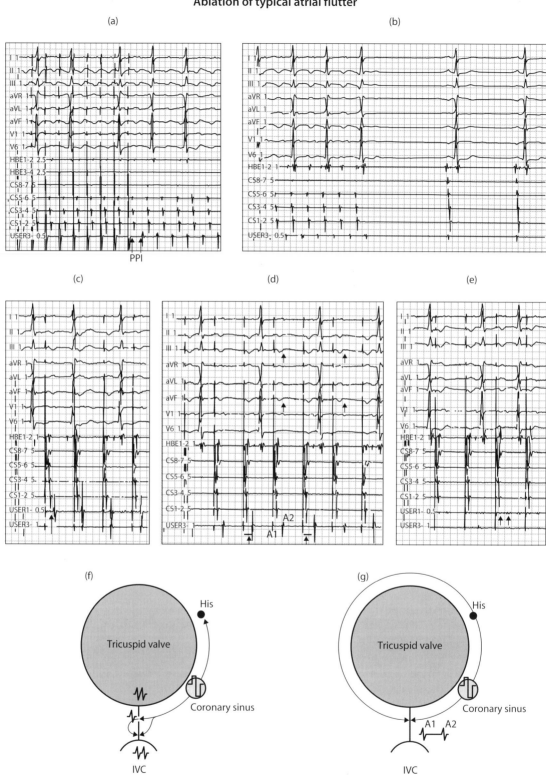

(a)

PPI

(b)

(c)

(d)

A1

A2

(e)

(f)

His

Tricuspid valve

Coronary sinus

IVC

(g)

His

Tricuspid valve

Coronary sinus

A1 A2

IVC

Fig. 20.11 Ablation of typical (isthmus-dependent) atrial flutter. After numerous radiofrequency energy applications between the tricuspid annulus and inferior vena cava, atrial flutter persisted, and isthmus participation in flutter mechanism was questioned. To confirm isthmus participation, overdrive atrial pacing was performed through the distal contact of ablation electrode (*a*). Pacing accelerates the arrhythmia (P-P intervals shorten from 265 to 250 ms), but flutter wave morphology perfectly matches spontaneous activity (concealed entrainment). Post-pacing interval (PPI) at the proximal pair of ablation electrode equals tachycardia cycle length. This also shows that the ablation electrode is in the tachycardia circuit. Isthmus excavation (pouch) with prominent A wave was found when manipulating with the electrode. Ablation was continued at this site, and flutter stopped (*b*). During coronary sinus pacing, however, the ablation electrode showed narrowly spaced double potentials (*c*) (*f*). Further ablation near this spot resulted in prolongation of the St-A interval on the proximal pair of ablation electrode (closed arrows, (*d*), and subtle yet definite changes in paced P-wave morphology (open arrows). Examinination of the ablation line showed widely spaced double potentials with an A1-A2 interval of 115 ms (arrows) (*e*) (*g*).

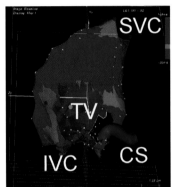
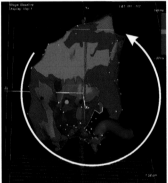
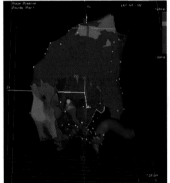

Fig. 20.12 Three-dimensional electroanatomical map of the right atrium constructed using the CARTO system. A single-chamber map of the RA is presented corresponding with the left anterior oblique fluoroscopy projection [tricuspid valve facing the investigator is seen, coronary sinus (red tube) is tagged]. Panels from left to right show propagation map of typical (counterclockwise) atrial flutter: excitation (red color) crosses the isthmus (*left panel*), climbs up the septal RA wall (*middle panel*) and proceeds to inferolateral RA (*right panel*).

Decrease of ventricular rate after radiofrequency catheter ablation of the 'slow' AV nodal pathway

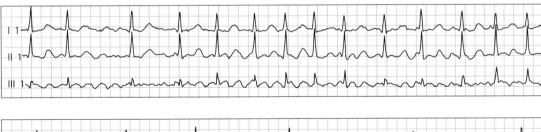

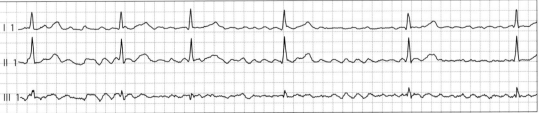

Fig. 20.13 Decrease of ventricular rate after radiofrequency catheter ablation of the 'slow' AV nodal pathway. (*Upper panel*) Tachysystolic AF with mean ventricular rate of 150 bpm. (*Lower panel*) After RF ablation in the 'slow' AV nodal pathway area, mean ventricular rate has dropped to 50 bpm. See text for discussion.

Idiopathic ventricular tachycardias

Tachycardias in this group are usually of focal origin, with a basic electrophysiological mechanism of triggered activity, abnormal automaticity or re-entry. Perpetuation of arrhythmia is desirable for localization of focus, and pace mapping is helpful if tachycardia is difficult to induce or sustain. However, in most cases premature ventricular complexes similar to that of tachycardia are appropriate ablation targets.[41,42] Criteria common for arrhythmias of focal origin are used to search for ablation targets:

- earliest ventricular activation during tachycardia;
- negative monopolar electrograms;
- pace-mapping is important if tachycardia is not sustained.

These local electrograms are usually discrete and not fractionated (no mid-diastolic potentials) during VT. Examples of these criteria for one of the most common forms of idiopathic VTs – right ventricular outflow tract tachycardia (RVOT), located below the pulmonary valve, in the septal or lateral part of RV infundibulum, is presented in Figures 20.14 and 20.15. Ablation is performed in sites satisfying the above-mentioned criteria, and sometimes several RF energy applications are required to cover several adjacent areas and reach deeper-located foci. A match of spontaneous and paced QRS complexes (pace mapping) is not always perfect in successful sites (as in re-entrant intrafascicular idiopathic left ventricular tachycardias), because tachycardia focus can be located somewhat deeper, but ablation of Purkinje fibers at some distance is enough to eliminate re-entry. During these LV tachycardias, prominent Purkinje potentials are seen at successful ablation sites, and ablation often results in a block of the corresponding fascicle (Fig. 20.16).

Localization of arrhythmogenic focus is difficult in some cases. For example, tachycardia showing outflow tract morphology similar to that of the right ventricular outflow tract, can be located in left ventricular outflow tract, either below or above the aortic valve (Fig. 20.17). A feature distinguishing this entity may be earlier precordial R wave transition (in lead V_3 instead of lead V_4, in contrast to RVOT arrhythmias).

Success rate of RVOT catheter ablation is 80–90%.[43–47] The same excellent results are reported in left ventricular verapamil-sensitive tachycardias – about 90%.[48,49]

Ventricular tachycardias related to structural heart diseases

Structurally-related VTs are often due to the re-entrant mechanism. The most common form of this group is VT related to scar after myocardial infarction. Ablation of these VTs is based on search of fragmented ventricular activity at the scar border, inducing the tachycardia and entrainment mapping. Catheter ablation of ischemic VTs is based upon results of surgical treatment including encircling ventriculotomy, endocardial resection and other techniques (Fig. 20.18). Fragmented electrical activity preceding the QRS complex is seen at appropriate ablation sites (Fig. 20.19), but entrainment mapping is also needed to identify the slow zone critical for tachycardia perpetuation[50] instead of 'dead-end' pathways. Ablation of ischemic VT and other structurally-related VTs is challenging for several reasons:

- multiple transition zones between the scar and viable myocardium may exist, and usually these patients have multiple tachycardias;
- tachycardias are poorly tolerated hemodynamically and often require cardioversion before mapping is completed;

Pace mapping before ablation of right ventricular outflow tract tachycardia

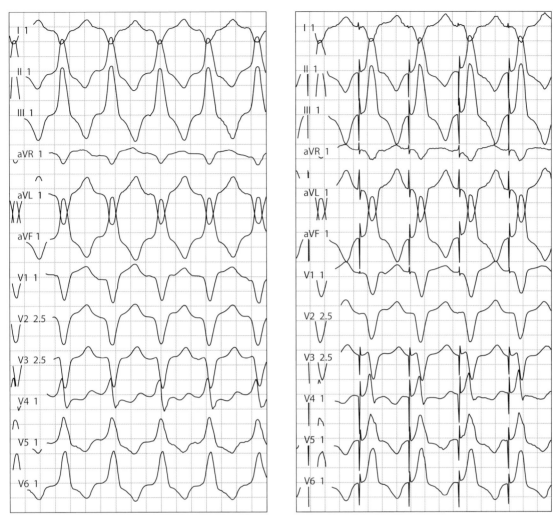

Fig. 20.14 Pace mapping before ablation of right ventricular outflow tract tachycardia. (*Left panel*) ECG during spontaneous tachycardia. (*Right panel*) Pacing from the ablation electrode shows perfect pace mapping match of spontaneous and paced QRS complexes. Ablation at this place completely eliminated the arrhythmia.

- thickness of LV wall and septum leads to the possibility of a three-dimensional circuit, and deeply penetrating energy is required (as 'cooled-tip' ablation).

Patients suffering from dilated cadiomyopathies also have inducible re-entrant ventricular tachycardias. Non-homogeneous (patchy) fibrosis leads to a possibility of multiple tachycardia circuits, with possible exits at different depths, including subepicardial layers. A particular form of VT related to dilated cardiomyopathy is bundle branch re-entrant tachycardia. An ECG during sinus rhythm often shows intraventricular conduction disturbances and a long PQ interval due to a long HV interval (infrahisian conduction abnormalities). These tachycardias are fast and poorly tolerated hemodynamically, but patients can be sometimes cured by ablation of the right branch of the His bundle.[51] An example is shown in Figure 20.20. However

Early ventricular activation before right ventricular outflow tract tachycardia ablation

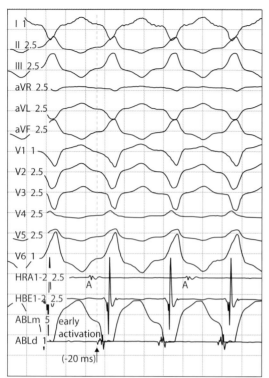

Fig. 20.15 Early ventricular activation at the successful ablation site during right ventricular outflow tract tachycardia. Local ventricular activation precedes the QRS complex by 20 ms.

other forms of VT may coexist with bundle branch re-entrant VT, and these patients are often candidates for ICD implantation.

Catheter ablation of arrhythmogenic RV dysplasia is also based upon evaluation of fragmented potentials, representing delayed conduction in myocardial isles surrounded by fatty and fibrous tissue. Although the acute success rate is 60–80%,[52,53] the relapse rate is as high as 60%,[53] possibly related to the progressing character of the disease.

Results of VT ablation

Idiopathic VTs have an ablation success rate approaching 90%. Ablation of structurally-related VT is far less effective (54–81% in VT related to ischemic heart disease[55,56] and 61% in dilated cardiomyopathy[22]) because structurally-related VTs are often multiple, and patients are at risk of sudden death in cases of recurrence. Therefore indications for ICD implantation exist in many of these patients. After ICD implantation there is sometimes a need to perform VT ablation because of frequent ICD discharges or the incessant character of VT. Techniques for VT ablation are still to be improved to achieve a higher success rate. In cases of poorly tolerated frequent attacks of VT, three-dimensional electroanatomical mapping systems are useful to perform ablation between scars, scar isolation, connect the scar to mitral annulus and therefore to obviate the possibility of impulse rotation around the scar.

INDICATIONS FOR PERFORMING RF CATHETER ABLATION

The decision to perform RF catheter ablation is individual for each patient. Guidelines to perform these procedures are proposed by The American College of Cardiology and American Heart Association.[57] Indications according to these guidelines are summarized in Table 20.3.

SURGERY FOR TACHYARRHYTHMIAS

Surgical treatment was the first non-pharmacological curative option for many kinds of tachyarrhythmias and gave the impulse for development of catheter techniques. These days surgery for WPW syndrome, AV nodal tachycardias, and a significant portion of atrial and ventricular arrhythmias is largely abandoned because of effective and less traumatic catheter treatment. Major areas now open for surgery are:

Typical left fascicular tachycardia

(a)

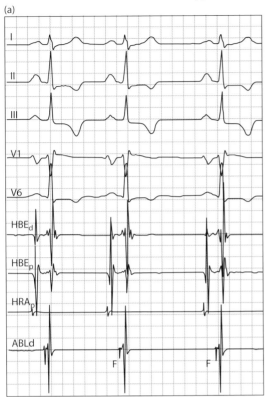

(b)

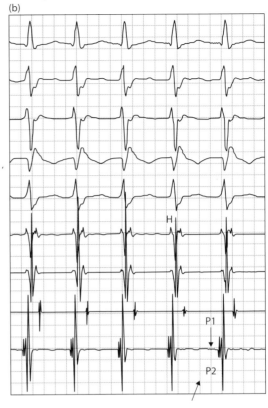

(c)

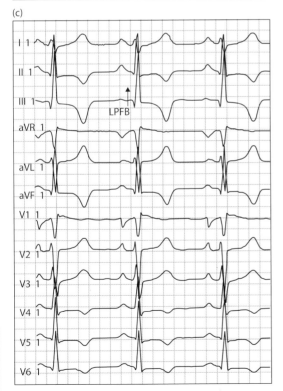

Fig. 20.16 Signals recorded from the successful ablation site during sinus rhythm and posterior left fascicular (typical) tachycardia. (a) Purkinje potential (F) during sinus rhythm. (b) Fascicular potentials (P1 and P2, arrow) suggesting slow conduction in the Purkinje system during tachycardia. (c) After successful ablation of VT, left posterior fascicular hemiblock (LPFB, arrow) appeared.

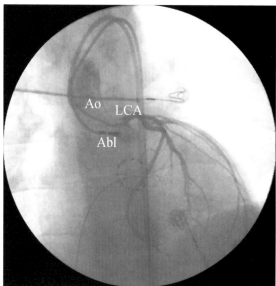

Ablation of left ventricular outflow tract tachycardia

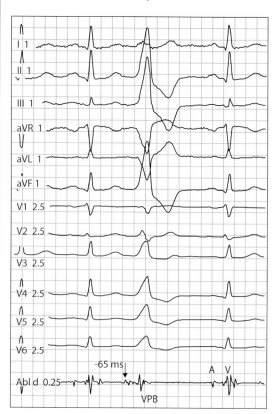

Fig. 20.17 Ablation of left ventricular outflow tract tachycardia (presenting as short runs and single premature beats, as on this figure). (*Left panel*) Left coronary angiography shows ablation electrode location in the aortic cusp (the latter is opacified). Distance from ablation catheter to LCA ostium is about 17 mm. (*Right panel*) Electrogram from the ablation catheter shows prominent atrial potential and early fragmented ventricular activity during ventricular premature beat (VPB), preceding the QRS complex by 65 ms. Note precordial R-wave transition in lead V_3 and compare to that in lead V_4 during RVOT arrhythmia (Fig. 20.14). Ao, aorta; LCA, left coronary artery; Abl, ablation electrode.

- treatment of ischemic ventricular tachycardias (usually together with revascularization);
- treatment of atrial fibrillation (maze procedure, with or without valve surgery);
- tachyarrhythmias resistant to other kinds of treatment (WPW syndrome, usually associated with Ebstein's anomaly, and other individual cases).

FUTURE DIRECTIONS

Alternative energy sources are being tested for specific applications. Catheter ablation of atrial fibrillation, if feasible, can improve quality of life in considerable numbers of patients. Future techniques have to be designed to avoid pulmonary venous stenosis. Another issue is variable anatomy of pulmonary vein ostia. For these reasons, catheter balloons heated by ultrasound are being tested. Cryothermal catheters (tip is cooled by evaporation of liquid nitrous oxide circulating inside the electrode) are also being studied for these applications. To create deep (transmural) lesions in the left ventricular wall, microwave energy can be delivered into tissues using electrode antennas. The problem with this kind of energy is that the physics of microwaves requires waveguides for energy delivery, resulting in stiff electrodes. Attempts at a pericardial approach to subepicardially located ventricular tachycardia circuits have been reported, and in the future the pericardial approach with thoracoscopy may have some role in arrhythmia ablation.

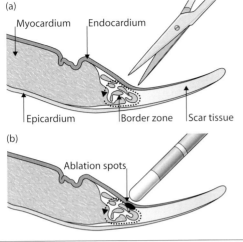

Non-pharmacological treatment of post-infarction ventricular tachycardia

(a)

Myocardium   Endocardium

Epicardium   Border zone   Scar tissue

(b)

Ablation spots

Fig. 20.18 Principles of non-pharmacological treatment of ventricular tachycardia related to scar after myocardial infarction. (a) During the operation extensive endocardial resection is necessary at the border zone, removing isles of viable myocardium that are substrate for VT. A possible part of the tachycardia circuit in the transitional zone (see Fig. 19.1) is shown by dashed arrowed line. (b) The purpose of catheter ablation is to eradicate these transitional zones. Because the transitional zone is often broad, multiple tachycardias often exist and extensive and deep ablation is necessary to eliminate arrhythmia substrate.

References

1. Sealy WC, Hattler BG Jr, Blumenschein SD, et al. Surgical treatment of Wolff-Parkinson-White syndrome. Ann Thorac Surg 1969; 8:1–11.
2. Horowitz LN, Harken AH, Kastor JA, et al. Ventricular resection guided by epicardial and endocardial mapping for treatment of recurrent ventricular tachycardia. N Engl J Med 1980; 302:589–593.
3. Scheinman MM, Morady F, Hess DS, et al. Catheter-induced ablation of the atrioventricular junction to control refractory supraventricular arrhythmias. JAMA 1982; 248:851–855.
4. Gallagher JJ, Svenson RH, Kasell JH, et al. Catheter technique for closed-chest ablation of the atrioventricular conduction system. N Engl J Med 1982; 306:194–200.
5. Weber H, Schmitz L. Catheter technique for closed-chest ablation of an accessory pathway. N Engl J Med 1983; 308:654.
6. Morady F, Scheinman MM. Transvenous catheter ablation of a posteroseptal accessory pathway in a patient with the Wolff-Parkinson-White syndrome. N Engl J Med 1984; 310:705–707.
7. Warin JF, Haissaguerre M, Lemetayer P, et al. Catheter ablation of accessory pathways with a direct approach. Results in 35 patients. Circulation 1988; 78:800–815.
8. Belhassen B, Miller HI, Geller E, et al. Transcatheter electrical shock ablation of ventricular tachycardia. J Am Coll Cardiol 1986; 7:1347–1355.
9. Borggrefe M, Breithardt G, Podczeck A. Catheter ablation of ventricular tachycardia using defibrillator pulses: Electrophysiological findings and long-term results. Eur Heart J 1989; 10:591–601.
10. Evans GT Jr, Scheinman MM, Scheinman MM, et al. The Percutaneous Cardiac Mapping and Ablation Registry: Final summary of results. Pacing Clin Electrophysiol 1988; 11:1621–1626.
11. Huang SK, Jordan N, Graham A. Closed-chest catheter desiccation of atrioventricular junction using radiofrequency energy—a new method of catheter ablation. Circulation 1985; 72:111–389.
12. Borggrefe M, Budde T, Podczeck A, et al. High frequency alternating current ablation of an accessory pathway in humans. J Am Coll Cardiol 1987; 10:576–582.
13. Wittkampf FH, Hauer RN, Robles de Medina EO. Control of radiofrequency lesion size by power regulation. Circulation 1989; 80:962–968.
14. Haines DE, Watson DD. Tissue heating during radiofrequency catheter ablation: A thermodynamic model and observations in isolated perfused and superfused canine right ventricular free wall. Pacing Clin Electrophysiol 1989; 12:962–976.
15. Jackman WM, Wang XZ, Friday KJ, et al. Catheter ablation of atrioventricular junction using radiofrequency current in 17 patients. Comparison of standard and large-tip catheter electrodes. Circulation 1991; 83:1562–1576.
16. Jackman WM, Wang X, Friday KJ, et al. Catheter ablation of accessory atrioventricular pathways (Wolff-Parkinson-White syndrome) by radiofrequency current. N Engl J Med 1991; 324:1605–1611.
17. Calkins H, Sousa J, el-Atassi R, et al. Diagnosis and cure of the Wolff-Parkinson-White syndrome or paroxysmal supraventricular tachycardias during a single electrophysiologic test. N Engl J Med 1991; 324:1612–1618.
18. Deshpande SS, Bremner S, Sra JS, et al. Ablation of left free-wall accessory pathways using radiofrequency energy at the atrial insertion site: transseptal versus transaortic approach. J Cardiovasc Electrophysiol 1994; 5:219–231.
19. Lesh MD, Van Hare GF, Scheinman MM, et al. Comparison of the retrograde and transseptal methods for ablation of left free wall accessory pathways. J Am Coll Cardiol 1993; 22:542–549.
20. Xie B, Heald SC, Bashir Y, et al. Radiofrequency catheter ablation of septal accessory atrioventricular pathways. Br Heart J 1994; 72:281–284.

Catheter ablation of post-infarction ventricular tachycardia

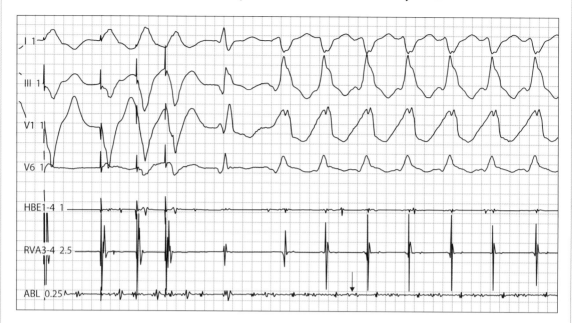

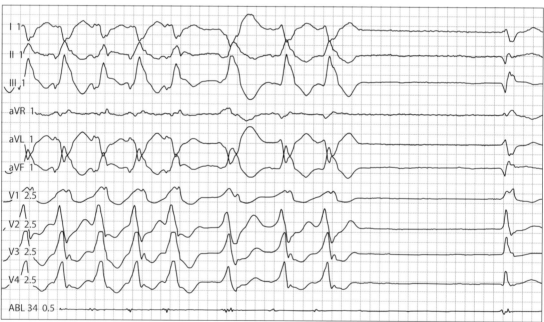

Fig. 20.19 Ablation of VT related to scar after myocardial infarction. (*Upper panel*) Tachycardia is induced with programmed ventricular pacing. Fragmented atrial activity is seen on the ablation electrode signal and is preceding the QRS complex during tachycardia (signals are fragmented and this activation of slow conduction zone near the scar occupies the diastole – 'continuous electrical activity', indicated by arrow). (*Lower panel*) Ablation at this site leads to slowing and cessation of tachycardia.

Catheter ablation of bundle branch re-entrant ventricular tachycardia

(a)

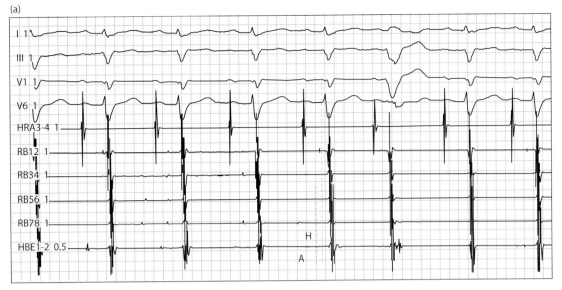

(b)

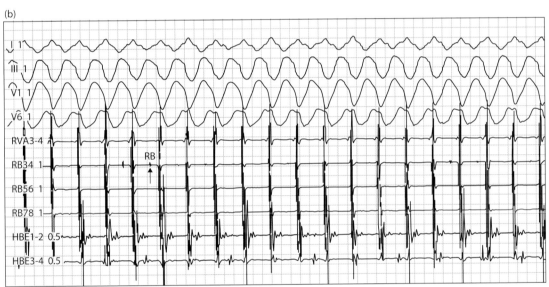

Fig. 20.20 Ablation of bundle branch re-entrant VT in a patient with dilated cardiomyopathy. (a) Sinus rhythm shows long PQ interval, prolonged HV interval of 75 ms and intraventricular conduction defect. (b) Ventricular pacing induces fast VT with LBBB pattern with right branch potential (RB, arrow) preceding the QRS complex and and RB-V interval longer than that during sinus rhythm. (c) RF energy application in the RB area causes RBBB (note QRS shape change in lead V_1, arrow) and renders VT non-inducible.

(c)

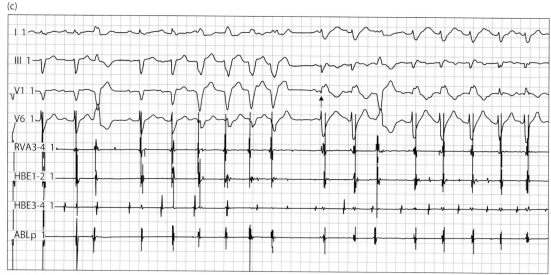

Fig. 20.20, cont'd

21. Dhala AA, Deshpande SS, Bremner S, et al. Transcatheter ablation of posteroseptal accessory pathways using a venous approach and radiofrequency energy. Circulation 1994; 90:1799–1810.

22. Scheinman, M M. Patterns of catheter ablation practice in the United States: Results of the 1992 NASPE survey. Pacing Clin Electrophysiol 1994; 17:873 [Abstract].

23. Hindricks, G on behalf of the Multicentre European Radiofrequency Survey (MERFS) Investigators of the Working Group on Arrhythmias of the European Society of Cardiology: The Multicentre European Radiofrequency Survey (MERFS): Complications of radiofequency catheter ablation of arrhythmias. Eur Heart J 1993; 14:1644.

24. Pritchett EL, Anderson RW, Benditt DG, et al. Reentry within the atrioventricular node: Surgical cure with preservation of atrioventricular conduction. Circulation 1979; 60:440–446.

25. Guiraudon GM, Klein GJ, Sharma AD, et al. Skeletonization of the atrioventricular node for AV node reentrant tachycardia: Experience with 32 patients. Ann Thorac Surg 1990; 49:565–572.

26. Davis LM, Johnson DC, Uther JB, et al. What is the best method for assessing the long-term outcome of surgery for accessory pathways and atrioventricular junctional reentrant tachycardias? Circulation 1991; 83:528–535.

27. Sra JS, Jazayeri MR, Blanck Z, et al. Slow pathway ablation in patients with atrioventricular node reentrant tachycardia and a prolonged PR interval. J Am Col Cardiol 1994; 24:1064–1068.

28. Marinskis G, Aidietis A, Jezov V, et al. Safety of the 'slow' pathway catheter ablation in patients with atriventricular nodal reentry tachycardia and decreased anterograde conduction through the 'fast' pathway. Semin Cardiol 2000; 6:65–67.

29. Jackman WM, Beckman KJ, McClelland JH, et al. Treatment of supraventricular tachycardia due to atrioventricular nodal reentry by radiofrequency catheter ablation of slow-pathway conduction. N Engl J Med 1992; 327:313–318.

30. Haissaguerre M, Haita F, Fischer B, et al. Elimination of atrioventricular nodal reentrant tachycardia using discrete slow potentials to guide application of radiofrequency energy. Circulation 1992; 85:2162–2175.

31. McGuire MA, de Bakker JM, Vermeulen JT, et al. Origin and significance of double potentials near the atrioventricular node. Correlation of extracellular potentials, intracellular potentials, and histology. Circulation 1994; 89:2351–2360.

32. Kalbfleisch SJ, Strickberger SA, Williamson B, et al. Randomized comparison of anatomic and electrogram mapping approaches to ablation of the slow pathway of atrioventricular node reentrant tachycardia. J Am Coll Cardiol 1994; 23:716–723.

33. Willems S, Weiss C, Shenasa M, et al. Optimized mapping of slow pathway ablation guided by subthreshold stimulation: a randomized prospective study in patients with recurrent atrioventricular nodal re-entrant tachycardia. J Am Coll Cardiol 2001; 37:1645–1650.

34. Haissaguerre M, Jais P, Shah DC, et al. Right and left atrial radiofrequency catheter ablation therapy of paroxysmal atrial fibrillation. J Cardiovasc Electrophysiol 1996; 7:1132–1144.

35. Jais P, Haissaguerre M, Shah DC, et al. A focal source of atrial fibrillation treated by discrete radiofrequency ablation. Circulation 1997; 95:572–576.

36. Pappone C, Rosanio S, Oreto G, et al. Circumferential radiofrequency ablation of pulmonary vein ostia. A new anatomic approach

Table 20.3 Indications to perform catheter ablation of various tachycardias (Modified from Zipes et al[57]).

Tachycardia group	Class I	Class II	Class III
Catheter ablation and modification of AV[a] junction	1. Patients with symptomatic atrial tachyarrhythmias who have inadequately controlled ventricular rates unless primary ablation of the atrial tachyarrhythmia is possible 2. Patients with symptomatic atrial tachyarrhythmias such as those above but when drugs are not tolerated or the patient does not wish to take them, even though the ventricular rate can be controlled 3. Patients with symptomatic non-paroxysmal junctional tachycardia that is drug resistant, drugs are not tolerated, or the patient does not wish to take them 4. Patients resuscitated from sudden cardiac death due to atrial flutter or atrial fibrillation with a rapid ventricular response in the absence of an accessory pathway	Patients with a dual-chamber pacemaker and pacemaker-mediated tachycardia that cannot be treated effectively by drugs or by reprogramming the pacemaker	Patients with atrial tachyarrhythmias responsive to drug therapy acceptable to the patient
Radiofrequency catheter ablation for atrioventricular nodal re-entrant tachycardia	Patients with symptomatic sustained AVNRT that is drug resistant or the patient is drug intolerant or does not desire long-term drug therapy	1. Patients with sustained AVNRT[a] identified during electrophysiological study or catheter ablation of another arrhythmia 2. The finding of dual AV nodal pathway physiology and atrial echoes but without AVNRT during electrophysiological study in patients suspected of having AVNRT clinically	1. Patients with AVNRT responsive to drug therapy that is well tolerated and preferred by the patient to ablation 2. The finding of dual AV nodal pathway physiology (with or without echo complexes) during electrophysiological study in patients in whom AVNRT is not suspected clinically
Radiofrequency catheter ablation of atrial tachycardia, flutter and fibrillation	1. Patients with atrial tachycardia that is drug resistant or the patient is drug intolerant or does not desire long-term drug therapy 2. Patients with atrial flutter that is drug resistant or the patient is drug intolerant or does not desire long-term drug therapy	1. Atrial flutter/atrial tachycardia associated with paroxysmal atrial fibrillation when the tachycardia is drug resistant or the patient is drug intolerant or does not desire long-term drug therapy	1. Patients with atrial arrhythmia that is responsive to drug therapy, well tolerated, and preferred by the patient to ablation 2. Patients with multiform atrial tachycardia

Table 20.3 Indications to perform catheter ablation of various tachycardias (Modified from Zipes et al[57]). (cont'd)

Tachycardia group	Class I	Class II	Class III
		2. Patients with atrial fibrillation and evidence of a localized site(s) of origin when the tachycardia is drug resistant or the patient is drug intolerant or does not desire long-term drug therapy	
Radiofrequency catheter ablation of accessory pathways	1. Patients with symptomatic AV re-entrant tachycardia that is drug resist or the patient is drug intolerant or does not desire long-term drug therapy 2. Patients with atrial fibrillation (or other atrial tachyarrhythmia) and a rapid ventricular response via the accessory pathway when the tachycardia is drug resistant or the patient is drug intolerant or does not desire long-term drug therapy	1. Patients with AV re-entrant tachycardia or atrial fibrillation with rapid ventricular rates identified during electrophysiological study of another arrhythmia 2. Asymptomatic patients with ventricular pre-excitation whose livelihood or profession, important activities, insurability, or mental well being or the public safety would be affected by spontaneous tachyarrhythmias or the presence of the ECG abnormality 3. Patients with atrial fibrillation and a controlled ventricular response via the accessory pathway 4. Patients with a family history of sudden cardiac death	Patients who have accessory pathway-related arrhythmias that are responsive to drug therapy, well tolerated, and preferred by the patient to ablation
Radiofrequency catheter ablation of ventricular tachycardia	1. Patients with symptomatic sustained monomorphic VT when the tachycardia is drug resistant or the patient is drug intolerant or does not desire long-term drug therapy 2. Patients with bundle branch re-entrant ventricular tachycardia 3. Patients with sustained monomorphic VT and an ICD who are receiving multiple shocks not manageable by reprogramming or concomitant drug therapy	Non-sustained VT[c] that is symptomatic when the tachycardia is drug resistant or the patient is drug intolerant or does not desire long-term drug therapy	1. Patients with VT that is responsive to drug, ICD[d], or surgical therapy and that therapy is well tolerated and preferred by the patient to ablation 2. Unstable, rapid, multiple, or polymorphic VT that cannot be adequately localized by current mapping techniques 3. Asymptomatic and clinically benign non-sustained VT

[a]AV, atrioventricular nodal; [b]AVNRT, atrioventricular nodal reentrant tachycardia; [c]VT, ventricular tachycardia; [d], implantable cardioverter defibrillator.

for curing atrial fibrillation. Circulation. 2000; 102:2619–2628.

37. Cosio FG, Arribas F, Barbero JM, et al. Validation of double-spike electrograms as markers of conduction delay or block in atrial flutter. Am J Cardiol 1994; 61:775–780.

38. Cosio FG, Goicolea A, Lopez-Gil M, et al. Atrial endocardial mapping in the rare form of atrial flutter. Am J Cardiol 1990; 66:715–720.

39. Cosio FG, Lopez-Gil M, Goicolea A, et al. Radiofrequency ablation of the inferior vena cava-tricuspid valve isthmus in common atrial flutter. Am J Cardiol 1993; 71:705–709.

40. Cox JL, Schuessler RB, D'Agostino HJ Jr, et al. The surgical treatment of atrial fibrillation. III. Development of a definitive surgical procedure. J Thorac Cardiovasc Surg 1991; 101:569-583.

41. Jadonath RL, Schwartzman DS, Preminger MW, et al. Utility of the 12-lead electrocardiogram in localizing the origin of right ventricular outflow tract tachycardia. Am Heart J 1995; 130(5):1107–1113.

42. Movsowitz C, Schwartzman D, Callans DJ, et al. Idiopathic right ventricular outflow tract tachycardia: Narrowing the anatomic location for successful ablation. Am Heart J 1996; 131(5):930–936.

43. Gumbrielle T, Bourke JP, Doig JC, et al. Electrocardiographic features of septal locations of right ventricular outflow tract tachycardia. Am J Cardiol 1997; 79:213–216.

44. Rodriguez LM, Smeets JL, Timmermans C, et al. Predictors for successful ablation of right- and left-sided idiopathic ventricular tachycardia. Am J Cardiol 1997; 79:309–314.

45. Morady F, Kadish AH, DiCarlo L, et al. Long-term results of catheter ablation of idiopathic right ventricular tachycardia. Circulation 1990; 82:2093–2099.

46. Vohra J, Shah A, Hua W, et al. Radiofrequency ablation of idiopathic ventricular tachycardia. Aust N Z J Med 1996; 26:186–194.

47. Chinushi M, Aizawa Y, Takahashi K, et al. Morphological variation of nonreentrant idiopathic ventricular tachycardia originating from the right ventricular outflow tract and effect of radiofrequency lesion. Pacing Clin Electrophysiol 1997; 20:325–336.

48. Wen MS, Yeh SJ. Wang CC, et al. Successful radiofrequency ablation of idiopathic left ventricular tachycardia at a site away from the tachycardia exit. J Am Coll Cardiol 1997; 30:1024–1031.

49. Wu D, Wen MS, Yeh SJ. Ablation of idiopathic left ventricular tachycardia. In: Huang SS, Wilber DJ, eds. Radiofrequency catheter ablation of cardiac arrhythmias. Armonk: Futura Publishing Company; 2000:601–619.

50. Stewenson WG, Khan H, Sager P, et al. Identification of reentry circuit sites during catheter mapping and radiofrequency ablation of ventricular tachycardia late after myocardial infarction. Circulation 1993; 88:1647–1670.

51. Blanck Z, Dhala A, Deshpande S, et al. Bundle branch reentrant ventricular tachycardia: cumulative experience in 48 patients. J Cardiovasc Electrophysiol 1993; 4:253–262.

52. Asso A, Farre J, Zayas R, et al. Radiofrequency catheter ablation of ventricular tachycardia in patients with arrhythmogenic right ventricular dysplasia [abstract]. J Am Coll Cardiol 1995; 25(suppl A):315A.

53. Stabile G, Pappone C, De Simone A, et al. Arrhythmogenic myocardiopathy: radiofrequency catheter ablation of ventricular tachycardia [abstract]. Pacing Clin Electrophysiol 1995; 18(part 2):1177.

54. Haverkamp W, Borgreffe M, Chen X, et al. Radiofrequency catheter ablation in patients with sustained ventricular tachycardia and arrhythmogenic right ventricular disease [abstract]. Circulation 1993; 88(suppl 1):I353.

55. Wilber DJ, Kopp DE, Glascock DN, et al. Catheter ablation of the mitral isthmus for ventricular tachycardia associated with inferior infarction. Circulation 1995; 92:3481–3489.

56. Rothman SA, Hsia HH, Cossii SF, et al. Radiofrequency catheter ablation of postin-farction ventricular tachycardia: long-term success and the significance of inducible nonclinical arrhythmias. Circulation 1997; 96: 3499–3508.

57. Zipes D, DiMarco JP, Gillette PC, et al. P. ACC/AHA Task force report. Guidelines for Clinical Intracardiac Electrophysiological Studies and Catheter Ablation Procedures. J Am Coll Cardiol 1995; 26:555–573

Implantable cardioverter-defibrillators

Audrius Aidietis PhD
Vilnius University Hospital, Vilnius, Lithuania

Germanas Marinskis PhD
Vilnius University Hospital, Vilnius, Lithuania

Implantable cardioverter-defibrillators (ICDs) are designed to promptly recognize and treat life-threatening ventricular tachyarrhythmias

Introduction

The chance of patient survival in life-threatening arrhythmia drops with every minute of ongoing arrhythmia. Implantable cardioverter-defibrillators (ICDs) are designed to promptly recognize and treat life-threatening ventricular tachyarrhythmias. Since first patient implant by Mirowski in 1980, progress in ICD size and functionality led to their wide clinical application. Bulky and straightforwardly defibrillating devices implanted in the abdominal area with epicardial lead patches have progressed to tiered-therapy devices of 60–70 g with transvenous leads allowing pectoral implantation. Main steps in ICD design are presented in Table 21.1.

> The principle of defibrillation therapy is to deliver a shock, depolarizing a critical amount of fibrillating ventricular muscle

PRINCIPLES OF ICD FUNCTION

To protect the patient from life-threatening ventricular arrhythmias, the ICD continuously monitors heart activity. Main criterion launching therapeutic interventions is ventricular rate being detected by the ICD. Different algorithms of signal processing are applied, including automated signal gain adjustment to escape oversensing of T waves during normal rhythm and to detect smaller ventricular signals during ventricular fibrillation (VF). To avoid inappropriate shock in fast supraventricular tachycardias (like tachysystolic atrial fibrillation not uncommon to ICD patients), various criteria may be applied (like interval stability, sudden onset, electrogram width and others). Dual-chamber detection allows better differentiation from supraventricular arrhythmias, but is not absolutely specific because ventricular tachycardia (VT) and atrial arrhythmias may coexist. Upon detection of VT or VF, various therapeutic measures may be applied. The ICD is capable of delivering interventions ranging from antitachycardia pacing (ATP) stimuli of 1–10 V to high energy shock of up to 40 J (750–800 V).

The principle of defibrillation therapy is to deliver current that depolarizes a critical amount of fibrillating ventricular muscle. In contemporary ICDs, current vector between the right ventricular coil and ICD housing is sufficient for most cases (Fig. 21.1).

The main advance in ICD was the introduction of tiered therapy that allows treatment of arrhythmia according to its severity therefore diminishing the number of shocks, and improving the patient's comfort and psychological status (Table 21.2). The possible number of tachycardia 'zones' and variants of antitachycardia interventions vary from model to model, and rate criterion of VF should invariably lead to high-energy shock.

Table 21.1 Progress in implantable cardioverter-defibrillator therapy

1980	First implant in patient
1982	Cardioversion capability added to defibrillation
1987	Transvenous lead system
1993	Pectoral implantation
1995	Dual-chamber detection

Transvenous defibrillation system

ICD

RV coil electrode

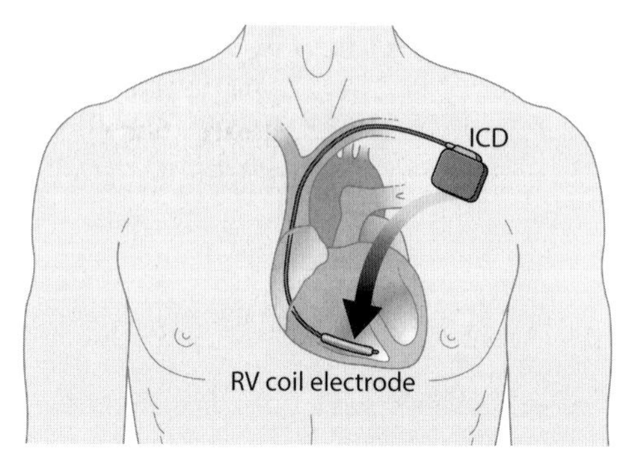

Fig. 21.1 Transvenous defibrillation system. In most cases of recent ICD implants, current between the electrode coil positioned in the right ventricle is enough for depolarizing the critical mass of fibrillating ventricular muscle and stopping fibrillatory activity.

Table 21.2 Variants of therapeutic interventions upon VT or VF detection (tiered therapy)

Arrhythmia	Intervention	Example of detection rate
Slower ventricular tachycardia	Antitachycardia pacing	120–160
Faster ventricular tachycardia	Antitachycardia pacing, low-energy shock	161–200
Ventricular fibrillation	High-energy shock	> 200

Selection of detection criteria and aggressiveness of intervention are highly individual. For example, in a patient with VT of 180 beats per min (bpm) that is tolerated for several minutes, antitachycardia pacing may be used, and in a patient with poorly tolerated tachycardia of 150 bpm, low-energy shock cardioversion should be applied as a initial therapy after some number of detected tachycardia intervals.

The electrogram storage feature allows analysis of arrhythmia episodes and tailoring of the most appropriate therapy. In many patients, arrhythmia starts from VT that degenerates into VF. It was shown during electrophysiological studies that many VT could be interrupted not only by low-energy shocks, but also by ventricular pacing at rates faster than tachycardia (an example of antitachycardia pacing is shown in Fig. 21.2). The first implantable ICDs proceeded to immediate defibrillation upon detection of the arrhythmia. In recent devices, tiered therapy may be used, but there is often a possibility that antitachycardia pacing may make the tachycardia faster and poorly tolerated. Therefore, defibrillation function must be always available.

INDICATIONS FOR ICD THERAPY

Studies on secondary sudden death prevention (AVID,[1] CASH,[2] several ongoing) and primary sudden death prevention (MADIT,[3] several ongoing) have shown that implantable defibrillators improve survival of patients who were resuscitated from cardiac arrest or are at risk of malignant ventricular tachyarrhythmias. Disillusion with drug therapy results for these patients (like CAST study) increased indications for ICD implantation. Guidelines for ICD implantation are presented in Table 21.3. Clear (class I) indications incorporate a smaller proportion of patients, and opinions on the need for ICD implantation differ for a considerable number of conditions (class II). Some indications considered to be class I in one country (or even institution) may be considered to be class II in another. These indications change according to the results of recent trials. According to the studies, strong opinions exist that even non-sustained VT in compromised left ventricular function, cardiomyopathy and other structural heart disease puts the patient at risk and ICD option is to be considered. Psychiatric issues and life expectancy may also be taken into account when deciding about class III (not indicated).

> Implantable defibrillators improve survival of patients resuscitated from cardiac arrest or at risk of recurrent malignant ventricular tachyarrhythmias

IMPLANTATION PROCEDURE

Size and weight of recent ICD models makes the implantation technique similar to that of a pacemaker, with periprocedural mortality of less than 1%. As well as

Antitachycardia pacing by ICD

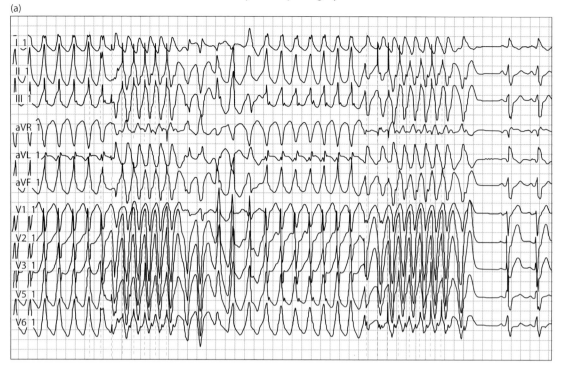

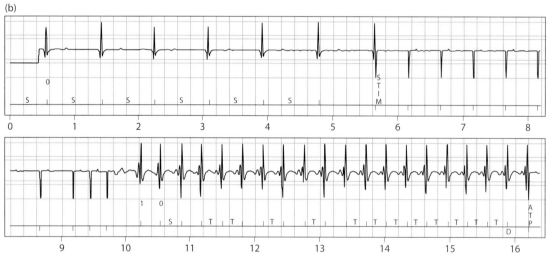

Fig. 21.2 Antitachycardia pacing delivered by ICD implantation. (a) The first antitachycardia pacing burst (cycle length 75% of tachycardia) is unsuccessful. Note slight changes in QRS morphology (better seen in lead V_2) that may reflect shift of tachycardia circuit or change of its exit site. Another burst at faster rate (first ATP burst – 20 ms) terminates the tachycardia. (b) An episode from the ICD electrogram storage memory. Tachycardia induction by programmed pacing is seen (upper strip) then followed by antitachycardia pacing shown on upper panel (two bottom strips).

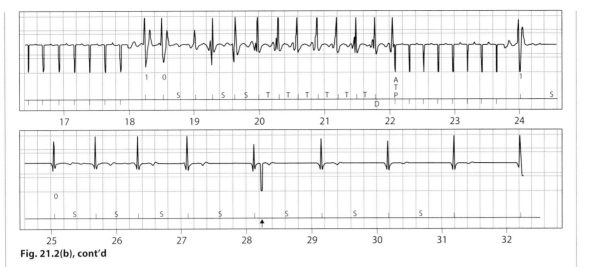

Fig. 21.2(b), cont'd

Table 21.3 Indications for implantable cardioverter-defibrillator therapy (Modified from Gregoratos[4]).

Class I	Class II	Class III
1. Cardiac arrest due to VF or VT not due to a transient or reversible cause. 3. Syncope of undetermined origin with clinically relevant, hemodynamically significant sustained VT or VF induced at electrophysiological study when drug therapy is ineffective, not tolerated, or not preferred. 4. Non-sustained VT with coronary disease, prior MI, LV dysfunction, and inducible VF or sustained VT at electrophysiological study that is not suppressible by a class I anti-arrhythmic drug.	1. Cardiac arrest presumed to be due to VF when electrophysiological testing is precluded by other medical conditions. 2. Severe symptoms attributable to sustained ventricular tachyarrhythmias while awaiting cardiac transplantation. 3. Familial or inherited conditions with a high risk for life-threatening ventricular tachyarrhythmias such as long QT syndrome or hypertrophic cardiomyopathy. 4. Non-sustained VT with coronary artery disease, prior MI, and LV dysfunction, and inducible sustained VT or VF at electrophysiological study. 5. Recurrent syncope of undetermined etiology in the presence of ventricular dysfunction and inducible ventricular arrhythmias at electrophysiological study when other causes of syncope have been excluded.	1. Syncope of undetermined cause in a patient without inducible ventricular 2. Incessant VT or VF 3. VF or VT resulting from arrhythmias amenable to surgical or catheter ablation; for example, atrial arrhythmias associated with the Wolff-Parkinson-White syndrome, right ventricular outflow tract VT, idiopathic left ventricular tachycardia, or fascicular VT. 4. Ventricular tachyarrhythmias due to a transient or reversible disorder (e.g. AMI, electrolyte imbalance, drugs, trauma).

AMI, acute myocardial infarction; LV, left ventricular; MI, myocardial infarction; VF, ventricular fibrillation; VT, ventricular tachycardia

procedure-related complications (such as hematoma and pneumothorax), there are more possible complications related to device testing. After the lead positioning, both pacing/detection and high voltage circuits are tested in order to expose device malfunction or inappropriate lead connection/position and the device's ability to detect and terminate the worst arrhythmia (ventricular fibrillation) is then tested. For this purpose short general anesthesia is initiated and VF is induced (usually twice, using special functions such as very fast pacing or shock-on-T wave feature – see Fig. 21.3). Since shocks of more than 2 J are almost as painful as 30 J, rarely is there a need to know the exact minimal amount of energy sufficient for defibrillation. Recent recommendations are to consider the defibrillation threshold (DFT) satisfactory at 10 J lower than maximal device output capability. In some cases this is a problem, and possible solutions are changing the shock polarity, adding another lead coil in superior vena cava, or subcutaneous patch electrode, or using the device with maximum output available at the market. Biphasic shocks have significantly lower DFTs than monophasic, and programming of positive and negative phase duration can have some influence on DFT. VT induction by pacing and antitachycardia pacing testing is not obligatory, and depends on the patient's clinical problem, but is often welcome to possibly diminish the need for shocks.

FOLLOW-UP AND PROBLEMS

Follow-up policy differs from institution to institution. Usually patients have their device checked every 3 to 6 months. Appropriate therapy is not an indication for immediate check, but is advisable to check for possible adjustments. Complaints are not uncommon because of the complex character of ICD treatment leading to the possibility of various problems (inappropriate therapy, multiple appropriate shocks, detection failure because of slower VT and so on). Changes in the patient's status such as deterioration of heart failure, adding other drugs and appearance of concomitant arrhythmias

Testing of ICD defibrillation function

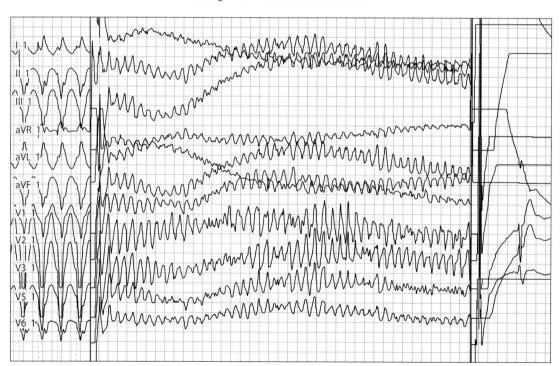

Fig. 21.3 Testing of ICD defibrillation function. During the implantation procedure, ventricular fibrillation is induced by a device emitting a 200 V shock on T wave after the ventricular pacing sequence. Then the device detects the arrhythmia, charges to 550 V (about 12 J) and in less than 8 s delivers shock, defibrillating the heart.

may lead to these problems (Fig. 21.4). Fortunately current ICDs have extensive diagnosis and programming capabilities, and these problems can be often solved.

FUTURE DIRECTIONS

Continuing progress in ICD engineering makes these devices appropriate for the

treatment of many patients suffering from life-threatening arrhythmias. Further improvements include lead design, detection optimization (like Holter monitor and multiple source electrogram function), better energy sources and circuit engineering allowing dual-chamber pacing and multisite ventricular pacing features to be incorporated. These steps, together with

Inappropriate ICD shock during tachysystolic atrial fibrillation

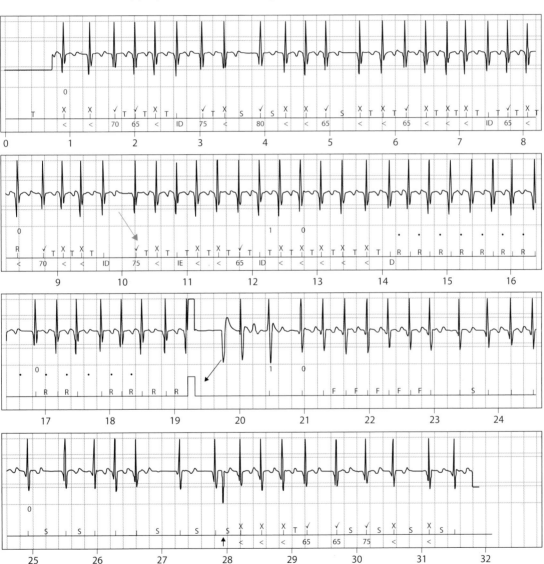

Fig. 21.4 Inappropriate ICD shock delivered in response to tachysystolic atrial fibrillation. Physical exertion in a patient with poor LV function led to an increase in the heart rate above tachycardia detection rate. After detection of 12 consecutive cycles with cut-off rate (start at open arrow), the device starts charging (dots). Continuation of tachyarrhythmia reconfirms the diagnosis (R), and a 12 J shock is delivered. AF does not stop, however. This problem had to be solved by administering AV-nodal blocking drugs and readjusting detection criteria.

ongoing and future clinical trials, will allow us to better recognize the role of this kind of therapy and possibly to use it widely for primary prevention of sudden cardiac death.

References

1. The Antiarrhythmics Versus Implantable Defibrillators (AVID) Investigators: A comparison of antiarrhythmic-drug therapy with implantable defibrillators in patients resuscitated from near-fatal ventricular arrhythmias. N Engl J Med 1997; 337:1576–1583.
2. Siebels J, Kuck KH, and the CASH Investigators. Implantable cardioverter defibrillator compared with antiarrhythmic drug treatment in cardiac arrest survivors (the Cardiac Arrest Study Hamburg). Am Heart J 1994; 127:1139–1144.
3. Moss AJ, Hall WJ, Cannom DS, et al, for the Multicenter Automatic Defibrillator Implantation Trial Investigators: Improved survival with an implanted defibrillator in patients with coronary disease at high risk for ventricular arrhythmia. N Engl J Med 1996, 335:1933–1940.
4. Gregoratos G, Cheitlin MD, Conill A, et al. ACC/AHA guidelines for implantation of cardiac pacemakers and antiarrhythmia devices: a report of the American College of Cardiology/American Heart Association Task Force on Practice Guidelines (Committee on Pacemaker Implantation). J Am Coll Cardiol 1998; 31:1175–1209.

Index